CONTENTS

Introduction

The busy schedule of our life doesn't leave much time for cooking. However, each of us wants to eat healthy and delicious meals. Getting this, you need a responsible approach. Why do you need to choose the Crock Pot? It perfectly copes both with complicated and simple recipes, while eliminating the need of controlling the cooking process and spending much time in the kitchen.

The device will never be superfluous, as it can cook almost all your favorite meals but in a healthier way. The most popular ingredients to cook in the Crock Pot are:

- meat and poultry;
- fish;
- vegetables;
- soups;
- stuffing;
- porridge
- jams
- broths
- desserts

You should bear in mind that the cooking process in the Crock Pot has to be started long before eating time. You can do all preparations at one certain time and forget about cooking for the rest of the day. Correctly using the Crock Pot in your kitchen and cooking according to the recipes from this cookbook, you are doomed to success!

The Crock Pot is a fairly easy-to-use kitchen equipment that doesn't require professional cooking skills. The process of cooking will be easy for all people: busy professionals, teenagers, etc.

How does it work? Everything is very easy. Firstly, you need to put food in a Crock Pot bowl. The hull of the Crock Pot is made of stainless steel, while inside it is supplemented with a ceramic bowl so that the food doesn't burn. After you put the food inside, cover it with a lid.

The next step will be the selection of the desired cooking mode: normal or high. After this, you can forget about cooking for a few hours and spend time for yourself. The Crock Pot will automatically turn off after the meal is completely cooked. As usual, the Crock Pot models have a timer that will give you an audible signal and notify when the meal is cooked.

The fact that during cooking it is allowed to open the lid at any time to add ingredients to the meal or, if desired, control the process, gives the extra points in favor of the Crock Pot. As usual, the Crock Pot lid is made of heat-resistant glass; so you can oversee the cooking process easily.

There are two types of Crock Pots: with sensor screen and with buttons. Both options don't change the main features of the Crock Pot significantly.

Cleaning the Crock Pot is a simple process. You will need minimal effort. Since the Crock Pot bowl is non-stick and cooking occurs with a small amount or without fat, cleaning will take a minimum of time. The Crock Pot bowl and lid can be washed in a dishwashing machine or with sponge and detergent by hands.

To sum up all the pros and cons of the Crock Pot, it is safe to say that the kitchen appliance has more positive sides than negative once. The few disadvantages that are possible to determine are short cord and lack of timer on some models of the Crock Pot. However, the advantages of a Crock Pot make it an indispensable tool in the kitchen. Let's sum the advantages up:

- You don't spend much time for cooking. You can calmly spend time with your beloved once, work, or take rest while the meal is cooking;
- The principle of the Crock Pot work doesn't let the meal overboil, overflow or burn out;
- Perfect for toddlers. Cooking the vitamin fruit puree without sugar is possible at home. The Crock Pot will care about every member of your family;
- due to the optimum temperature and long cooking time, the Crock Pot will save all the useful vitamins and minerals. It also helps preserve the taste and aroma of the cooked meal;
- suitable for cooking broths, condensed milk, jams, confitures, and preserves.

According to the pros of the Crock Pot that were listed above, it is possible to conclude that it is a unique kitchen appliance with an unusual way of cooking. The Crock Pot is a modern substitutor of the old stove where food was cooked on the firewood. Looks amazing, doesn't it? You can stew the ingredients in the Crock Pot for many hours and at the same time, your meal will be succulent and save the soft texture. The kitchen appliance is a wonderful discovery for people who follow a healthy lifestyle, a strict diet or have some health problems. It can be good also for cooking food for toddlers and making desserts. As you can see the kitchen appliance is perfect for everyone!

A Crock Pot will be an indispensable assistant in your kitchen and this cookbook will help you to impress your beloved with new gorgeous meals day by day!

TOP 10 Crock Pot Tips

1.Shorten cooking time by preparation ingredients in advance.

Most of the ingredients for a Crock Pot can be prepared (cut, peeled, chopped, diced) in advance. Put all prepared ingredients in the zip log bag and store it in the fridge. Doing this you will save the vital minerals and vitamins of the products and spend less your time for cooking.

2.Use fat from meat instead of using an additional amount of fats and oils.

Cut the fat from the meat cuts and put them in the bottom of the Crock Pot. Then add all remaining ingredients. Doing this you will avoid overcooking and reduce the amount of needed oil.

3.Get rid of extra liquid.

Sometimes you cannot calculate the needed amount of liquid or vegetables/fruits produce extra juice. There is a trick that will help you easily eliminate the unnecessary liquid: mix 1 tablespoon of flour with 3 tablespoons of water and whisk it until smooth. Then add the liquid in the meal during cooking and stir well. In a few minutes, the liquid will be thicker and less. If the trick doesn't work, add more flour or mix it with cornstarch.

4.Save your time by adding all ingredients in one time.

As usual Crock Pot recipes ask to add all ingredients gradually; nevertheless, it will not be crucial if you add all components in once. Bear in mind that such a method sometimes does not work with a mix of meat and vegetables.

5.More time for achieving the gorgeous taste.

Some meals such as stews, soups, ragout, porridges, and pies need time fore resting to have better taste. Even if it is not mentioned in the recipes. Leave the cooked meal for 4-5 hours or overnight and you will feel the difference.

6.Cooker liners.

Cooker liners are like a panacea for those who hate cleaning the Crock Pot after cooking. Put it over the Crock Pot bowl and then close the lid. Doing this, you will forget about soaking the Crock Pot during the night and the problem with eliminating the burnt fat.

7.Add milk at the end of cooking.

The milk has features of curdling while a long time of cooking. Furthermore, it can cause high foam while boiling. That is why it is recommended to add milk at the end of the cooking process or mix it with water (1:2).

8.Open the lid only when the meal is cooked.

If there are no mentions in the directions – never open the lid of the Crock Pot. The Crock Pot lid keeps the heat and after opening it, it will take some time to reach a proper cooking temperature again.

9.Cheap cuts of meat are the best.

Use the cheap cuts of meat such as brisket, chuck, shoulder, etc. As usual, they take a long time for cooking to achieve soft and melted texture, but the Crock Pot makes miracle and even the toughest type of meat will be tender and succulent.

10. Increase or decrease the cooking time by yourself.

Sometimes we need to hurry up with dinner or conversely. The special conversion will help you to make no mistake in cooking time:

LOW	HIGH
7 hours	3 hours
8 hours	4 hours
9 hours	5 hours
10 hours	6 hours
11 hours	7 hours
12 hours	8 hours

Breakfast Recipes

Chocolate Toast

Yield: 4 servings | **Prep time:** 15 minutes | **Cook time:** 40 minutes

- 4 white bread slices
- 1 tablespoon vanilla extract
- 2 tablespoons Nutella
- 1 banana, mashed
- 1 tablespoon coconut oil
- ¼ cup full-fat milk

1. Mix vanilla extract, Nutella, mashed banana, coconut oil, and milk.
2. Pour the mixture in the Crock Pot and cook on High for 40 minutes.
3. Make a quick pressure release and cool the chocolate mixture.
4. Spread the toasts with cooked mixture.

per serving: 148 calories, 2g protein, 18.2g carbohydrates, 7.1g fat, 1.5g fiber, 2mg cholesterol, 73mg sodium, 182mg potassium.

Breakfast Casserole

Yield: 5 servings | **Prep time:** 15 minutes | **Cook time:** 7 hours

- 1 cup Cheddar cheese, shredded
- 1 potato, peeled, diced
- ½ cup carrot, grated
- 1 teaspoon ground turmeric
- ½ teaspoon cayenne pepper
- 5 eggs, beaten
- 5 oz ham, chopped
- ½ cup bell pepper, chopped

1. Make the layer from potato in the Crock Pot mold.
2. Then put the layer of carrot over the potatoes.
3. Sprinkle the vegetables with ground turmeric and cayenne pepper.
4. Then add ham and bell pepper.
5. Pour the beaten eggs over the casserole and top with shredded cheese.
6. Cook the meal on LOW for 7 hours.

per serving: 237 calories, 16.8g protein, 10g carbohydrates, 14.4g fat, 1.7g fiber, 204mg cholesterol, 582mg sodium, 378mg potassium.

Egg Casserole

Yield: 4 servings | **Prep time:** 10 minutes | **Cook time:** 2.5 hours

- 8 oz ham, cut into strips
- 5 eggs, beaten
- 2 tablespoons fresh dill, chopped
- ½ cup heavy cream
- 2 oz Parmesan, grated
- 1 teaspoon ground paprika
- ½ teaspoon avocado oil

1. Brush the Crock Pot with avocado oil from inside.
2. The mix eggs with dill, heavy cream, Parmesan, and ground paprika.
3. After this, put the ham in the bottom of the Crock Pot and top with egg mixture.
4. Close and seal the lid.
5. Cook the casserole on High for 2.5 hours.

per serving: 275 calories, 21.6g protein, 4.7g carbohydrates, 19.2g fat, 1.2g fiber, 268mg cholesterol, 957mg sodium, 313mg potassium.

Milk Oatmeal

Yield: 4 servings | **Prep time:** 10 minutes | **Cook time:** 2 hours

- 2 cups oatmeal
- 1 cup of water
- 1 cup milk
- 1 tablespoon liquid honey
- 1 teaspoon vanilla extract
- 1 tablespoon coconut oil
- ¼ teaspoon ground cinnamon

1. Put all ingredients except liquid honey in the Crock Pot and mix.
2. Close the lid and cook the meal on High for 2 hours.
3. Then stir the cooked oatmeal and transfer in the serving bowls.
4. Top the meal with a small amount of liquid honey.

per serving: 234 calories, 7.4g protein, 35.3g carbohydrates, 7.3g fat, 4.2g fiber, 5mg cholesterol, 33mg sodium, 189mg potassium.

Creamy Quinoa with Nuts

Yield: 5 servings | **Prep time:** 10 minutes | **Cook time:** 3 hours

- 1 oz nuts, crushed
- 2 cup quinoa
- 1 cup heavy cream
- 1 cup of water
- 1 teaspoon salt
- ¼ teaspoon chili flakes
- 1 oz Parmesan, grated

1. Put quinoa, heavy cream, water, salt, and chili flakes in the Crock Pot.
2. Cook the ingredients on High for 3 hours.
3. Then add grated cheese and crushed nuts.
4. Stir the meal well and transfer in the serving plates.

per serving: 385 calories, 12.9g protein, 46g carbohydrates, 17.1g fat, 5.3g fiber, 37mg cholesterol, 570mg sodium, 436mg potassium.

Butternut Squash Pate

Yield: 7 servings | **Prep time:** 7 minutes | **Cook time:** 4 hours

- 8 oz butternut squash puree
- 1 tablespoon honey
- 1 teaspoon cinnamon
- ¼ teaspoon ground clove
- 1 tablespoon lemon juice
- 2 tablespoons coconut oil

1. Put all ingredients in the Crock Pot, gently stir, and cook on Low for 4 hours.

per serving: 63 calories, 0g protein, 6.9g carbohydrates, 3.9g fat, 0.8g fiber, 0mg cholesterol, 3mg sodium, 7mg potassium.

Strawberry Yogurt

Yield: 7 servings | **Prep time:** 15 hours | **Cook time:** 3 hours

- 4 cup milk
- 1 cup Greek yogurt
- 1 cup strawberries, sliced
- 1 teaspoon coconut shred

1. Pour the milk into the Crock Pot and cook it on HIGH for 3 hours. Cool the milk till it reaches the temperature of 100F. Add Greek yogurt, mix the liquid carefully, and cover with a towel.
2. Leave the yogurt for 10 hours in a warm place.
3. Pour the thick yogurt mixture in the colander or cheese mold and leave for 5 hours to avoid the extra liquid.
4. Transfer the cooked yogurt in the ramekins and top with sliced strawberries and coconut shred.

per serving: 105 calories,7.6g protein, 9.9g carbohydrates, 4.2g fat, 0.6g fiber, 13mg cholesterol, 76mg sodium, 152mg potassium.

Chocolate Oatmeal

Yield: 5 servings | **Prep time:** 10 minutes | **Cook time:** 4 hours

- 1 oz dark chocolate, chopped
- 1 teaspoon vanilla extract
- 2 cups of coconut milk
- 2 cup oatmeal
- ½ teaspoon ground cardamom

1. Put all ingredients in the Crock Pot and stir carefully with the help of the spoon.
2. Close the lid and cook the meal for 4 hours on Low.

per serving: 386 calories, 7.1g protein, 32.5g carbohydrates, 27.2g fat, 6.1g fiber,1mg cholesterol, 19mg sodium; 374mg potassium.

Zucchini Quinoa

Yield: 3 servings | **Prep time:** 10 minutes | **Cook time:** 3 hours

- ½ zucchini, grated
- 1 teaspoon coconut oil
- 1 cup quinoa
- 2 cup chicken stock
- 1 teaspoon salt
- 1 tablespoon cream cheese
- 1 oz goat cheese, crumbled

1. Mix grated zucchini with coconut oil, quinoa, and chicken stock and transfer in the Crock Pot.
2. Then add cream cheese and salt.
3. Cook the meal on High for 3 hours.
4. Then stir the cooked quinoa well and transfer in the serving plates.
5. Top the meal with crumbled goat cheese.

per serving: 288 calories, 12g protein, 38.3g carbohydrates, 9.9g fat, 4.3g fiber, 14mg cholesterol, 1333mg sodium, 423mg potassium.

Apple Crumble

Yield: 2 servings | **Prep time:** 10 minutes | **Cook time:** 5 hours

- 1 tablespoon liquid honey
- 2 Granny Smith apples
- 4 oz granola
- 4 tablespoons water
- 1 tablespoon almond butter
- 1 teaspoon vanilla extract

1. Cut the apple into small wedges.
2. Remove the seeds from the apples and chop them into small pieces. Put them in the Crock Pot.
3. Add water, almond butter, vanilla extract, and honey.
4. Cook the apples for 5 hours on Low.
5. Then stir them carefully.
6. Put the cooked apples and granola one-by-one in the serving glasses.

per serving: 268 calories, 10.8g protein, 71.4g carbohydrates, 18.5g fat, 11.3g fiber, 0mg cholesterol, 17mg sodium, 613mg potassium.

Morning Pie

Yield: 6 servings | **Prep time:** 10 minutes | **Cook time:** 3 hours

- ½ cup oatmeal
- 1 cups full-fat milk
- 1 cup butternut squash, diced
- 1 teaspoon vanilla extract
- ½ teaspoon ground cinnamon
- 1 teaspoon sesame oil
- 4 pecans, crushed

1. Mix oatmeal and milk in the Crock Pot.
2. Add diced butternut squash, vanilla extract, and ground cinnamon.
3. Then add sesame oil and pecans.
4. Carefully mix the ingredients and close the lid.
5. Cook the pie on Low for 3 hours.
6. Then cool the pie and cut it into servings.

per serving: 203 calories, 5.2g protein, 16.4g carbohydrates, 13.8g fat, 3.4g fiber, 9mg cholesterol, 33mg sodium, 321mg potassium.

Broccoli Omelet

Yield: 4 servings | **Prep time:** 10 minutes | **Cook time:** 2 hours

- 5 eggs, beaten
- 1 tablespoon cream cheese
- 3 oz broccoli, chopped
- 1 tomato, chopped
- 1 teaspoon avocado oil

1. Mix eggs with cream cheese and transfer in the Crock Pot.
2. Add avocado oil, broccoli, and tomato.
3. Close the lid and cook the omelet on High for 2 hours.

per serving: 99 calories, 7.9g protein, 2.6g carbohydrates, 6.6g fat, 0.8g fiber, 207mg cholesterol, 92mg sodium, 184mg potassium.

Spinach Frittata

Yield: 6 servings | **Prep time:** 10 minutes | **Cook time:** 2 hours

- 2 cups spinach, chopped

- 1 teaspoon smoked paprika
- 1 teaspoon sesame oil
- 7 eggs, beaten
- 2 tablespoons coconut oil
- ¼ cup heavy cream
1. Mix eggs with heavy cream.
2. Then grease the Crock Pot with coconut oil and pour the egg mixture inside.
3. Add smoked paprika, sesame oil, and spinach.
4. Carefully mix the ingredients and close the lid.
5. Cook the frittata on High for 2 hours.
per serving: 140 calories, 6.9g protein, 1.1g carbohydrates, 12.3g fat, 0.4g fiber, 198mg cholesterol, 82mg sodium, 137mg potassium.

Broccoli Quiche
Yield: 8 servings | **Prep time:** 10 minutes | **Cook time:** 5 hours
- 2 tablespoons oatmeal
- 1 cup broccoli, chopped
- ½ cup fresh cilantro, chopped
- ¼ cup Mozzarella, shredded
- 1 teaspoon olive oil
- 8 eggs, beaten
- 1 teaspoon ground paprika
1. Brush the Crock Pot bowl with olive oil.
2. In the mixing bowl mix oatmeal, eggs, and ground paprika.
3. Pour the mixture in the Crock Pot.
4. Add all remaining ingredients, gently stir the mixture.
5. Close the lid and cook the quiche for 5 hours on High.
per serving: 80 calories, 6.3g protein, 2.2g carbohydrates, 5.3g fat, 0.6g fiber, 164mg cholesterol, 71mg sodium, 111mg potassium.

Romano Cheese Frittata
Yield: 4 servings | **Prep time:** 10 minutes | **Cook time:** 3 hours
- 4 oz Romano cheese, grated
- 5 eggs, beaten
- ¼ cup of coconut milk
- ½ cup bell pepper, chopped
- ½ teaspoon ground white pepper
- 1 teaspoon olive oil
- ½ teaspoon ground coriander
1. Mix eggs with coconut milk, ground white pepper, bell pepper, and ground coriander.
2. Then brush the Crock Pot bowl with olive oil.
3. Pour the egg mixture in the Crock Pot.
4. Cook the frittata on High for 2.5 hours.
5. Then top the frittata with Romano cheese and cook for 30 minutes on High.
per serving: 238 calories, 16.5g protein, 3.6g carbohydrates, 17.9g fat, 0.6g fiber, 234mg cholesterol, 420mg sodium, 169mg potassium.

Corn Casserole
Yield: 6 servings | **Prep time:** 10 minutes | **Cook time:** 8 hours
- 1 cup sweet corn kernels

- 1 chili pepper, chopped
- 1 tomato, chopped
- 1 cup Mozzarella, shredded
- 2 tablespoons cream cheese
- 5 oz ham, chopped
- 1 teaspoon garlic powder
- 2 eggs, beaten
1. Mix sweet corn kernels, with chili pepper, tomato, and ham.
2. Add minced garlic and stir the ingredients.
3. Transfer it in the Crock Pot and flatten gently.
4. Top the casserole with eggs, cream cheese, and Mozzarella.
5. Cook the casserole on LOW for 8 hours.
per serving: 110 calories, 8.3g protein, 7.2g carbohydrates, 5.8g fat, 1g fiber, 74mg cholesterol, 449mg sodium, 159mg potassium.

Butter Oatmeal
Yield: 4 serving | **Prep time:** 5 minutes | **Cook time:** 10 minutes
- 1 tablespoon liquid honey
- 1 tablespoon coconut shred
- 1 teaspoon vanilla extract
- 1 cup of water
- ½ cup heavy cream
- 1 cup oatmeal
- 2 tablespoons butter
1. Put butter, oatmeal, heavy cream, water, vanilla extract, and coconut shred in the Crock Pot.
2. Carefully stir the ingredients and close the lid.
3. Cook the meal on Low for 5 hours.
4. Then add liquid honey, stir it, and transfer in the serving bowls.
per serving: 212 calories, 3.1g protein, 19.2g carbohydrates, 13.9g fat, 2.3g fiber, 36mg cholesterol, 51mg sodium, 92mg potassium.

Egg Sandwich
Yield: 4 servings | **Prep time:** 10 minutes | **Cook time:** 2.5 hours
- 4 bread slices
- 4 eggs, beaten
- 4 ham slices
- 1 teaspoon smoked paprika
- ½ teaspoon ground turmeric
- ½ teaspoon minced garlic
- 1 tablespoon coconut oil
1. In the bowl mix eggs, smoked paprika, ground turmeric, and minced garlic.
2. Then dip every bread slice in the egg mixture.
3. Put the coconut oil in the Crock Pot.
4. Arrange the bread slices in the Crock Pot in one layer and top with ham.
5. Close the lid and cook the meal on HIGH for 2.5 hours.
per serving: 165 calories, 11g protein, 6.6g carbohydrates, 10.6g fat, 0.9g fiber, 180mg cholesterol, 488mg sodium, 169mg potassium.

Cream Grits
Yield: 2 servings | **Prep time:** 10 minutes | **Cook time:** 5 hours

- ½ cup grits
- ½ cup heavy cream
- 1 cup of water
- 1 tablespoon cream cheese

1. Put grits, heavy cream, and water in the Crock Pot.
2. Cook the meal on LOW for 5 hours.
3. When the grits are cooked, add cream cheese and stir carefully.
4. Transfer the meal in the serving bowls.

per serving: 151 calories, 1.6g protein, 6.9g carbohydrates, 13.2g fat, 1g fiber, 47mg cholesterol, 116mg sodium, 33mg potassium.

Sausage Frittata

Yield: 5 servings | **Prep time:** 10 minutes | **Cook time:** 4 hours

- ½ onion, diced
- 8 oz sausages, chopped
- 1 teaspoon coconut oil
- 1 cup Mozzarella, shredded
- 6 eggs, beaten
- ½ teaspoon cayenne pepper

1. Put sausages in the Crock Pot.
2. Add onion and coconut oil.
3. Close the lid and cook the ingredients on high for 2 hours.
4. Then stir them well.
5. Add eggs, cayenne pepper, and shredded mozzarella.
6. Carefully stir the meal and close the lid.
7. Cook it on high for 2 hours.

per serving: 258 calories, 17.2g protein, 1.7g carbohydrates, 20.1g fat, 0.3g fiber, 238mg cholesterol, 448mg sodium, 224mg potassium.

Milk Pudding

Yield: 2 servings | **Prep time:** 10 minutes | **Cook time:** 7 hours

- 1 cup milk
- 3 eggs, beaten
- 2 tablespoons cornstarch
- 1 teaspoon vanilla extract
- 1 tablespoon white sugar

1. Mix milk with eggs and cornstarch.
2. Whisk the mixture until smooth and add vanilla extract and white sugar.
3. Pour the liquid in the Crock Pot and close the lid.
4. Cook it on Low for 7 hours.

per serving: 214 calories, 12.3g protein, 20.1g carbohydrates, 9.1g fat, 9.7g fiber, 0.1mg cholesterol, 151mg sodium, 162mg potassium.

Poppy Seeds Buns

Yield: 8 servings | **Prep time:** 20 minutes | **Cook time:** 5 hours

- 3 tablespoon poppy seeds
- 1 teaspoon baking powder
- 1 egg, beaten
- 6 oz cottage cheese

- 1 cup flour
- 1 teaspoon ground cardamom
- 2 tablespoons olive oil

1. Mix poppy seeds with baking powder, egg, cottage cheese, flour, and ground cardamom.
2. Knead the homogenous dough.
3. Add olive oil and keep kneading the dough for 4 minutes more.
4. After this, make the small buns from the dough and put them in the Crock Pot bowl.
5. Close the lid and cook them on High for 5 hours.

per serving: 133 calories, 5.9g protein, 14g carbohydrates, 6.1g fat, 0.8g fiber, 22mg cholesterol, 96mg sodium, 134mg potassium.

Bacon Potatoes

Yield: 4 servings | **Prep time:** 10 minutes | **Cook time:** 5 hours

- 4 russet potatoes
- 1 teaspoon dried thyme
- 4 teaspoons olive oil
- 4 bacon slices

1. Cut the potatoes into halves and sprinkle with dried thyme and olive oil.
2. After this, cut every bacon slice into halves.
3. Put the potatoes in the Crock Pot bowl and top with bacon slices.
4. Close the lid and cook them for 5 hours on High.

per serving: 290 calories, 10.6g protein, 33.9g carbohydrates, 12.8g fat, 5.2g fiber, 21mg cholesterol, 452mg sodium, 976mg potassium.

Morning Muesli

Yield: 6 servings | **Prep time:** 10 minutes | **Cook time:** 4 hours

- 1 cup oatmeal
- 1 tablespoon raisins
- 1 teaspoon sesame seeds
- 1 teaspoon dried cranberries
- 1 banana, chopped
- 1 teaspoon ground cinnamon
- 2 cups of coconut milk

1. Mix coconut milk with oatmeal, raisins, sesame seeds, dried cranberries, and ground cinnamon.
2. Transfer the ingredients in the Crock Pot and cook on Low for 4 hours.
3. Then stir carefully and transfer in the serving bowls.
4. Top the muesli with chopped banana.

per serving: 262 calories, 4g protein, 19.8g carbohydrates, 20.3g fat, 4g fiber, 0mg cholesterol, 13mg sodium, 346mg potassium.

Giant Pancake

Yield: 4 servings | **Prep time:** 10 minutes | **Cook time:** 4 hours

- 1 cup pancake mix
- ½ cup milk
- 2 eggs, beaten
- 1 tablespoon coconut oil, melted

1. Whisk pancake mix with milk, and eggs.
2. Then brush the Crock Pot mold with coconut oil from inside.

3. Pour the pancake mixture in the Crock Pot and close the lid.
4. Cook it on High for 4 hours.
 per serving: 225 calories, 7.8g protein, 29.9g carbohydrates, 8.1g fat, 1g fiber, 94mg cholesterol, 529mg sodium, 7.8mg potassium.

Breakfast Monkey Bread
Yield: 6 servings | **Prep time:** 15 minutes | **Cook time:** 6 hours

- 10 oz biscuit rolls
- 1 tablespoon ground cardamom
- 1 tablespoon sugar
- 2 tablespoons coconut oil
- 1 egg, beaten
1. Chop the biscuit roll roughly.
2. Mix sugar with ground cardamom.
3. Melt the coconut oil.
4. Put the ½ part of chopped biscuit rolls in the Crock Pot in one layer and sprinkle with melted coconut oil and ½ part of all ground cinnamon mixture.
5. Then top it with remaining biscuit roll chops and sprinkle with cardamom mixture and coconut oil.
6. Then brush the bread with a beaten egg and close the lid.
7. Cook the meal on High for 6 hours.
8. Cook the cooked bread well.
 per serving: 178 calories, 6.1g protein, 26.4g carbohydrates, 7g fat, 2g fiber, 27mg cholesterol, 238mg sodium, 21mg potassium.

Egg Scramble
Yield: 4 servings | **Prep time:** 10 minutes | **Cook time:** 2.5 hours

- 4 eggs, beaten
- 1 tablespoon butter, melted
- 2 oz Cheddar cheese, shredded
- ¼ teaspoon cayenne pepper
- 1 teaspoon ground paprika
1. Mix eggs with butter, cheese, cayenne pepper, and ground paprika.
2. Then pour the mixture in the Crock Pot and close the lid.
3. Cook it on high for 2 hours.
4. Then open the lid and scramble the eggs.
5. Close the lid and cook the meal on high for 30 minutes.
 per serving: 147 calories, 9.2g protein, 0.9g carbohydrates, 12g fat, 0.2g fiber, 186mg cholesterol, 170mg sodium, 88mg potassium.

Bacon Eggs
Yield: 2 servings | **Prep time:** 10 minutes | **Cook time:** 2 hours

- 2 bacon slices
- 2 eggs, hard-boiled, peeled
- ¼ teaspoon ground black pepper
- 1 teaspoon olive oil
- ½ teaspoon dried thyme
1. Sprinkle the bacon with ground black pepper and dried thyme.

2. Then wrap the eggs in the bacon and sprinkle with olive oil.
3. Put the eggs in the Crock Pot and cook on High for 2 hours.
 per serving: 187 calories, 12.6g protein, 0.9g carbohydrates, 14.7g fat, 0.2g fiber, 185mg cholesterol, 501mg sodium, 172mg potassium.

Breakfast Muffins
Yield: 4 servings | **Prep time:** 10 minutes | **Cook time:** 3 hours

- 7 eggs, beaten
- 1 bell pepper, diced
- ½ teaspoon salt
- ½ teaspoon cayenne pepper
- 2 tablespoons almond meal
- 1 teaspoon avocado oil
1. Brush the muffin molds with avocado oil.
2. In the mixing bowl, mix eggs, bell pepper, salt, cayenne pepper, and almond meal.
3. Pour the muffin mixture in the muffin molds and transfer in the Crock Pot.
4. Cook the muffins on high for 3 hours.
 per serving: 139 calories, 10.7g protein, 3.7g carbohydrates, 9.4g fat, 0.9g fiber, 286mg cholesterol, 399mg sodium, 189mg potassium

Apricot Butter
Yield: 4 servings | **Prep time:** 10 minutes | **Cook time:** 7 hours

- 1 cup apricots, pitted, chopped
- 3 tablespoons butter
- 1 teaspoon ground cinnamon
- 1 teaspoon brown sugar
1. Put all ingredients in the Crock Pot and stir well
2. Close the lid and cook them on Low for 7 hours.
3. Then blend the mixture with the help of the immersion blender and cool until cold.
 per serving: 99 calories, 0.6g protein, 5.5g carbohydrates, 8.9g fat, 1.1g fiber, 23mg cholesterol, 62mg sodium, 106mg potassium.

Baby Carrots in Syrup
Yield: 5 servings | **Prep time:** 5 minutes | **Cook time:** 7 hours

- 3 cups baby carrots
- 1 cup apple juice
- 2 tablespoons brown sugar
- 1 teaspoon vanilla extract
1. Mix apple juice, brown sugar, and vanilla extract.
2. Pour the liquid in the Crock Pot.
3. Add baby carrots and close the lid.
4. Cook the meal on Low for 7 hours.
 per serving: 81 calories, 0g protein, 18.8g carbohydrates, 0.1g fat, 3.7g fiber, 0mg cholesterol, 363mg sodium, 56mg potassium.

Bacon Muffins
Yield: 5 servings | **Prep time:** 10 minutes | **Cook time:** 4 hours

- ½ cup flour

- 2 tablespoons coconut oil
- 2 eggs, beaten
- 1 teaspoon baking powder
- 2 oz bacon, chopped, cooked
- ¼ cup milk
1. Mix flour, milk, and eggs.
2. Add coconut oil, baking powder, and bacon. Stir the mixture carefully.
3. Then pour the batter in the muffin molds.
4. Transfer them in the Crock Pot and close the lid.
5. Cook the muffins on High for 4 hours.

per serving: 186 calories, 8.1g protein, 10.9g carbohydrates, 12.3g fat, 0.4g fiber, 79mg cholesterol, 293mg sodium, 209mg potassium.

Breakfast Meat Rolls

Yield: 12 servings | **Prep time:** 20 minutes | **Cook time:** 4.5 hours

- 1-pound puff pastry
- 1 cup ground pork
- 1 tablespoon garlic, diced
- 1 egg, beaten
- 1 tablespoon sesame oil
1. Roll up the puff pastry.
2. Then mix ground pork with garlic and egg.
3. Then spread the puff pastry with ground meat mixture and roll.
4. Cut the puff pastry rolls on small rolls.
5. Then sprinkle the rolls with sesame oil.
6. Arrange the meat rolls in the Crock Pot and close the lid.
7. Cook breakfast on High for 4.5 hours.

per serving: 244 calories, 4.9g protein, 17.3g carbohydrates, 17.2g fat, 0.6g fiber, 20mg cholesterol, 106mg sodium, 31mg potassium.

Breakfast Meatballs

Yield: 8 servings | **Prep time:** 15 minutes | **Cook time:** 7 hours

- 2 cups ground pork
- 1 egg, beaten
- 1 teaspoon garlic powder
- 1 tablespoon semolina
- ½ cup heavy cream
- 1 teaspoon cayenne pepper
1. Mix ground pork with egg, garlic powder, and semolina,
2. Then make the meatballs and put them in the Crock Pot.
3. Sprinkle them with cayenne pepper.
4. After this, add heavy cream and close the lid.
5. Cook the meatballs on low for 7 hours.

per serving: 98 calories, 6.1g protein, 1.6g carbohydrates, 7.4g fat, 0.1g fiber, 49mg cholesterol, 31mg sodium, 24mg potassium.

Ham Pockets

Yield: 4 servings | **Prep time:** 10 minutes | **Cook time:** 1 hour

- 4 pita bread
- ½ cup Cheddar cheese, shredded
- 4 ham slices
- 1 tablespoon mayonnaise

- 1 teaspoon dried dill
1. Mix cheese with mayonnaise and dill.
2. Then fill the pita bread with sliced ham and cheese mixture.
3. Wrap the stuffed pitas in the foil and place it in the Crock Pot.
4. Cook them on High for 1 hour.

per serving: 283 calories, 13.7g protein, 35.7g carbohydrates, 9.1g fat, 1.7g fiber, 32mg cholesterol, 801mg sodium, 175mg potassium.

Sweet Pepper Eggs

Yield: 2 servings | **Prep time:** 10 minutes | **Cook time:** 2.5 hours

- 1 sweet pepper
- 4 eggs
- ¼ teaspoon ground black pepper
- 1 teaspoon butter, melted
1. Slice the sweet pepper into 4 rounds.
2. Then brush the Crock Pot with butter from inside.
3. Put the sweet pepper rounds in the Crock Pot in one layer.
4. Then crack the eggs in the sweet pepper rounds.
5. Sprinkle the eggs with ground black pepper and close the lid.
6. Cook the meal on High for 2.5 hours.

per serving: 162 calories, 11.7g protein, 5.4g carbohydrates, 10.8g fat, 0.9g fiber, 332mg cholesterol, 138mg sodium, 234mg potassium.

Baguette Boats

Yield: 4 servings | **Prep time:** 10 minutes | **Cook time:** 3 hours

- 6 oz baguette (2 baguettes)
- 4 ham slices
- 1 teaspoon minced garlic
- ½ cup Mozzarella, shredded
- 1 teaspoon olive oil
- 1 egg, beaten
1. Cut the baguettes into the halves and remove the flesh from the bread. Chop the ham and mix it with egg, Mozzarella, and minced garlic.
2. Fill the baguettes with ham mixture.
3. Then brush the Crock Pot bowl with olive oil from inside.
4. Put the baguette boats in the Crock Pot and close the lid.
5. Cook them for 3 hours on High.

per serving: 205 calories, 12.1g protein, 25.5g carbohydrates, 6.1g fat, 1.4g fiber, 59mg cholesterol, 678mg sodium, 152mg potassium.

Honey Pumpkin

Yield: 4 servings | **Prep time:** 10 minutes | **Cook time:** 7 hours

- 2 tablespoons honey
- 1 tablespoon ground cinnamon
- 1 tablespoon ground cardamom
- 1-pound pumpkin, cubed
- ¼ cup of water
1. Put pumpkin in the Crock Pot.

2. Add honey, ground cinnamon, cardamom, and water. Mix the ingredients and close the lid.
3. Cook the pumpkin on Low for 7 hours.
per serving: 79 calories, 1.5g protein, 20.2g carbohydrates, 0.4g fat, 4.6g fiber, 0mg cholesterol, 7mg sodium, 263mg potassium.

Chicken Meatballs
Yield: 4 servings | **Prep time:** 15 minutes | **Cook time:** 4 hours
- 3 tablespoons bread crumbs
- 1 teaspoon cream cheese
- 10 oz ground chicken
- 1 tablespoon coconut oil
- 1 teaspoon Italian seasonings
1. Mix bread crumbs with cream cheese, ground chicken, and Italian seasonings.
2. Make the meatballs and put them in the Crock Pot.
3. Add coconut oil and close the lid.
4. Cook the chicken meatballs for 4 hours on High.
per serving: 190 calories, 21.2g protein, 3.8g carbohydrates, 9.6g fat, 0.2g fiber, 65mg cholesterol, 101mg sodium, 184mg potassium.

Sage Chicken Strips
Yield: 6 servings | **Prep time:** 15 minutes | **Cook time:** 4 hours
- ½ cup coconut cream
- 1-pound chicken fillet, cut into the strips
- 2 tablespoons cornflour
- 1 teaspoon ground black pepper
- 1 teaspoon dried sage
- 2 tablespoons sour cream
1. Sprinkle the chicken strips with ground black pepper, dried sage, and sour cream.
2. Then coat every chicken strip in the cornflour and arrange it in the Crock Pot.
3. Top the chicken with coconut cream and close the lid.
4. Cook the chicken strips on High for 4 hours.
per serving: 208 calories, 22.7g protein, 3.5g carbohydrates, 11.3g fat, 0.8g fiber, 69mg cholesterol, 70mg sodium, 255mg potassium.

Cheddar Eggs
Yield: 4 servings | **Prep time:** 10 minutes | **Cook time:** 2 hours
- 1 teaspoon butter, softened
- 4 eggs
- ½ teaspoon salt
- 1/3 cup Cheddar cheese, shredded
1. Grease the Crock Pot bowl with butter and crack the eggs inside.
2. Sprinkle the eggs with salt and shredded cheese.
3. Close the lid and cook on High for 2 hours.
per serving: 109 calories, 7.9g protein, 0.5g carbohydrates, 8.5g fat, 0g fiber, 176mg cholesterol, 418mg sodium, 69mg potassium.

Baked Eggs
Yield: 5 servings | **Prep time:** 10 minutes | **Cook time:** 8 hours

- 5 oz tater tots
- 2 white onion, diced
- 3 oz bacon, chopped, cooked
- 3 oz provolone cheese, shredded
- 4 eggs, beaten
- 1 teaspoon ground black pepper
- ½ cup milk
1. Make the layer of tater tots in the Crock Pot bowl.
2. Then top it with onion, bacon, and cheese.
3. After this, mix milk, ground black pepper, and eggs.
4. Pour the liquid over the cheese and close the lid.
5. Cook the meal on Low for 8 hours.
per serving: 287 calories, 17g protein, 14.3g carbohydrates, 18.1g fat, 1.8g fiber, 163mg cholesterol, 741mg sodium, 339mg potassium.

Tender Granola
Yield: 4 servings | **Prep time:** 10 minutes | **Cook time:** 30 minutes
- 4 oz rolled oats
- 1 tablespoon coconut oil
- 1 tablespoon liquid honey
- 3 oz almonds, chopped
- ½ teaspoon ground cinnamon
- 2 tablespoons dried cranberries
- Cooking spray
1. In the mixing bowl mix rolled oats, coconut oil, almonds, ground cinnamon, and dried cranberries.
2. Then make the tiny balls from the mixture.
3. Spray the Crock Pot with the cooking spray and put the oat balls inside.
4. Close the lid and cook the granola for 30 minutes on High.
per serving: 278 calories, 8.3g protein, 28.6g carbohydrates, 15.9g fat, 5.8g fiber, 0mg cholesterol, 2mg sodium, 268mg potassium.

Sweet Quinoa
Yield: 4 servings | **Prep time:** 10 minutes | **Cook time:** 3 hours
- 1 cup quinoa
- ¼ cup dates, chopped
- 3 cups of water
- 1 apricot, chopped
- ½ teaspoon ground nutmeg
1. Put quinoa, dates, and apricot in the Crock Pot.
2. Add ground nutmeg and mix the mixture.
3. Cook it on high for 3 hours.
per serving: 194 calories, 6.4g protein, 36.7g carbohydrates, 2.8g fat, 4.1g fiber, 0mg cholesterol, 8g sodium, 338mg potassium.

Vanilla Quinoa
Yield: 2 servings | **Prep time:** 10 minutes | **Cook time:** 4 hours
- ½ cup quinoa
- 2 cups of milk
- 1 teaspoon vanilla extract
- 1 tablespoon butter

1. Put quinoa, milk, and vanilla extract in the Crock Pot.
2. Cook it for 4 hours on Low.
3. Then add butter and stir the quinoa carefully.
 per serving: 335 calories, 14.1g protein, 39.5g carbohydrates, 13.3g fat, 3g fiber, 35mg cholesterol, 158mg sodium, 384mg potassium.

Raspberry Chia Pudding
Yield: 2 servings | **Prep time:** 10 minutes | **Cook time:** 2 hours
- 4 tablespoons chia seeds
- 1 cup of coconut milk
- 2 teaspoons raspberries
1. Put chia seeds and coconut milk in the Crock Pot and cook it for 2 hours on Low.
2. Then transfer the cooked chia pudding in the glasses and top with raspberries.
 per serving: 423 calories, 7.7g protein, 19.6g carbohydrates, 37.9g fat, 13.1g fiber, 0mg cholesterol, 23mg sodium, 442mg potassium.

Chicken Omelet
Yield: 4 servings | **Prep time:** 10 minutes | **Cook time:** 3 hours
- 4 oz chicken fillet, boiled, shredded
- 1 tomato, chopped
- 4 eggs, beaten
- 1 tablespoon cream cheese
- 1 teaspoon olive oil
1. Brush the Crock Pot bowl with olive oil from inside.
2. In the mixing bowl mix shredded chicken, tomato, eggs, and cream cheese.
3. Then pour the mixture in the Crock Pot bowl and close the lid.
4. Cook the omelet for 3 hours on Low.
 per serving: 138 calories, 14.1g protein, 1g carbohydrates, 8.5g fat, 0.2g fiber, 192mg cholesterol, 94mg sodium, 168mg potassium.

Orange Pudding
Yield: 4 servings | **Prep time:** 10 minutes | **Cook time:** 4 hours
- 1 cup carrot, grated
- 2 cups of milk
- 1 tablespoon cornstarch
- 1 teaspoon vanilla extract
- ½ teaspoon ground nutmeg
1. Put the carrot in the Crock Pot.
2. Add milk, vanilla extract, and ground nutmeg.
3. Then add cornstarch and stir the ingredients until cornstarch is dissolved.
4. Cook the pudding on low for 4 hours.
 per serving: 84 calories, 4.3g protein, 10.8g carbohydrates, 2.6g fat, 0.8g fiber, 10mg cholesterol, 77mg sodium, 161mg potassium.

Omelet with Greens
Yield: 2 servings | **Prep time:** 10 minutes | **Cook time:** 2 hours
- 3 eggs, beaten
- ¼ cup milk

- 1 cup baby arugula, chopped
- ½ teaspoon salt
- 1 teaspoon avocado oil
1. In the bowl mix eggs with milk, salt, and arugula.
2. Then sprinkle the Crock Pot with avocado oil from inside.
3. Pour the omelet egg mixture in the Crock Pot and close the lid.
4. Cook the meal on High for 2 hours.
 per serving: 115 calories, 9.6g protein, 2.5g carbohydrates, 7.6g fat, 0.3g fiber, 248mg cholesterol, 691mg sodium, 150mg potassium.

Cauliflower Pudding
Yield: 3 servings | **Prep time:** 10 minutes | **Cook time:** 2 hours
- 1 teaspoon liquid honey
- ½ teaspoon ground cardamom
- 7 oz cauliflower rice
- 1 teaspoon butter
- 1 cup of coconut milk
- 1 teaspoon cornstarch
1. Mix cornstarch with coconut milk and pour it in the Crock Pot.
2. Add ground cardamom, butter, and cauliflower rice.
3. Close the lid and cook the pudding on high for 2 hours.
4. When the pudding is cooked, stir it, and add liquid honey.
 per serving: 244 calories, 4.5g protein, 11.8g carbohydrates, 21.6g fat, 1.9g fiber, 3mg cholesterol, 101mg sodium, 216mg potassium.

Tomato Hot Eggs
Yield: 3 serving | **Prep time:** 10 minutes | **Cook time:** 2.5 hours
- 3 eggs, beaten
- 2 tomatoes, chopped
- 1 teaspoon coconut oil
- 1 bell pepper, diced
- 1 tablespoon hot sauce
1. Grease the Crock Pot with coconut oil from inside.
2. Then mix hot sauce with beaten eggs.
3. Add chopped tomatoes and bell pepper.
4. Pour the mixture in the Crock Pot and close the lid.
5. Cook the meal on high for 2.5 hours.
 per serving: 104 calories, 6.7g protein, 6.6g carbohydrates, 6.2g fat, 1.5g fiber, 164mg cholesterol, 193mg sodium, 335mg potassium.

Italian Style Scrambled Eggs
Yield: 4 servings | **Prep time:** 10 minutes | **Cook time:** 4 hours
- 4 eggs, beaten
- 3 oz Mozzarella, shredded
- ¼ cup milk
- 1 teaspoon Italian seasonings
- ¼ teaspoon salt
- 1 teaspoon butter, melted

1. Mix eggs with milk, Italian seasonings, and salt.
2. Pour butter and milk mixture in the Crock Pot and close the lid.
3. Cook the meal on high for 1 hour.
4. Then open the lid and scramble the eggs.
5. After this, top the meal with cheese and cook the eggs on low for 3 hours more.

per serving: 143 calories, 12.1g protein, 2g carbohydrates, 9.7g fat, 0g fiber, 180mg cholesterol, 351mg sodium, 69mg potassium.

Egg Quiche

Yield: 4 servings | **Prep time:** 5 minutes | **Cook time:** 7 hours

- 4 eggs, beaten
- 1 bell pepper, diced
- 1 onion, diced
- 1 teaspoon chili flakes
- ½ teaspoon ground paprika
- 2 tablespoons flax meal

1. Mix eggs with flax meal.
2. Add bell pepper, chili flakes, onion, and ground paprika.
3. Pour the quiche mixture in the Crock Pot and close the lid.
4. Cook the meal on low for 7 hours.

per serving: 99 calories, 6.9g protein, 6.3g carbohydrates, 5.8g fat, 2.1g fiber, 164mg cholesterol, 64mg sodium, 190mg potassium.

Basil Sausages

Yield: 5 servings | **Prep time:** 10 minutes | **Cook time:** 4 hours

- 1-pound Italian sausages, chopped
- 1 teaspoon dried basil
- 1 tablespoon olive oil
- 1 teaspoon ground coriander
- ¼ cup of water

1. Sprinkle the chopped sausages with ground coriander and dried basil and transfer in the Crock Pot.
2. Add olive oil and water.
3. Close the lid and cook the sausages on high for 4 hours.

per serving: 338 calories, 12.9g protein, 0.6g carbohydrates, 31.2g fat, 0g fiber, 69mg cholesterol, 664mg sodium, 231mg potassium.

Leek Bake

Yield: 3 servings | **Prep time:** 10 minutes | **Cook time:** 8 hours

- 2 cups leek, chopped
- 3 oz Cheddar cheese, shredded
- ¼ cup ground chicken
- 1 teaspoon dried thyme
- ½ cup chicken stock

1. Pour the chicken stock in the Crock Pot.
2. Put the leek in the chicken stock and sprinkle it with dried thyme and ground chicken.
3. Then top the chicken with Cheddar cheese and close the lid.
4. Cook the leek bake on low for 8 hours.

per serving: 175 calories, 11.5g protein, 9.1g carbohydrates, 10.6g fat, 1.2g fiber, 40mg cholesterol, 325mg sodium, 168mg potassium.

Sausage Bake

Yield: 5 servings | **Prep time:** 10 minutes | **Cook time:** 8 hours

- 1 cup potato, grated
- ½ white onion, minced
- 1-pound smoked andouille sausage, sliced
- 1 cup cheddar cheese, shredded
- ½ cup heavy cream
- 1 teaspoon sesame oil

1. In the bowl mix grated potato, onion, smoked sausages, cheese, and heavy cream.
2. Then brush the Crock Pot with sesame oil.
3. Put the sausage mixture in the Crock Pot.
4. Close the lid and cook the bake on Low for 8 hours.

per serving: 381 calories, 21.2g protein, 5.3g carbohydrates, 29.9g fat, 1.6g fiber, 99mg cholesterol, 744mg sodium, 110mg potassium.

French Toast

Yield: 2 servings | **Prep time:** 10 minutes | **Cook time:** 3.5 hours

- 2 white bread slices
- 1 teaspoon cream cheese
- 1 teaspoon white sugar
- 1 egg, beaten
- ¼ cup milk
- 1 tablespoon butter

1. Put butter in the Crock Pot.
2. Add cream cheese, white sugar, egg, and milk. Stir the mixture.
3. Then put the bread slices in the Crock Pot and close the lid.
4. Cook the toasts for 3.5 hours on High.

per serving: 135 calories, 4.7g protein, 8.3g carbohydrates, 9.5g fat, 0.2g fiber, 101mg cholesterol, 152mg sodium, 60mg potassium.

Peach Oats

Yield: 3 servings | **Prep time:** 7 minutes | **Cook time:** 7 hours

- ½ cup steel cut oats
- 1 cup milk
- ½ cup peaches, pitted, chopped
- 1 teaspoon ground cardamom

1. Mix steel-cut oats with milk and pour the mixture in the Crock Pot.
2. Add ground cardamom and peaches. Stir the ingredients gently and close the lid.
3. Cook the meal on low for 7 hours.

per serving: 159 calories, 7g protein, 24.8g carbohydrates, 3.8g fat, 3.2g fiber, 7mg cholesterol, 38mg sodium, 200mg potassium

Shrimp Omelet

Yield: 4 servings | **Prep time:** 8 minutes | **Cook time:** 3.5 hours

- 4 eggs, beaten
- 4 oz shrimps, peeled

- ½ teaspoon ground turmeric
- ½ teaspoon ground paprika
- ¼ teaspoon salt
- Cooking spray

1. Mix eggs with shrimps, turmeric, salt, and paprika.
2. Then spray the Crock Pot bowl with cooking spray.
3. After this, pour the egg mixture inside. Flatten the shrimps and close the lid.
4. Cook the omelet for 3.5 hours on High.

per serving: 98 calories, 12.1g protein, 1.1g carbohydrates, 4.9g fat, 0.2g fiber, 223mg cholesterol, 278mg sodium, 120mg potassium.

Raisins and Rice Pudding

Yield: 4 servings | **Prep time:** 5 minutes | **Cook time:** 6 hours

- 1 cup long-grain rice
- 2.5 cups organic almond milk
- 2 tablespoons cornstarch
- 1 teaspoon vanilla extract
- 2 tablespoons raisins, chopped

1. Put all ingredients in the Crock Pot and carefully mix.
2. Then close the lid and cook the pudding for 6 hours on Low.

per serving: 238 calories, 4.1g protein, 49.4g carbohydrates, 1.9g fat, 0.8g fiber, 0mg cholesterol, 91mg sodium, 89mg potassium

Turkey Omelet

Yield: 4 servings | **Prep time:** 10 minutes | **Cook time:** 5 hours

- ½ teaspoon garlic powder
- 6 oz ground turkey
- 4 eggs, beaten
- 1 tablespoon coconut oil
- ½ teaspoon salt
- ¼ cup milk

1. Mix milk with salt, eggs, and garlic powder. Then add ground turkey.
2. Grease the Crock Pot bowl bottom with coconut oil.
3. Put the egg mixture in the Crock Pot, flatten it, and close the lid.
4. Cook the omelet on Low for 5 hours.

per serving: 184 calories, 17.7g protein, 1.3g carbohydrates, 12.8g fat, 0g fiber, 208mg cholesterol, 405mg sodium, 186mg potassium

Spicy Arugula Quiche

Yield: 4 servings | **Prep time:** 10 minutes | **Cook time:** 2.5 hours

- 2 cups arugula, chopped
- ½ cup cremini mushrooms, chopped
- 4 eggs, beaten
- ½ cup heavy cream
- 2 tablespoons coconut flour
- 1 teaspoon Italian seasonings
- 1 teaspoon sesame oil

1. Mix coconut flour with Italian seasonings, heavy cream, eggs, and mushrooms.
2. Then add arugula and mix the mixture.
3. After this, brush the Crock Pot bottom with sesame oil.
4. Pour the egg mixture in the Crock Pot and close the lid.
5. Cook the quiche on High for 2.5 hours.
6. Then cool the quiche and cut into servings.

per serving: 163 calories, 7.3g protein, 5.6g carbohydrates, 12.5g fat, 2.7g fiber, 0mg cholesterol, 86mg sodium, 148mg potassium

Scallions and Bacon Omelet

Yield: 4 servings | **Prep time:** 10 minutes | **Cook time:** 2 hours

- 5 eggs, beaten
- 2 oz bacon, chopped, cooked
- 1 oz scallions, chopped
- 1 teaspoon olive oil
- ½ teaspoon ground black pepper
- ¼ teaspoon cayenne pepper

1. Brush the Crock Pot bowl bottom with olive oil.
2. After this, in the bowl mix eggs with bacon, scallions, ground black pepper, and cayenne pepper.
3. Pour the liquid in the Crock Pot and close the lid.
4. Cook the meal on high for 2 hours.

per serving: 169 calories, 12.3g protein, 1.4g carbohydrates, 12.6g fat, 0.3g fiber, 220mg cholesterol, 406mg sodium, 179mg potassium

Goat Cheese Frittata

Yield: 4 servings | **Prep time:** 10 minutes | **Cook time:** 2.5 hours

- 2 oz goat cheese, crumbled
- 5 eggs, beaten
- 1 tablespoon flour
- 2 oz bell pepper, chopped
- 1 teaspoon butter, softened
- 1 oz cilantro, chopped

1. Mix flour with eggs and bell pepper.
2. Then grease the Crock Pot bottom with butter and pour the egg mixture inside.
3. Then top the mixture with crumbled goat cheese and cilantro.
4. Close the lid and cook the meal on High for 2.5 hours.

per serving: 179 calories, 12.2g protein, 7g carbohydrates, 11.7g fat, 1.1g fiber, 222mg cholesterol, 138mg sodium, 232mg potassium

Light Egg Scramble

Yield: 2 servings | **Prep time:** 15 minutes | **Cook time:** 4 hours

- 1 tablespoon butter, melted
- 6 eggs, beaten
- 1 teaspoon salt
- 1 teaspoon ground paprika

1. Pour the melted butter in the Crock Pot.
2. Add eggs and salt and stir.
3. Cook the eggs on Low for 4 hours. Stir the eggs every 15 minutes.

4. When the egg scramble is cooked, top it with ground paprika.

per serving: 243 calories, 16.8g protein, 1.6g carbohydrates, 19g fat, 0.4g fiber, 506mg cholesterol, 1389mg sodium, 203mg potassium

Asparagus Egg Casserole
Yield: 4 servings | **Prep time:** 10 minutes | **Cook time:** 2.5 hours

- 7 eggs, beaten
- 4 oz asparagus, chopped, boiled
- 1 oz Parmesan, grated
- 1 teaspoon sesame oil
- 1 teaspoon dried dill
1. Pour the sesame oil in the Crock Pot.
2. Then mix dried dill with parmesan, asparagus, and eggs.
3. Pour the egg mixture in the Crock Pot and close the lid.
4. Cook the casserole on high for 2.5 hours.

per serving: 149 calories, 12.6g protein, 2.1g carbohydrates, 10.3g fat, 0.6g fiber, 292mg cholesterol, 175mg sodium, 169mg potassium

Tomato Eggs
Yield: 4 servings | **Prep time:** 10 minutes | **Cook time:** 2.5 hours

- 2 cups tomatoes, chopped
- ¼ cup tomato juice
- 1 onion, diced
- 1 teaspoon olive oil
- ½ teaspoon ground black pepper
- 4 eggs
1. Pour olive oil in the Crock Pot.
2. Add onion, tomato juice, and tomatoes.
3. Close the lid and cook the mixture on High for 1 hour.
4. Then mix the tomato mixture and crack the eggs inside.
5. Close the lid and cook them on High for 1.5 hours more.

per serving: 103 calories, 6.8g protein, 7.2g carbohydrates, 5.8g fat, 1.8g fiber, 164mg cholesterol, 108mg sodium, 350mg potassium

Feta Eggs
Yield: 4 servings | **Prep time:** 10 minutes | **Cook time:** 5 hours

- 4 eggs, beaten
- ¼ cup milk
- 4 oz Feta, crumbled
- 1 teaspoon olive oil
- 1 teaspoon dried thyme
- ¼ teaspoon salt
1. Mix eggs with milk, salt, and thyme.
2. Then add olive oil and pour the mixture in the Crock Pot.
3. Top it with crumbled eggs and close the lid.
4. Cook the meal on Low for 5 hours.

per serving: 156 calories, 10.1g protein, 2.4g carbohydrates, 11.9g fat, 0.1g fiber, 190mg cholesterol, 533mg sodium, 87mg potassium

Cheese and Turkey Casserole
Yield: 4 servings | **Prep time:** 10 minutes | **Cook time:** 6 hours

- 8 oz ground turkey
- 1 teaspoon butter
- 5 oz Monterey jack cheese, shredded
- 1 tablespoon dried parsley
- 1 teaspoon chili powder
- 1 red onion, diced
- ¼ cup of water
1. Put all ingredients in the Crock Pot and mix carefully.
2. Close the lid and cook the casserole on low for 6 hours.

per serving: 265 calories, 24.6g protein, 3.2g carbohydrates, 18.1g fat, 0.8g fiber, 92mg cholesterol, 266mg sodium, 240mg potassium

Kale Cups
Yield: 4 servings | **Prep time:** 10 minutes | **Cook time:** 2.5 hours

- 1 cup kale, chopped
- 4 eggs, beaten
- 1 teaspoon olive oil
- 1 teaspoon chili powder
- ½ cup Cheddar cheese, shredded
1. Mix kale with eggs, olive oil, and chili powder.
2. Transfer the mixture in the ramekins and top with Cheddar cheese.
3. Place the ramekins in the Crock Pot.
4. Close the lid and cook the meal on high for 2.5 hours.

per serving: 140 calories, 9.6g protein, 2.6g carbohydrates, 10.3g fat, 0.5g fiber, 179mg cholesterol, 163mg sodium, 168mg potassium

Smoked Salmon Omelet
Yield: 4 servings | **Prep time:** 10 minutes | **Cook time:** 2 hours

- 4 oz smoked salmon, sliced
- 5 eggs, beaten
- 1 teaspoon ground coriander
- 1 teaspoon butter, melted
1. Brush the Crock Pot bottom with melted butter.
2. Then mix eggs with ground coriander and pour the liquid in the Crock Pot.
3. Add smoked salmon and close the lid.
4. Cook the omelet on High for 2 hours.

per serving: 120 calories, 12.1g protein, 0.4g carbohydrates, 7.7g fat, 0g fiber, 214mg cholesterol, 651mg sodium, 124mg potassium

Breakfast Pork Ground
Yield: 4 servings | **Prep time:** 15 minutes | **Cook time:** 7 hours

- 1 cup ground pork
- 1 teaspoon tomato paste
- 1 red onion, diced
- ½ cup Mozzarella, shredded
- ½ cup corn kernels
- 1 tablespoon butter

1. Mix ground pork with tomato paste, mozzarella, butter, and corn kernels.
2. Transfer the mixture in the Crock Pot and cook on low for 7 hours.
3. Then transfer the cooked meal in the serving plates and top with diced onion.
per serving: 122 calories, 7g protein, 6.6g carbohydrates, 7.8g fat, 1.2g fiber, 28mg cholesterol, 67mg sodium, 106mg potassium

Chorizo Eggs
Yield: 4 servings | **Prep time:** 10 minutes | **Cook time:** 1.5 hours
- 5 oz chorizo, sliced
- 4 eggs, beaten
- 2 oz Parmesan, grated
- 1 teaspoon butter, softened
1. Grease the Crock Pot bottom with butter.
2. Add chorizo and cook them on high for 30 minutes.
3. Then flip the sliced chorizo and add eggs and Parmesan.
4. Close the lid and cook the meal on High for 1 hour more.
per serving: 278 calories, 18.6g protein, 1.5g carbohydrates, 21.9g fat, 0g fiber, 208mg cholesterol, 638mg sodium, 200mg potassium

Salami Eggs
Yield: 4 servings | **Prep time:** 10 minutes | **Cook time:** 2.5 hours
- 4 oz salami, sliced
- 4 eggs
- 1 teaspoon butter, melted
- 1 tablespoon chives, chopped
1. Pour the melted butter in the Crock Pot.
2. Crack the eggs inside.
3. Then top the eggs with salami and chives.
4. Close the lid and cook them on High for 2.5 hours.
per serving: 146 calories, 9.1g protein, 0.9g carbohydrates, 11.6g fat, 0g fiber, 186mg cholesterol, 392mg sodium, 115mg potassium

Coconut Oatmeal
Yield: 6 servings | **Prep time:** 10 minutes | **Cook time:** 5 hours
- 2 cups oatmeal
- 2 cups of coconut milk
- 1 cup of water
- 2 tablespoons coconut shred
- 1 tablespoon maple syrup
1. Put all ingredients in the Crock Pot and carefully mix.
2. Then close the lid and cook the oatmeal on low for 5 hours.
per serving: 313 calories, 5.4g protein, 25.8g carbohydrates, 22.5g fat, 4.8g fiber, 0mg cholesterol, 16mg sodium, 316mg potassium

Radish Bowl
Yield: 4 servings | **Prep time:** 10 minutes | **Cook time:** 1.5 hours
- 2 cups radish, halved
- 1 tablespoon dried dill
- 1 tablespoon olive oil
- 4 eggs, beaten
- ¼ teaspoon salt
- ¼ cup milk
1. Mix radish with dried dill, olive oil, salt, and milk and transfer in the Crock Pot.
2. Cook the radish on High for 30 minutes.
3. Then shake the vegetables well and add eggs. Mix the mixture gently and close the lid.
4. Cook the meal on High for 1 hour.
per serving: 112 calories, 6.6g protein, 3.5g carbohydrates, 8.3g fat, 1g fiber, 165mg cholesterol, 240mg sodium, 229mg potassium

Eggs with Brussel Sprouts
Yield: 4 servings | **Prep time:** 10 minutes | **Cook time:** 6 hours
- 1 cup Brussel sprouts, halved
- ½ cup Mozzarella, shredded
- 5 eggs, beaten
- 1 teaspoon chili powder
- 1 teaspoon olive oil
1. Pour olive oil in the Crock Pot.
2. Then add the layer of the Brussel sprouts.
3. Sprinkle the vegetables with chili powder and eggs.
4. Then add mozzarella and close the lid.
5. Cook the meal on Low for 6 hours.
per serving: 110 calories, 8.8g protein, 2.9g carbohydrates, 7.5g fat, 1.1g fiber, 206mg cholesterol, 110mg sodium, 172mg potassium

Raspberry Chia Porridge
Yield: 4 servings | **Prep time:** 15 minutes | **Cook time:** 4 hours
- 1 cup raspberry
- 3 tablespoons maple syrup
- 1 cup chia seeds
- 4 cups of milk
1. Put chia seeds and milk in the Crock Pot and cook the mixture on low for 4 hours.
2. Meanwhile, mix raspberries and maple syrup in the blender and blend the mixture until smooth.
3. When the chia porridge is cooked, transfer it in the serving bowls and top with blended raspberry mixture.
per serving: 315 calories, 13.1g protein, 37.7g carbohydrates, 13.9g fat, 11.7g fiber, 20mg cholesterol, 121mg sodium, 332mg potassium

Tomato Ground Chicken
Yield: 4 servings | **Prep time:** 10 minutes | **Cook time:** 6 hours
- 10 oz ground chicken
- 1 cup tomatoes, chopped
- ¼ cup cream
- 1 teaspoon chili powder
1. Mix ground chicken with cream and chili powder and transfer in the Crock Pot.
2. Add tomatoes and close the lid.
3. Cook the meal on Low for 6 hours.

4.   Then carefully mix the chicken.
per serving: 154 calories, 21.1g protein, 2.6g carbohydrates, 6.3g fat, 0.8g fiber, 66mg cholesterol, 75mg sodium, 297mg potassium

Olive Eggs
Yield: 4 servings | **Prep time:** 10 minutes | **Cook time:** 2 hours
- 10 kalamata olives, sliced
- 8 eggs, beaten
- 1 teaspoon cayenne pepper
- 1 tablespoon butter
1.   Grease the Crock Pot bottom with butter.
2.   Then add beaten eggs and cayenne pepper.
3.   After this, top the eggs with olives and close the lid.
4.   Cook the eggs on High for 2 hours.
per serving: 165 calories, 11.2g protein, 1.6g carbohydrates, 12.9g fat, 0.5g fiber, 335mg cholesterol, 240mg sodium, 129mg potassium

Sweet Vegetable Rice Pudding
Yield: 4 servings | **Prep time:** 10 minutes | **Cook time:** 1 hour
- 2 cups cauliflower, shredded
- 3 cups of milk
- 1 tablespoon potato starch
- 2 tablespoons maple syrup
1.   Mix potato starch with milk and pour in the Crock Pot.
2.   Add maple syrup and cauliflower shred. Cook the mixture on High for 1 hour.
per serving: 140 calories, 7g protein, 20.9g carbohydrates, 3.8g fat, 1.3g fiber, 15mg cholesterol, 102mg sodium, 277mg potassium

Leek Eggs
Yield: 4 servings | **Prep time:** 10 minutes | **Cook time:** 2.5 hours
- 10 oz leek, sliced
- 4 eggs, beaten
- 1 teaspoon olive oil
- ½ teaspoon cumin seeds
- 3 oz Cheddar cheese, shredded
1.   Mix leek with olive oil and eggs.
2.   Then transfer the mixture in the Crock Pot.
3.   Sprinkle the egg mixture with Cheddar cheese and cumin seeds.
4.   Close the lid and cook the meal on High for 2.5 hours.
per serving: 203 calories, 11.9g protein, 10.8g carbohydrates, 12.9g fat, 1.3g fiber, 186mg cholesterol, 208mg sodium, 212mg potassium

Cheese Meat
Yield: 4 servings | **Prep time:** 10 minutes | **Cook time:** 7 hours
- 10 oz ground beef
- 1 teaspoon minced garlic
- 1 cup Cheddar cheese, shredded
- ½ cup tomato juice
- 1 teaspoon chili powder
- 1 teaspoon olive oil

1.   Pour olive oil in the Crock Pot.
2.   Add ground beef, minced garlic, tomato juice, and chili powder. Carefully mix the mixture.
3.   Then top the meal with cheddar cheese and close the lid.
4.   Cook the meal on low for 7 hours.
5.   Carefully mix the meat before serving.
per serving: 264 calories, 28.9g protein, 2.2g carbohydrates, 15.1g fat, 0.4g fiber, 93mg cholesterol, 311mg sodium, 398mg potassium

Breakfast Salad
Yield: 4 servings | **Prep time:** 10 minutes | **Cook time:** 2.5 hours
- 1 cup ground beef
- 1 teaspoon chili powder
- 1 onion, diced
- 1 tablespoon olive oil
- 2 cups arugula, chopped
- 1 cup tomatoes, chopped
1.   Mix ground beef with chili powder, diced onion, and olive oil.
2.   Put the mixture in the Crock Pot and close the lid.
3.   Cook it on High for 2.5 hours.
4.   Then transfer the mixture in the salad bowl, cool gently.
5.   Add tomatoes and arugula. Mix the salad.
per serving: 128 calories, 12.3g protein, 5.1g carbohydrates, 6.7g fat, 1.5g fiber, 34mg cholesterol, 45mg sodium, 373mg potassium

Carrot Oatmeal
Yield: 4 servings | **Prep time:** 10 minutes | **Cook time:** 6 hours
- 1 cup oatmeal
- 1 cup carrot, shredded
- 1 tablespoon raisins
- 1 tablespoon maple syrup
- 2 cups of water
- 1 teaspoon butter
1.   Put all ingredients in the Crock Pot.
2.   Close the lid and cook the oatmeal on low for 6 hours.
3.   Carefully mix the cooked meal.
per serving: 117 calories, 3g protein, 21.7g carbohydrates, 2g fat, 2.8g fiber, 3mg cholesterol, 31mg sodium, 191mg potassium

Seafood Eggs
Yield: 4 servings | **Prep time:** 10 minutes | **Cook time:** 2.5 hours
- 4 eggs, beaten
- 2 tablespoons cream cheese
- 1 teaspoon Italian seasonings
- 6 oz shrimps, peeled
- 1 teaspoon olive oil
1.   Mix cream cheese with eggs.
2.   Add Italian seasonings and shrimps.
3.   Then brush the ramekins with olive oil and pour the egg mixture inside.
4.   Transfer the ramekins in the Crock Pot.
5.   Cook the eggs on High for 2.5 hours.

per serving: 144 calories, 15.6g protein, 1.3g carbohydrates, 8.4g fat, 0g fiber, 260mg cholesterol, 181mg sodium, 138mg potassium

Carrot Pudding
Yield: 4 servings | **Prep time:** 10 minutes | **Cook time:** 5 hours

- 3 cups carrot, shredded
- 1 tablespoon potato starch
- 3 tablespoons maple syrup
- 1 teaspoon ground cinnamon
- 4 cups of milk

1. Mix potato starch with milk and pour the liquid in the Crock Pot.
2. Add ground cinnamon, maple syrup, and carrot.
3. Close the lid and cook the pudding on Low for 5 hours.

per serving: 206 calories, 8.7g protein, 33.1g carbohydrates, 5g fat, 2.3g fiber, 20mg cholesterol, 173mg sodium, 437mg potassium

Sausage Pie
Yield: 5 servings | **Prep time:** 10 minutes | **Cook time:** 3 hours

- 7 oz potato, cooked, mashed
- 3 eggs, beaten
- 4 oz sausages, chopped
- 1 teaspoon Italian seasonings
- 2 oz Mozzarella, shredded
- 1 teaspoon olive oil

1. Mix eggs with mashed potato and Italian seasonings.
2. Then brush the Crock Pot bottom with olive oil.
3. Put the mashed potato mixture inside and flatten it.
4. Then add sausages and Mozzarella.
5. Close the lid and cook the pie on High for 3 hours.

per serving: 188 calories, 11.7g protein, 7.6g carbohydrates, 12.3g fat, 0.9g fiber, 124mg cholesterol, 278mg sodium, 270mg potassium

Squash Butter
Yield: 4 servings | **Prep time:** 10 minutes | **Cook time:** 2 hours

- 1 cup butternut squash puree
- 1 teaspoon allspices
- 4 tablespoons applesauce
- 2 tablespoons butter
- 1 teaspoon cornflour

1. Put all ingredients in the Crock Pot and mix until homogenous.
2. Then close the lid and cook the butter on High for 2 hours.
3. Transfer the cooked squash butter in the plastic vessel and cool it well.

per serving: 78 calories, 0.2g protein, 6.3g carbohydrates, 5.8g fat, 0.8g fiber, 15mg cholesterol, 44mg sodium, 20mg potassium

Sweet Eggs
Yield: 4 servings | **Prep time:** 10 minutes | **Cook time:** 4 hours

- 4 oz white bread, chopped
- 2 tablespoons sugar
- 6 eggs, beaten
- ¼ cup milk
- 1 teaspoon vanilla extract
- 1 teaspoon avocado oil

1. Mix eggs with sugar and milk. Add vanilla extract and bread.
2. Then brush the Crock Pot bottom with avocado oil.
3. Pour the egg mixture inside and close the lid.
4. Cook the meal on Low for 4 hours.

per serving: 204 calories, 11g protein, 21.8g carbohydrates, 8g fat, 0.7g fiber, 247mg cholesterol, 293mg sodium, 131mg potassium

Peach Puree
Yield: 2 servings | **Prep time:** 10 minutes | **Cook time:** 7 hours

- 2 cups peaches, chopped
- 1 tablespoon sugar
- 1 teaspoon ground cinnamon
- ¼ cup of water

1. Put all ingredients in the Crock Pot.
2. Close the lid and cook them on low for 7 hours.
3. Then make the puree with the help of the immersion blender.
4. Store the puree in the fridge for up to 1 day.

per serving: 84 calories, 1.5g protein, 20.9g carbohydrates, 0.4g fat, 2.9g fiber, 0mg cholesterol, 1mg sodium, 290mg potassium

Breakfast Spinach Pie
Yield: 4 servings | **Prep time:** 15 minutes | **Cook time:** 2 hours

- 5 flour tortillas
- 2 eggs, beaten
- ¼ cup milk
- 3 cups spinach, chopped
- ½ cup mozzarella, shredded
- Cooking spray

1. Spray the Crock Pot with cooking spray.
2. Then put 3 flour tortilla in the bottom of the Crock Pot.
3. Mix milk with eggs.
4. Sprinkle the small amount of the milk mixture over the flour tortilla.
5. Add chopped spinach and mozzarella.
6. Cover the mixture with remaining tortillas and add milk mixture.
7. Close the lid and cook the pie on High for 2 hours.

per serving: 120 calories, 6.6g protein, 15.3g carbohydrates, 4.1g fat, 2.4g fiber, 85mg cholesterol, 91mg sodium, 220mg potassium

Tofu Eggs
Yield: 4 servings | **Prep time:** 10 minutes | **Cook time:** 7 hours

- 4 eggs, beaten
- 4 oz tofu, chopped
- ½ teaspoon curry paste
- 2 tablespoons coconut milk

- 1 teaspoon olive oil
- ½ teaspoon butter, melted
1. Mix coconut milk with curry paste.
2. Then sprinkle the tofu with curry mixture.
3. After this, pour butter in the Crock Pot.
4. Add eggs, olive oil, and tofu mixture.
5. Close the lid and cook the meal on Low for 7 hours.

per serving: 118 calories, 8.1g protein, 1.4g carbohydrates, 9.4g fat, 0.4g fiber, 165mg cholesterol, 70mg sodium, 121mg potassium

Sweet Toasts

Yield: 4 servings | **Prep time:** 10 minutes | **Cook time:** 5 hours

- 4 slices of white bread
- 3 eggs, beaten
- 1 tablespoon sugar
- 1 teaspoon olive oil
- 1 teaspoon vanilla extract
1. Mix eggs with sugar and vanilla extract.
2. Then pour the mixture in the Crock Pot.
3. Add olive oil and bread slices.
4. Close the lid and cook the meal on Low for 5 hours.

per serving: 95 calories, 4.8g protein, 7.9g carbohydrates, 4.8g fat, 0.2g fiber, 123mg cholesterol, 108mg sodium, 55mg potassium

Cilantro Shrimp Bake

Yield: 4 servings | **Prep time:** 10 minutes | **Cook time:** 2.5 hours

- 1 cup potato, mashed, cooked
- ¼ cup fresh cilantro, chopped
- ¼ cup cream
- 1 teaspoon butter, melted
- 6 oz shrimps, peeled, chopped
- 4 eggs, beaten
1. Mix mashed potatoes with cream and eggs.
2. Add butter and transfer the mixture in the Crock Pot.
3. Then add cilantro and shrimps.
4. Close the lid and cook the meal on High for 2.5 hours.
5. Cool the cooked meal well and then cut into servings.

per serving: 146 calories, 15.8g protein, 4.8g carbohydrates, 6.9g fat, 0.4g fiber, 259mg cholesterol, 179mg sodium, 221mg potassium

Potato Omelet

Yield: 4 servings | **Prep time:** 10 minutes | **Cook time:** 6 hours

- 1 cup potatoes, sliced
- 1 onion, sliced
- 6 eggs, beaten
- 2 tablespoons olive oil
- 1 teaspoon salt
- ½ teaspoon ground black pepper
1. Mix potatoes with ground black pepper and salt.
2. Transfer them in the Crock Pot, add olive oil and cook on high for 30 minutes.

3. Then mix the potatoes and add onion and eggs.
4. Stir the mixture and cook the omelet on Low for 6 hours.

per serving: 192 calories, 9.3g protein, 9.1g carbohydrates, 13.6g fat, 1.6g fiber, 246mg cholesterol, 677mg sodium, 285mg potassium

Jalapeno Muffins

Yield: 4 servings | **Prep time:** 10 minutes | **Cook time:** 3 hours

- 4 tablespoons flour
- 4 jalapeno pepper, diced
- 2 eggs, beaten
- 2 tablespoons cream cheese
- 1 oz Parmesan, grated
- 1 teaspoon olive oil
1. Brush the silicone muffin molds with olive oil.
2. Then mix all remaining ingredients in the mixing bowl. In the end, you will get a smooth batter.
3. Transfer the batter in the prepared muffin molds.
4. Then put the molds in the Crock Pot and close the lid.
5. Cook the muffins on High for 3 hours.

per serving: 114 calories, 6.4g protein, 7.3g carbohydrates, 6.8g fat, 0.6g fiber, 92mg cholesterol, 112mg sodium, 74mg potassium

Feta and Eggs Muffins

Yield: 2 servings | **Prep time:** 12 minutes | **Cook time:** 6 hours

- 2 eggs, beaten
- 2 teaspoons cream cheese
- 1 oz feta, crumbled
- 1 oz fresh cilantro, chopped
- ½ teaspoon chili powder
- 1 teaspoon butter, melted
1. Mix all ingredients and pour in the silicone muffin molds.
2. After this, transfer the muffin molds in the Crock Pot.
3. Cook the breakfast on Low for 6 hours.

per serving: 134 calories, 8.2g protein, 1.9g carbohydrates, 10.6g fat, 0.6g fiber, 185mg cholesterol, 256mg sodium, 159mg potassium

Morning Ham Muffins

Yield: 4 servings | **Prep time:** 15 minutes | **Cook time:** 2.5 hours

- 4 eggs, beaten
- 3 oz Mozzarella, shredded
- 3 oz ham, chopped
- 1 teaspoon olive oil
- 1 teaspoon dried parsley
- ½ teaspoon salt
1. Mix eggs with dried parsley, salt, and ham.
2. Add mozzarella and stir the muffin mixture carefully.
3. Sprinkle the silicone muffin molds with olive oil.
4. After this, pour the egg and ham mixture in the muffin molds and transfer in the Crock Pot.
5. Cook the muffins on High for 2.5 hours.

per serving: 168 calories, 15.1g protein, 1.9g carbohydrates, 11.1g fat, 0.3g fiber, 187mg cholesterol, 757mg sodium, 122mg potassium

Potato Muffins

Yield: 4 servings | **Prep time:** 15 minutes | **Cook time:** 2 hours

- 4 teaspoons flax meal
- 1 bell pepper, diced
- 1 cup potato, cooked, mashed
- 2 eggs, beaten
- 1 teaspoon ground paprika
- 2 oz Mozzarella, shredded

1. Mix flax meal with potato and eggs.
2. Then add ground paprika and bell pepper. Stir the mixture with the help of the spoon until homogenous.
3. After this, transfer the potato mixture in the muffin molds. Top the muffins with Mozzarella and transfer in the Crock Pot.
4. Close the lid and cook the muffins on High for 2 hours.

per serving: 107 calories, 8g protein, 7.2g carbohydrates, 5.7g fat, 1.7g fiber, 89mg cholesterol, 118mg sodium, 196mg potassium

Walnut and Cheese Balls

Yield: 5 servings | **Prep time:** 15 minutes | **Cook time:** 1.5 hours

- 1 cup walnuts, grinded
- 2 eggs, beaten
- 3 oz Parmesan, grated
- ¼ cup breadcrumbs
- 2 tablespoons coconut oil, melted

1. Mix grinded walnuts and breadcrumbs.
2. Then add eggs and Parmesan.
3. Carefully mix the mixture and make the medium size balls from them.
4. Then pour melted coconut oil in the Crock Pot.
5. Add walnuts balls. Arrange them in one layer and close the lid.
6. Cook the balls on high for 1 hour.
7. Then flip them on another side and cook for 30 minutes more.

per serving: 303 calories, 14.4g protein, 7.1g carbohydrates, 25.9g fat, 1.9g fiber, 78mg cholesterol, 223mg sodium, 165mg potassium

Meat Buns

Yield: 4 servings | **Prep time:** 15 minutes | **Cook time:** 6 hours

- 1 cup ground pork
- ½ cup ground chicken
- 1 tablespoon semolina
- 1 teaspoon dried oregano
- 1 teaspoon butter, melted
- 1 teaspoon salt

1. Mix ground pork with ground chicken.
2. Add semolina, dried oregano, and salt.
3. Then add butter and stir the meat mixture until homogenous.
4. Transfer it in the silicon bun molds.
5. Put the molds with buns in the Crock Pot.

6. Close the lid and cook them on Low for 6 hours.

per serving: 110 calories, 10.4g protein, 2.1g carbohydrates, 6.3g fat, 0.3g fiber, 37mg cholesterol, 623mg sodium, 54mg potassium

Celery Stalk Muffins

Yield: 4 servings | **Prep time:** 15 minutes | **Cook time:** 3 hours

- 4 teaspoons flour
- 1 egg, beaten
- 2 tablespoons cream cheese
- ½ teaspoon baking powder
- 4 oz celery stalk, diced
- 1 teaspoon cayenne pepper
- 2 oz Cheddar cheese, shredded

1. Mix flour with eggs, cream cheese, baking powder, and cayenne pepper.
2. Then add cheese and celery stalk. Stir the mixture with the help of the spoon.
3. After this, put it in the muffin molds and transfer in the Crock Pot.
4. Cook the muffins on High for 3 hours.

per serving: 106 calories, 5.8g protein, 3.8g carbohydrates, 7.7g fat, 0.7g fiber, 61mg cholesterol, 142mg sodium, 184mg potassium

Apricot Oatmeal

Yield: 4 servings | **Prep time:** 10 minutes | **Cook time:** 4 hours

- 1 ½ cup oatmeal
- 1 cup of water
- 3 cups of milk
- 1 cup apricots, pitted, sliced
- 1 teaspoon butter

1. Put oatmeal in the Crock Pot.
2. Add water, milk, and butter.
3. Close the lid and cook the mixture on high for 1 hour.
4. Then add apricots, carefully mix the oatmeal and close the lid.
5. Cook the meal on Low for 3 hours.

per serving: 235 calories, 10.5g protein, 34g carbohydrates, 7g fat, 3.9g fiber, 18mg cholesterol, 97mg sodium, 317mg potassium

Sausage Pie

Yield: 4 servings | **Prep time:** 15 minutes | **Cook time:** 3 hours

- ½ cup flour
- ¼ cup skim milk
- 1 teaspoon baking powder
- 1 teaspoon salt
- ½ teaspoon chili flakes
- 4 sausages, chopped
- 1 egg, beaten
- Cooking spray

1. Mix flour with skin milk and baking powder.
2. Then add salt, chili flakes, and egg. Stir the mixture until smooth. You will get the batter.
3. Spray the Crock Pot with cooking spray from inside.
4. Then pour the batter in the Crock Pot.
5. Add chopped sausages and close the lid.

6.   Cook the pie on High for 3 hours.
per serving: 171 calories, 8.7g protein, 13.4g carbohydrates, 8.9g fat, 0.5g fiber, 64mg cholesterol, 809mg sodium, 262mg potassium

Shredded Chicken Muffins
Yield: 4 servings | **Prep time:** 15 minutes | **Cook time:** 2.5 hours
- 6 oz chicken fillet, boiled
- 4 eggs, beaten
- 1 teaspoon salt
- 1 teaspoon ground black pepper
- 1 teaspoon olive oil

1.   Shred the chicken fillet with the help of the fork and mix with eggs, salt, and ground black pepper.
2.   Then brush the muffin molds with olive oil and transfer the shredded chicken mixture inside.
3.   Put the muffins in the Crock Pot.
4.   Close the lid and cook them on High for 2.5 hours.
per serving: 155 calories, 17.9g protein, 0.7g carbohydrates, 8.7g fat, 0.1g fiber, 202mg cholesterol, 680mg sodium, 169mg potassium

Soups, Chilies & Stews

Chicken and Noodles Soup
Yield: 8 servings | **Prep time:** 10 minutes | **Cook time:** 7 hours
- 1-pound chicken breast, skinless, boneless, chopped
- 1 teaspoon salt
- 1 teaspoon chili flakes
- 1 teaspoon coriander
- 1 cup bell pepper, chopped
- 4 oz egg noodles
- 8 cups chicken stock

1.   Mix chicken breast with salt, chili flakes, coriander, and place in the Crock Pot.
2.   Add chicken stock and close the lid.
3.   Cook the ingredients on Low for 6 hours.
4.   Then add egg noodles and bell pepper and cook the soup for 1 hour on High.
per serving: 99 calories, 13.5g protein, 5.4g carbohydrates, 2.3g fat, 0.4g fiber, 40mg cholesterol, 1084mg sodium, 259mg potassium.

Light Zucchini Soup
Yield: 4 servings | **Prep time:** 15 minutes | **Cook time:** 30 minutes
- 1 large zucchini
- 1 white onion, diced
- 4 cups beef broth
- 1 teaspoon dried thyme
- ½ teaspoon dried rosemary

1.   Pour the beef broth in the Crock Pot.
2.   Add onion, dried thyme, and dried rosemary.
3.   After this, make the spirals from the zucchini with the help of the spiralizer and transfer them in the Crock Pot.

4.   Close the lid and cook the sou on High for 30 minutes.
per serving: 64 calories, 6.2g protein, 6.5g carbohydrates, 1.6g fat, 1.6g fiber, 0mg cholesterol, 773mg sodium, 462mg potassium.

Garlic Bean Soup
Yield: 4 servings | **Prep time:** 10 minutes | **Cook time:** 8 hours
- 1 teaspoon minced garlic
- 1 cup celery stalk, chopped
- 1 cup white beans, soaked
- 5 cups of water
- 1 teaspoon salt
- 1 teaspoon ground paprika
- 1 tablespoon tomato paste

1.   Put all ingredients in the Crock Pot and carefully stir until tomato paste is dissolved.
2.   Then close the lid and cook the soup on low for 8 hours.
per serving: 178 calories, 12.3g protein, 32.5g carbohydrates, 0.6g fat, 8.5g fiber, 0mg cholesterol, 623mg sodium, 1031mg potassium.

French Soup
Yield: 5 servings | **Prep time:** 10 minutes | **Cook time:** 7 hours
- 5 oz Gruyere cheese, shredded
- 2 cups of water
- 2 cups chicken stock
- 2 cups white onion, diced
- ½ teaspoon cayenne pepper
- ½ cup heavy cream

1.   Pour chicken stock, water, and heavy cream in the Crock Pot.
2.   Add onion, cayenne pepper, and close the lid.
3.   Cook the ingredients on high for 4 hours.
4.   When the time is finished, open the lid, stir the mixture, and add cheese.
5.   Carefully mix the soup and cook it on Low for 3 hours.
per serving: 181 calories, 9.5g protein, 5.1g carbohydrates, 13.9g fat, 1g fiber, 48mg cholesterol, 410mg sodium, 110mg potassium.

Mexican Style Soup
Yield: 6 servings | **Prep time:** 10 minutes | **Cook time:** 5 hours
- 1-pound chicken fillet, cut into strips
- 2 tablespoons enchilada sauce
- 6 cups chicken stock
- 1 cup black beans, soaked
- 1 cup tomatoes, chopped
- 1 teaspoon garlic powder
- ¼ cup fresh cilantro, chopped

1.   Put all ingredients in the Crock Pot and close the lid.
2.   Cook the soup on high for 5 hours.
3.   When the time is finished, open the lid and carefully mix the soup with the help of the ladle.
per serving: 276 calories, 30.1g protein, 23.8g carbohydrates, 6.8g fat, 5.9g fiber, 67mg cholesterol, 833mg sodium, 784mg potassium.

Paprika Noddle Soup

Yield: 4 servings | **Prep time:** 10 minutes | **Cook time:** 4 hours

- 3 oz egg noodles
- 3 cups chicken stock
- 1 teaspoon butter
- 1 teaspoon ground paprika
- ½ teaspoon salt
- 2 tablespoons fresh parsley, chopped

1. Put egg noodles in the Crock Pot.
2. Add chicken stock, butter, ground paprika, and salt.
3. Close the lid and cook the soup on High for 4 hours.
4. Then open the lid, add parsley, and stir the soup.

per serving: 47 calories, 1.6g protein, 6.3g carbohydrates, 1.9g fat, 0.5g fiber, 9mg cholesterol, 873mg sodium, 42mg potassium.

Butternut Squash Soup

Yield: 5 servings | **Prep time:** 15 minutes | **Cook time:** 7 hours

- 2 cups butternut squash, chopped
- 1 cup carrot, chopped
- 3 cups chicken stock
- 1 cup heavy cream
- 1 teaspoon ground cardamom
- 1 teaspoon ground cinnamon

Put the butternut squash in the Crock Pot.
Sprinkle it with ground cardamom and ground cinnamon.
Then add carrot and chicken stock.
Close the lid and cook the soup on High for 5 hours.
Then blend the soup until smooth with the help of the immersion blender and add heavy cream.
Cook the soup on high for 2 hours more.

per serving: 125 calories, 1.7g protein, 10.5g carbohydrates, 9.3g fat, 2g fiber, 33mg cholesterol, 485mg sodium, 301mg potassium.

Taco Soup

Yield: 3 servings | **Prep time:** 10 minutes | **Cook time:** 8 hours

- 1 cup ground chicken
- 3 cup chicken stock
- 1 tomato, chopped
- ¼ cup corn kernels
- 1 jalapeno pepper, sliced
- 1 tablespoon taco seasoning
- ¼ cup black olives, sliced
- 3 corn tortillas, chopped

1. Put the ground chicken in the Crock Pot.
2. Add chicken stock, tomato, corn kernels, jalapeno pepper, taco seasoning, and black olives.
3. Close the lid and cook the soup on low for 8 hours.
4. When the soup is cooked, ladle it in the bowls and top with chopped tortillas.

per serving: 193 calories, 16.3g protein, 18.3g carbohydrates, 6.1g fat, 2.6g fiber, 42mg cholesterol, 1196mg sodium, 267mg potassium.

Cream of Chicken Soup

Yield: 5 servings | **Prep time:** 10 minutes | **Cook time:** 6 hours

- 1-pound chicken fillet
- 5 cups chicken stock
- 1 cup heavy cream
- 1 tablespoon smoked paprika
- ½ cup Cheddar cheese, shredded
- ½ cup cauliflower, chopped
- 1 teaspoon ground black pepper

1. Put the chicken in the Crock Pot.
2. Add chicken stock, heavy cream, smoked paprika, cauliflower, and ground black pepper.
3. Close the lid and cook the mixture for 5 hours on High.
4. After this, remove the chicken from the Crock Pot.
5. Blend the remaining Crock Pot mixture until smooth.
6. Then return the shredded chicken in the Crock Pot.
7. Add Cheddar cheese and cook the soup on High for 1 hour.

per serving: 318 calories, 30.7g protein, 3.1g carbohydrates, 20.1g fat, 0.9g fiber, 125mg cholesterol, 925mg sodium, 332mg potassium.

Celery Soup with Ham

Yield: 8 servings | **Prep time:** 10 minutes | **Cook time:** 5 hours

- 8 oz ham, chopped
- 8 cups chicken stock
- 1 teaspoon white pepper
- ½ teaspoon cayenne pepper
- 2 cups celery stalk, chopped
- ½ cup corn kernels

Put all ingredients in the Crock Pot and gently stir.
Close the lid and cook the soup on High for 5 hours.
When the soup is cooked, cool it to the room temperature and ladle into the bowls.

per serving: 69 calories, 5.9g protein, 4.6g carbohydrates, 3.2g fat, 1.1g fiber, 16mg cholesterol, 1155mg sodium, 193mg potassium.

Spiced Lasagna Soup

Yield: 6 servings | **Prep time:** 20 minutes | **Cook time:** 6 hours

- 2 sheets of lasagna noodles, crushed
- 1 oz Parmesan, grated
- 1 teaspoon ground turmeric
- 1 yellow onion, diced
- 2 cups ground beef
- 6 cups beef broth
- ½ cup tomatoes, chopped
- 1 tablespoon dried basil

1. Roast the ground beef in the hot skillet for 4 minutes. Stir it constantly and transfer in the Crock Pot.
2. Add turmeric, onion, tomatoes, basil, and beef broth.
3. Stir the soup, add lasagna noodles, and close the lid.

4. Cook the soup on High for 6 hours.
5. Top the cooked soup with Parmesan.
per serving: 208 calories, 17.8g protein, 14.6g carbohydrates, 8.3g fat, 0.7g fiber, 40mg cholesterol, 840mg sodium, 390mg potassium.

Barley Soup
Yield: 5 servings | **Prep time:** 10 minutes | **Cook time:** 8 hours

- ¼ cup barley
- 5 cups chicken stock
- 4 oz pork tenderloin, chopped
- 1 tablespoon dried cilantro
- 1 tablespoon tomato paste
- 3 oz carrot, grated
- ½ cup heavy cream

1. Put pork tenderloin in the Crock Pot.
2. Add barley, chicken stock, tomato paste, carrot, and heavy cream.
3. Carefully stir the soup mixture and close the lid.
4. Cook it on Low for 8 hours.
per serving: 126 calories, 8.3g protein, 10.1g carbohydrates, 6g fat, 2.2g fiber, 33mg cholesterol, 797mg sodium, 249mg potassium.

Lobster Soup
Yield: 4 servings | **Prep time:** 10 minutes | **Cook time:** 2 hours

- 4 cups of water
- 1-pound lobster tail, chopped
- ½ cup fresh cilantro, chopped
- 1 cup coconut cream
- 1 teaspoon ground coriander
- 1 garlic clove, diced

1. Pour water and coconut cream in the Crock Pot.
2. Add a lobster tail, cilantro, and ground coriander.
3. Then add the garlic clove and close the lid.
4. Cook the lobster soup on High for 2 hours.
per serving: 241 calories, 23g protein, 3.6g carbohydrates, 15.2g fat, 1.4g fiber, 165mg cholesterol, 568mg sodium, 435mg potassium.

Red Kidney Beans Soup
Yield: 6 servings | **Prep time:** 10 minutes | **Cook time:** 5 hours

- 2 cups red kidney beans, canned
- 1 cup cauliflower, chopped
- 1 cup carrot, diced
- 1 teaspoon chili powder
- 1 teaspoon Italian seasonings
- 1 cup tomatoes, canned
- 4 cups chicken stock

1. Put all ingredients except red kidney beans in the Crock Pot.
2. Close the lid and cook the soup on High for 4 hours.
3. Then add red kidney beans and stir the soup carefully with the help of the spoon.
4. Close the lid and cook it on high for 1 hour more.

per serving: 234 calories, 15.1g protein, 42.3g carbohydrates, 1.4g fat, 10.7g fiber, 1mg cholesterol, 540mg sodium, 1032mg potassium.

Light Minestrone Soup
Yield: 4 servings | **Prep time:** 7 minutes | **Cook time:** 4 hours

- 1 cup green beans, chopped
- 1 small zucchini, chopped
- ¼ cup garbanzo beans
- 5 cups chicken stock
- 1 teaspoon curry powder
- 2 tablespoons tomato paste
- ½ cup ground pork

1. Put all ingredients in the Crock Pot bowl.
2. Close the lid and cook the soup on High for 4 hours.
per serving: 195 calories, 14.6g protein, 13.3g carbohydrates, 9.8g fat, 3.9g fiber, 37mg cholesterol, 999mg sodium, 493mg potassium.

Orange Soup
Yield: 6 servings | **Prep time:** 15 minutes | **Cook time:** 4 hours

- 1 cup sweet potato, chopped
- 1 cup carrot, chopped
- 1 teaspoon ground turmeric
- 1 teaspoon curry powder
- 1 cup heavy cream
- 4 cups of water

1. Put sweet potato and carrot in the Crock Pot.
2. Add ground turmeric and water.
3. Then mix the curry powder and heavy cream and pour the liquid over the vegetables.
4. Close the lid and cook the soup for 4 hours on High.
5. Blend the soup with the help of the immersion blender if desired.
per serving: 109 calories, 1.3g protein, 9.7g carbohydrates, 7.6g fat, 1.8g fiber, 27mg cholesterol, 37mg sodium, 248mg potassium.

Green Peas Chowder
Yield: 6 servings | **Prep time:** 10 minutes | **Cook time:** 8 hours

- 1-pound chicken breast, skinless, boneless, chopped
- 6 cups of water
- 1 cup green peas
- ¼ cup Greek Yogurt
- 1 tablespoon dried basil
- 1 teaspoon ground black pepper
- ½ teaspoon salt

1. Mix salt, chicken breast, ground black pepper, and dried basil.
2. Transfer the ingredients in the Crock Pot.
3. Add water, green peas, yogurt, and close the lid.
4. Cook the chowder on Low for 8 hours.
per serving: 113 calories, 18.2g protein, 4.1g carbohydrates, 2.2g fat, 1.3g fiber, 49mg cholesterol, 244mg sodium, 359mg potassium.

German Style Soup

Yield: 6 servings | **Prep time:** 10 minutes | **Cook time:** 8.5 hours

- 1-pound beef loin, chopped
- 6 cups of water
- 1 cup sauerkraut
- 1 onion, diced
- 1 teaspoon cayenne pepper
- ½ cup greek yogurt
1. Put beef and onion in the Crock Pot.
2. Add yogurt, water, and cayenne pepper.
3. Cook the mixture on low for 8 hours.
4. When the beef is cooked, add sauerkraut and stir the soup carefully.
5. Cook the soup on high for 30 minutes.

per serving: 137 calories, 16.1g protein, 4.3g carbohydrates, 5.8g fat, 1.1g fiber, 41mg cholesterol, 503mg sodium, 93mg potassium.

Chorizo Soup
Yield: 6 servings | **Prep time:** 10 minutes | **Cook time:** 5 hours

- 9 oz chorizo, chopped
- 7 cups of water
- 1 cup potato, chopped
- 1 teaspoon minced garlic, chopped
- 1 zucchini, chopped
- ½ cup spinach, chopped
- 1 teaspoon salt
1. Put the chorizo in the skillet and roast it for 2 minutes per side on high heat.
2. Then transfer the chorizo in the Crock Pot.
3. Add water, potato, minced garlic, zucchini, spinach, and salt.
4. Close the lid and cook the soup on high for 5 hours.
5. Then cool the soup to the room temperature.

per serving: 210 calories, 11g protein, 4.3g carbohydrates, 16.4g fat, 0.7g fiber, 37mg cholesterol, 927mg sodium, 326mg potassium.

Shrimp Chowder
Yield: 4 servings | **Prep time:** 5 minutes | **Cook time:** 1 hour

- 1-pound shrimps
- ½ cup fennel bulb, chopped
- 1 bay leaf
- ½ teaspoon peppercorn
- 1 cup of coconut milk
- 3 cups of water
- 1 teaspoon ground coriander
1. Put all ingredients in the Crock Pot.
2. Close the lid and cook the chowder on High for 1 hour.

per serving: 277 calories, 27.4g protein, 6.1g carbohydrates, 16.3g fat, 1.8g fiber, 239mg cholesterol, 297mg sodium, 401mg potassium.

Snow Peas Soup
Yield: 4 servings | **Prep time:** 10 minutes | **Cook time:** 3.5 hours

- 1 tablespoon chives, chopped
- 1 teaspoon ground ginger
- 8 oz salmon fillet, chopped

- 5 oz bamboo shoots, canned, chopped
- 2 cups snow peas
- 1 teaspoon hot sauce
- 5 cups of water
1. Put bamboo shoots in the Crock Pot.
2. Add ground ginger, salmon, snow peas, and water.
3. Close the lid and cook the soup for 3 hours on high.
4. Then add hot sauce and chives. Stir the soup carefully and cook for 30 minutes on high.

per serving: 120 calories, 14.6g protein, 7.9g carbohydrates, 3.8g fat, 3.1g fiber, 25mg cholesterol, 70mg sodium, 612mg potassium

Clam Soup
Yield: 2 servings | **Prep time:** 10 minutes | **Cook time:** 1.5 hours

- ¼ teaspoon ground black pepper
- ¼ teaspoon chili flakes
- 3 cups fish stock
- 8 oz clams, canned
- 1 oz scallions, chopped
- 2 tablespoons sour cream
- ½ teaspoon dried thyme
1. Pour fish stock in the Crock Pot.
2. Add canned clams, chili flakes, ground black pepper, scallions, and dried thyme.
3. Add sour cream and dried thyme.
4. Cook the soup on High for 1.5 hours.

per serving: 145 calories, 9.3g protein, 14.3g carbohydrates, 5.6g fat, 1g fiber, 9mg cholesterol, 965mg sodium, 667mg potassium.

Turmeric Squash Soup
Yield: 6 servings | **Prep time:** 10 minutes | **Cook time:** 9 hours

- 3 chicken thighs, skinless, boneless, chopped
- 3 cups butternut squash, chopped
- 1 teaspoon ground turmeric
- 1 onion, sliced
- 1 oz green chilies, chopped, canned
- 6 cups of water
1. Put chicken thighs in the bottom of the Crock Pot and top them with green chilies.
2. Then add the ground turmeric, butternut squash, and water.
3. Add sliced onion and close the lid.
4. Cook the soup on low for 9 Hours.

per serving: 194 calories, 22.6g protein, 13.4g carbohydrates, 5.8g fat, 3.2g fiber, 65mg cholesterol, 78mg sodium, 551mg potassium.

Ground Pork Soup
Yield: 4 servings | **Prep time:** 10 minutes | **Cook time:** 5.5 hour

- 1 cup ground pork
- ½ cup red kidney beans, canned
- 1 cup tomatoes, canned
- 4 cups of water
- 1 tablespoon dried cilantro
- 1 teaspoon salt

1. Put ground pork in the Crock Pot.
2. Add tomatoes, water, dried cilantro, and salt.
3. Close the lid and cook the ingredients on High for 5 hours.
4. Then add canned red kidney beans and cook the soup on high for 30 minutes more.

per serving: 318 calories, 25.7g protein, 15.9g carbohydrates, 16.6g fat, 4.1g fiber, 74mg cholesterol, 651mg sodium, 706mg potassium.

White Mushroom Soup
Yield: 6 servings | **Prep time:** 15 minutes | **Cook time:** 8 hours

- 9 oz white mushrooms, chopped
- 6 chicken stock
- 1 teaspoon dried cilantro
- ½ teaspoon ground black pepper
- 1 teaspoon butter
- 1 cup potatoes, chopped
- ½ carrot, diced

1. Melt butter in the skillet.
2. Add white mushrooms and roast them for 5 minutes on high heat. Stir the mushrooms constantly.
3. Transfer them in the Crock Pot.
4. Add chicken stock, cilantro, ground black pepper, and potato.
5. Add carrot and close the lid.
6. Cook the soup on low for 8 hours.

per serving: 44 calories, 2.5g protein, 6.7g carbohydrates, 1.4g fat, 1.2g fiber, 2mg cholesterol, 776mg sodium, 271mg potassium.

Yogurt Soup
Yield: 4 servings | **Prep time:** 10 minutes | **Cook time:** 5 hours

- 1 cup Greek yogurt
- ½ teaspoon dried mint
- ½ teaspoon ground black pepper
- 1 onion, diced
- 1 tablespoon coconut oil
- 3 cups chicken stock
- 7 oz chicken fillet, chopped

1. Melt the coconut oil in the skillet.
2. Add onion and roast it until light brown.
3. After this, transfer the roasted onion in the Crock Pot.
4. Add dried mint, ground black pepper, chicken stock, and chicken fillet.
5. Add Greek yogurt and carefully mix the soup ingredients.
6. Close the lid and cook the soup on High for 5 hours.

per serving: 180 calories, 20.2g protein, 5.3g carbohydrates, 8.6g fat, 0.7g fiber, 47mg cholesterol, 633mg sodium, 247mg potassium.

Russet Potato Soup
Yield: 6 servings | **Prep time:** 15 minutes | **Cook time:** 7 hours

- 1 cup onion, diced
- 5 cups of water
- 2 cups russet potatoes, chopped
- 1 teaspoon dried parsley

- 1 garlic clove
- ½ cup carrot, grated
- 1 oz Parmesan, grated
- 1 cup heavy cream

1. Put the onion in the Crock Pot.
2. Add water, potatoes, parsley, peeled garlic clove, carrot, and heavy cream.
3. Close the lid and cook the soup on low for 7 hours.
4. When the time is finished, mash the soup gently with the help of the potato mash.
5. Add Parmesan and stir the soup.

per serving: 131 calories, 3.1g protein, 11.5g carbohydrates, 8.5g fat, 1.9g fiber, 31mg cholesterol, 68mg sodium, 281mg potassium.

Lamb Stew
Yield: 5 servings | **Prep time:** 15 minutes | **Cook time:** 5 hours

- 1 pound lamb meat, cubed
- 1 red onion, sliced
- 1 teaspoon cayenne pepper
- 1 teaspoon dried rosemary
- ½ teaspoon dried thyme
- 1 cup potatoes, chopped
- 4 cups of water

1. Sprinkle the lamb meat with cayenne pepper, dried rosemary, and dried thyme.
2. Transfer the meat in the Crock Pot.
3. Add water, onion, and potatoes.
4. Close the lid and cook the stew on high for 5 hours.

per serving: 216 calories, 17.7g protein, 7.2g carbohydrates, 12.2g fat, 1.4g fiber, 64mg cholesterol, 73mg sodium, 166mg potassium.

Tomato Chickpeas Stew
Yield: 4 servings | **Prep time:** 10 minutes | **Cook time:** 7 hours

- 2 tablespoons tomato paste
- 1 cup chickpeas, soaked
- 5 cups of water
- 1 yellow onion, chopped
- ½ cup fresh parsley, chopped
- 1 teaspoon ground black pepper
- 1 carrot, chopped

1. Mix tomato paste with water and pour in the Crock Pot.
2. Add chickpeas, onion, parsley, ground black pepper, and carrot.
3. Close the lid and cook the stew on Low for 7 hours.

per serving: 210 calories, 10.7g protein, 36.7g carbohydrates, 3.2g fat, 10.4g fiber, 0mg cholesterol, 45mg sodium, 659mg potassium.

Hot Lentil Soup
Yield: 4 servings | **Prep time:** 15 minutes | **Cook time:** 24.5 hours

- 1 potato, peeled, diced
- 1 cup lentils
- 5 cups chicken stock

- 1 onion, diced
- 1 teaspoon chili powder 1 teaspoon cayenne pepper
- 1 teaspoon olive oil
- 1 tablespoon tomato paste

1. Roast the onion in the olive oil until light brown and transfer in the Crock Pot.
2. Add lentils, chicken stock, potato, chili powder, cayenne pepper, and tomato paste.
3. Carefully stir the soup mixture until the tomato paste is dissolved.
4. Close the lid and cook the soup on High for 4.5 hours.

per serving: 242 calories, 14.7g protein, 41.1g carbohydrates, 2.7g fat, 16.7g fiber, 0mg cholesterol, 972mg sodium, 758mg potassium.

Coconut Cod Stew
Yield: 6 servings | **Prep time:** 15 minutes | **Cook time:** 6.5 hours

- 1-pound cod fillet, chopped
- 2 oz scallions, roughly chopped
- 1 cup coconut cream
- 1 teaspoon curry powder
- 1 teaspoon garlic, diced

1. Mix curry powder with coconut cream and garlic.
2. Add scallions and gently stir the liquid.
3. After this, pour it in the Crock Pot and add cod fillet.
4. Stir the stew mixture gently and close the lid.
5. Cook the stew on low for 6.5 hours.

per serving: 158 calories, 14.7g protein, 3.3g carbohydrates, 10.3g fat, 1.3g fiber, 37mg cholesterol, 55mg sodium, 138mg potassium.

Celery Stew
Yield: 4 servings | **Prep time:** 15 minutes | **Cook time:** 6 hours

- 3 cups of water
- 1-pound beef stew meat, cubed
- 2 cups celery, chopped
- ½ cup cremini mushrooms, sliced
- 2 tablespoons sour cream
- 1 teaspoon smoked paprika
- 1 teaspoon cayenne pepper
- 1 tablespoon sesame oil

1. Mix beef stew meat with cayenne pepper and put in the hot skillet.
2. Add sesame oil and roast the meat for 1 minute per side on high heat.
3. Transfer the meat in the Crock Pot.
4. Add celery, cremini mushrooms, sour cream, smoked paprika, and water.
5. Close the lid and cook the stew on high for 6 hours.

per serving: 267 calories, 35.3g protein, 2.7g carbohydrates, 12g fat, 1.2g fiber, 104g cholesterol, 124mg sodium, 660mg potassium.

Tender Mushroom Stew
Yield: 6 servings | **Prep time:** 10 minutes | **Cook time:** 8 hours

- 1-pound cremini mushrooms, chopped
- 1 cup carrot, grated
- 1 yellow onion, diced
- 2 teaspoons dried basil
- ½ cup greek yogurt
- ½ cup rutabaga, chopped
- 5 cups beef broth

1. Put all ingredients in the Crock Pot.
2. Close the lid and cook the stew on Low for 8 hours.

per serving: 84 calories, 8.1g protein, g carbohydrates, 1.6g fat, 1.6g fiber, 1mg cholesterol, 662mg sodium, 660mg potassium

Beans Stew
Yield: 3 servings | **Prep time:** 10 minutes | **Cook time:** 5 hours

- ½ cup sweet pepper, chopped
- ¼ cup onion, chopped
- 1 cup edamame beans
- 1 cup tomatoes
- 1 teaspoon cayenne pepper
- 5 cups of water
- 2 tablespoons cream cheese

1. Mix water with cream cheese and pour the liquid in the Crock Pot.
2. Add cayenne pepper, edamame beans, and onion.
3. Then chop the tomatoes roughly and add in the Crock Pot.
4. Close the lid and cook the stew on high for 5 hours.

per serving: 74 calories, 3.4g protein, 7.9g carbohydrates, 3.6g fat, 2.4g fiber, 7mg cholesterol, 109mg sodium, 218mg potassium.

Lentil Stew
Yield: 4 servings | **Prep time:** 10 minutes | **Cook time:** 6 hours

- 2 cups chicken stock
- ½ cup red lentils
- 1 eggplant, chopped
- 1 tablespoon tomato paste
- 1 cup of water
- 1 teaspoon Italian seasonings

1. Mix chicken stock with red lentils and tomato paste.
2. Pour the mixture in the Crock Pot.
3. Add eggplants and Italian seasonings.
4. Cook the stew on low for 6 hours.

per serving: 125 calories, 7.8g protein, 22.4g carbohydrates, 1.1g fat, 11.5g fiber, 1mg cholesterol, 392mg sodium, 540mg potassium.

Ground Beef Stew
Yield: 5 servings | **Prep time:** 10 minutes | **Cook time:** 7 hours

- 1 cup bell pepper, diced
- 2 cups ground beef
- 1 teaspoon minced garlic
- 1 teaspoon dried rosemary
- 1 cup tomatoes, chopped

- 1 teaspoon salt
- 3 cups of water
1. Put all ingredients in the Crock Pot and stir them.
2. Close the lid and cook the stew on Low for 7 hours.

per serving: 135 calories, 18.6g protein, 3.5g carbohydrates, 4.8g fat, 0.9g fiber, 55mg cholesterol, 524mg sodium, 419mg potassium.

Chicken Chili
Yield: 4 servings | **Prep time:** 10 minutes | **Cook time:** 5 hours

- 2 cups ground chicken
- 1 chili pepper, chopped
- 1 yellow onion, chopped
- 2 tablespoons tomato paste
- 1 teaspoon dried basil
- ½ teaspoon ground coriander
- 3 cups of water
1. Mix ground chicken with dried basil and ground coriander.
2. Then transfer the chicken in the Crock Pot.
3. Add onion, chili pepper, tomato paste, and water. Carefully stir the mixture and close the lid.
4. Cook the chili on high for 5 hours.

per serving: 151 calories, 20.9g protein, 4.2g carbohydrates, 5.3g fat, 1g fiber, 62mg cholesterol, 75mg sodium, 296mg potassium.

Haddock Stew
Yield: 6 servings | **Prep time:** 15 minutes | **Cook time:** 3 hours

- ½ cup clam juice
- 2 teaspoons tomato paste
- 2 celery stalks, chopped
- ½ teaspoon ground coriander
- 14 oz haddock fillet, chopped
- 1 cup of water
- 1 teaspoon butter
1. Melt the butter in the skillet and add chopped fish fillets.
2. Roast them for 1 minute per side and transfer in the Crock Pot.
3. Add celery stalk, ground coriander, clam juice, and tomato paste.
4. Then add water and close the lid.
5. Cook the stew on high for 3 hours.
6. Carefully stir the stew before serving.

per serving: 92 calories, 16.3g protein, 2.7g carbohydrates, 1.3g fat, 0.2g fiber, 51mg cholesterol, 142mg sodium, 315mg potassium.

Autumn Stew
Yield: 4 servings | **Prep time:** 10 minutes | **Cook time:** 6 hours

- 1 cup potatoes, chopped
- ½ cup broccoli, chopped
- 1 cup baby spinach
- 1 teaspoon curry paste
- 2 tablespoons heavy cream
- 1 carrot, chopped

- 3 cups chicken stock
1. In the shallow bowl mix curry paste and heavy cream. Pour the liquid in the Crock Pot.
2. Add potatoes, broccoli, baby spinach, carrot, and chicken stock.
3. Close the lid and cook the stew on Low for 6 hours.

per serving: 79 calories, 2g protein, 9.5g carbohydrates, 4g fat, 1.7g fiber, 10mg cholesterol, 598mg sodium, 296mg potassium.

French Stew
Yield: 4 servings | **Prep time:** 10 minutes | **Cook time:** 6 hours

- 1 zucchini, cubed
- 1 eggplant, cubed
- 1 cup tomatoes, canned
- 1 teaspoon dried oregano
- 3 oz Provolone cheese, chopped
- 7 oz beef sirloin, chopped
- 1 teaspoon ground black pepper
- 3 cups of water
1. Put chopped beef sirloin in the Crock Pot.
2. Add water, ground black pepper, dried oregano, and tomatoes.
3. Cook the ingredients on High for 4 hours.
4. Then add zucchini, eggplant, and all remaining ingredients.
5. Close the lid and cook the stew on high for 2 hours.

per serving: 214 calories, 22.7g protein, 11.2g carbohydrates, 9.2g fat, 5.4g fiber, 59mg cholesterol, 234mg sodium, 741mg potassium.

Ginger and Sweet Potato Stew
Yield: 3 servings | **Prep time:** 10 minutes | **Cook time:** 7 hours

- 1 cup sweet potatoes, chopped
- ½ teaspoon ground ginger
- 1 cup bell pepper, cut into the strips
- 1 apple, chopped
- 1 teaspoon ground cumin
- 2 cups beef broth
1. Mix ingredients in the Crock Pot.
2. Close the lid and cook the stew on Low for 7 hours.

per serving: 140 calories, 4.8g protein, 28.3g carbohydrates, 1.4g fat, 4.5g fiber, 0mg cholesterol, 516mg sodium, 716mg potassium.

Tomato and Turkey Chili
Yield: 6 servings | **Prep time:** 10 minutes | **Cook time:** 7 hours

- 1-pound turkey fillet, chopped
- 2 cup tomatoes, chopped
- 1 jalapeno pepper, chopped
- 1 onion, diced
- 1 cup chicken stock
1. Put turkey and tomatoes in the Crock Pot.
2. Add jalapeno pepper, onion, and chicken stock.
3. Close the lid and cook the chili on low for 7 hours.

per serving: 164 calories, 22.7g protein, 4.3g carbohydrates, 5.8g fat, 1.2g fiber, 67mg cholesterol, 196mg sodium, 360mg potassium.

Bacon Stew

Yield: 4 servings | **Prep time:** 10 minutes | **Cook time:** 5 hours

- 3 oz bacon, chopped, cooked
- 1/3 teaspoon ground black pepper
- ½ teaspoon garlic powder
- 2 cups vegetable stock
- 1 tablespoon cornstarch
- 1 cup turnip, peeled, chopped
- ½ cup carrot, chopped

1. Mix cornstarch with vegetable stock and whisk until smooth.
2. Pour the liquid in the Crock Pot.
3. Add all remaining ingredients and close the lid.
4. Cook the stew on low for 5 hours.

per serving: 142 calories, 8.6g protein, 6.4g carbohydrates, 9g fat, 1.3g fiber, 23mg cholesterol, 548mg sodium, 232mg potassium.

Butternut Squash Chili

Yield: 4 servings | **Prep time:** 10 minutes | **Cook time:** 3.5 hours

- 1 cup butternut squash, chopped
- 2 tablespoons pumpkin puree
- ½ cup red kidney beans, canned
- 1 teaspoon smoked paprika
- ½ teaspoon chili flakes
- 1 tablespoon cocoa powder
- ½ teaspoon salt
- 2 cups chicken stock

1. Mix cocoa powder with chicken stock and stir it until smooth.
2. Then pour the liquid in the Crock Pot.
3. Add all remaining ingredients and carefully mix the chili.
4. Close the lid and cook the chili on high for 3.5 hours.

per serving: 105 calories, 6.3g protein, 20.2g carbohydrates, 0.8g fat, 5g fiber, 0mg cholesterol, 678mg sodium, 506mg potassium.

Beef Liver Stew

Yield: 3 servings | **Prep time:** 15 minutes | **Cook time:** 7 hours

- 6 oz beef liver, cut into strips
- 2 tablespoons all-purpose flour
- 1 tablespoon olive oil
- ½ cup sour cream
- ½ cup of water
- 1 onion, roughly chopped
- 1 teaspoon ground black pepper

1. Mix beef liver with flour and roast it in the olive oil on high heat for 2 minutes per side.
2. Then transfer the liver in the Crock Pot.
3. Add all remaining ingredients and close the lid.
4. Cook the stew on low for 7 hours.

per serving: 257 calories, 17.3g protein, 12.4g carbohydrates, 15.5g fat, 1.1g fiber, 233mg cholesterol, 67mg sodium, 323mg potassium.

Paprika Hominy Stew

Yield: 4 servings | **Prep time:** 10 minutes | **Cook time:** 4 hours

- 2 cups hominy, canned
- 1 tablespoon smoked paprika
- 1 teaspoon hot sauce
- ½ cup full-fat cream
- ½ cup ground chicken
- 1 cup of water

1. Carefully mix all ingredients in the Crock Pot and close the lid.
2. Cook the stew on high for 4 hours.

per serving: 126 calories, 10.7g protein, 14.4g carbohydrates, 2.6g fat, 2.7g fiber, 18mg cholesterol, 380mg sodium, 140mg potassium.

Barley Stew

Yield: 4 servings | **Prep time:** 7 minutes | **Cook time:** 9 hours

- ½ cup barley
- 4 cups chicken stock
- 1 cup zucchini, chopped
- 1 tablespoon tomato paste
- ½ carrot, diced
- 1 teaspoon salt

1. Put all ingredients in the Crock Pot and carefully stir.
2. Cook the stew on low for 9 hours.

per serving: 102 calories, 4.1g protein, 20.1g carbohydrates, 1.2g fat, 4.6g fiber, 0mg cholesterol, 1360mg sodium, 258mg potassium.

Fennel Stew

Yield: 6 servings | **Prep time:** 15 minutes | **Cook time:** 5 hours

- 1-pound beef sirloin, chopped
- 1 cup fennel bulb, chopped
- 3 cups of water
- 1 yellow onion, chopped
- 1 tablespoon dried dill
- 1 teaspoon olive oil

1. Roast beef sirloin in the skillet for 2 minutes per side.
2. Then transfer the meat in the Crock Pot.
3. Add olive oil, a fennel bulb, water, onion, and dried dill.
4. Close the lid and cook the stew on high for 5 hours.

per serving: 160 calories, 23.4g protein, 3.1g carbohydrates, 5.6g fat, 0.9g fiber, 68mg cholesterol, 63mg sodium, 410mg potassium.

Cabbage Stew

Yield: 2 servings | **Prep time:** 7 minutes | **Cook time:** 3 hours

- 2 cups white cabbage, shredded
- ½ cup tomato juice
- 1 teaspoon ground white pepper

- 1 cup cauliflower, chopped
- ½ cup potato, chopped
- 1 cup of water
1. Put cabbage, potato, and cauliflower in the Crock Pot.
2. Add tomato juice, ground white pepper, and water. Stir the stew ingredients and close the lid.
3. Cook the stew on high for 3 hours.
per serving: 57 calories, 2.8g protein, 13.3g carbohydrates, 0.2g fat, 3.9g fiber, 0mg cholesterol, 196mg sodium, 503mg potassium.

Smoked Sausage Stew
Yield: 5 servings | **Prep time:** 10 minutes | **Cook time:** 3.5 hours
- 1-pound smoked sausages, chopped
- 1 cup broccoli, chopped
- 1 cup tomato juice
- 1 cup of water
- 1 teaspoon butter
- 1 teaspoon dried thyme
- ¼ cup Cheddar cheese, shredded
1. Grease the Crock Pot bowl with butter from inside.
2. Put the smoked sausages in one layer in the Crock Pot.
3. Add the layer of broccoli and Cheddar cheese.
4. Then mix water with tomato juice and dried thyme.
5. Pour the liquid over the sausage mixture and close the lid.
6. Cook the stew on high for 3.5 hours.
per serving: 352 calories, 20g protein, 3.5g carbohydrates, 28.5g fat, 0.7g fiber, 84mg cholesterol, 858mg sodium, 443mg potassium

Meat Baby Carrot Stew
Yield: 3 servings | **Prep time:** 10 minutes | **Cook time:** 8 hours
- 1 cup baby carrot
- 6 oz lamb loin, chopped
- 1 tablespoon tomato paste
- 1 teaspoon peppercorns
- 3 cups of water
- 1 bay leaf
1. Put all ingredients in the Crock Pot.
2. Close the lid and cook the stew on Low for 8 hours.
3. Carefully stir the stew and cool it to the room temperature.
per serving: 187 calories, 10.5g protein, 6.1g carbohydrates, 13.1g fat, 1.7g fiber, 40mg cholesterol, 85mg sodium, 65mg potassium.

Jamaican Stew
Yield: 8 servings | **Prep time:** 15 minutes | **Cook time:** 1 hour
- 1 tablespoon coconut oil
- 1 teaspoon garlic powder
- ½ cup bell pepper, sliced
- ½ cup heavy cream
- 1-pound salmon fillet, chopped
- 1 teaspoon ground coriander

- ½ teaspoon ground cumin
1. Put the coconut oil in the Crock Pot.
2. Then mix the salmon with ground cumin and ground coriander and put in the Crock Pot.
3. Add the layer of bell pepper and sprinkle with garlic powder.
4. Add heavy cream and close the lid.
5. Cook the stew on High for 1 hour.
per serving: 120 calories, 11.3g protein, 1.1g carbohydrates, 8g fat, 6.9g fiber, 35mg cholesterol, 28mg sodium, 244mg potassium.

Pumpkin Stew with Chicken
Yield: 2 servings | **Prep time:** 10 minutes | **Cook time:** 4 hours
- ½ cup pumpkin, chopped
- 6 oz chicken fillet, cut into strips
- 1 tablespoon curry powder
- ¼ cup coconut cream
- ½ teaspoon ground cinnamon
- 1 onion, chopped
1. Mix pumpkin with chicken fillet strips in the mixing bowl.
2. Add curry powder, coconut cream, ground cinnamon, and onion.
3. Mix the stew ingredients and transfer them in the Crock Pot.
4. Cook the meal on high for 4 hours.
per serving: 291 calories, 16.2g protein, 25g carbohydrates, 15.8g fat, 5.7g fiber, 40mg cholesterol, 586mg sodium, 336mg potassium.

Lobster Stew
Yield: 4 servings | **Prep time:** 10 minutes | **Cook time:** 1 hour
- 7 oz lobster tail, peeled, chopped
- 3 tomatoes, chopped
- 1 onion, roughly chopped
- 1 cup fish stock
- ½ teaspoon dried lemongrass
- 2 tablespoons cream cheese
1. Put all ingredients in the Crock Pot and gently stir.
2. Close the lid and cook the stew on High for 1 hour.
per serving: 100 calories, 12.2g protein, 6.3g carbohydrates, 2.8g fat, 1.7g fiber, 78mg cholesterol, 352mg sodium, 464mg potassium.

Ginger Fish Stew
Yield: 5 servings | **Prep time:** 10 minutes | **Cook time:** 6 hours
- 1 oz fresh ginger, peeled, chopped
- 1 cup baby carrot
- 1-pound salmon fillet, chopped
- 1 teaspoon fish sauce
- ½ teaspoon ground nutmeg
- ½ cup green peas
- 3 cups of water
1. Put all ingredients in the Crock Pot bowl.
2. Gently stir the stew ingredients and close the lid.
3. Cook the stew on low for 6 hours.

per serving: 159 calories, 19.1g protein, 7.7g carbohydrates, 6.1g fat, 2g fiber, 40mg cholesterol, 153mg sodium, 506mg potassium.

Mexican Style Stew
Yield: 6 servings | **Prep time:** 10 minutes | **Cook time:** 6 hours

- 1 cup corn kernels
- 1 cup green peas
- ¼ cup white rice
- 4 cups chicken stock
- 1 teaspoon taco seasoning
- 1 teaspoon dried cilantro
- 1 tablespoon butter

1. Put butter and wild rice in the Crock Pot.
2. Then add corn kernels, green peas, chicken stock, taco seasoning, and dried cilantro.
3. Close the lid and cook the stew on Low for 6 hours.

per serving: 97 calories, 3.2g protein, 15.6g carbohydrates, 2.7g fat, 2g fiber, 5mg cholesterol, 599mg sodium, 148mg potassium.

Mussel Stew
Yield: 4 servings | **Prep time:** 5 minutes | **Cook time:** 55 minutes

- 1-pound mussels
- 2 garlic cloves, diced
- 1 teaspoon smoked paprika
- ½ teaspoon chili powder
- 1 eggplant, chopped
- 1 cup coconut cream
- 1 tablespoon sesame seeds
- 1 teaspoon tomato paste

1. Put all ingredients from the list above in the Crock Pot and gently stir.
2. Close the lid and cook the mussel stew for 55 minutes on High.

per serving: 283 calories, 16.7g protein, 16g carbohydrates, 18.3g fat, 6g fiber, 32mg cholesterol, 341mg sodium, 832mg potassium.

Chinese Style Cod Stew
Yield: 2 servings | **Prep time:** 10 minutes | **Cook time:** 5 hours

- 6 oz cod fillet
- 1 teaspoon sesame seeds
- 1 teaspoon olive oil
- 1 garlic clove, chopped
- ¼ cup of soy sauce
- ¼ cup fish stock
- 4 oz fennel bulb, chopped

1. Pour fish stock in the Crock Pot.
2. Add soy sauce, olive oil, garlic, and sesame seeds.
3. Then chop the fish roughly and add in the Crock Pot.
4. Cook the meal on Low for 5 hours.

per serving: 139 calories, 18.9g protein, 7.4g carbohydrates, 4.2g fat, 2.2g fiber, 42mg cholesterol, 1926mg sodium, 359mg potassium.

Taco Spices Stew

Yield: 4 servings | **Prep time:** 10 minutes | **Cook time:** 8 hours

- 1-pound beef sirloin
- 1 teaspoon liquid honey
- 3 cups of water
- 1 cup sweet potato, chopped
- 1 teaspoon salt
- 1 teaspoon taco seasonings

1. Cut the beef sirloin into the strips and sprinkle with taco seasonings.
2. Then transfer the beef strips in the Crock Pot.
3. Add salt, sweet potato, water, and liquid honey.
4. Close the lid and cook the stew for 8 hours on Low.

per serving: 264 calories, 35.4g protein, 12.3g carbohydrates, 7.2g fat, 1.7g fiber, 101mg cholesterol, 732mg sodium, 697mg potassium.

Crab Stew
Yield: 4 servings | **Prep time:** 10 minutes | **Cook time:** 5 hours

- 8 oz crab meat, chopped
- ½ cup mango, chopped
- 1 teaspoon dried lemongrass
- 1 teaspoon ground turmeric
- 1 potato, peeled chopped
- 1 cup of water
- ½ cup of coconut milk

1. Put all ingredients in the Crock Pot.
2. Gently stir them with the help of the spoon and close the lid.
3. Cook the stew on low for 5 hours.
4. Then leave the cooked stew for 10-15 minutes to rest.

per serving: 167 calories, 8.9g protein, 13.6g carbohydrates, 8.3g fat, 2.1g fiber, 30mg cholesterol, 364mg sodium, 310mg potassium.

Rice, Grains & Beans

Sweet Peppers with Rice

Yield: 6 servings | **Prep time:** 15 minutes | **Cook time:** 6 hours

- 6 sweet peppers
- ½ cup white rice, half-cooked
- ½ onion, minced
- 1 teaspoon ground black pepper
- 1 teaspoon ground coriander
- ½ cup tomato juice
- 1 tablespoon cream cheese

1. In the mixing bowl mix rice, onion, ground black pepper, and ground coriander.
2. Then remove the seeds from the sweet peppers.
3. Fill the sweet peppers with rice mixture ad transfer in the Crock Pot one-by-one.
4. Pour the tomato juice over the Crock Pot. Add cream cheese.
5. Close the lid and cook the meal on Low for 6 hours.

per serving: 108 calories, 2.7g protein, 23.3g carbohydrates, 1g fat, 2.2g fiber, 2mg cholesterol, 64mg sodium, 308mg potassium.

Beans-Rice Mix

Yield: 4 servings | **Prep time:** 15 minutes | **Cook time:** 3 hours

- 5 oz red kidney beans, canned
- 1 teaspoon garlic powder
- ¼ teaspoon ground coriander
- ½ cup long-grain rice
- 2 cups chicken stock

1. Put long-grain rice in the Crock Pot.
2. Add chicken stock, ground coriander, and garlic powder.
3. Close the lid and cook the rice for 2.5 hours on High.
4. Then add red kidney beans, stir the mixture, and cook for 30 minutes in High.

per serving: 211 calories, 10.1g protein, 41.1g carbohydrates, 0.8g fat, 5.8g fiber, 0mg cholesterol, 387mg sodium, 523mg potassium.

Fragrant Turmeric Beans

Yield: 4 servings | **Prep time:** 8 minutes | **Cook time:** 8 hours

- 1 jalapeno pepper, sliced
- 1 oz fresh ginger, grated
- 1 teaspoon ground turmeric
- 2 cups black beans, soaked
- 5 cups chicken stock

1. Put black beans in the Crock Pot.
2. Add jalapeno pepper, ginger, ground turmeric, and chicken stock.
3. Cook the meal on low for 8 hours.

per serving: 371 calories, 22.5g protein, 67g carbohydrates, 2.6g fat, 15.9g fiber, 0mg cholesterol, 962mg sodium, 1573mg potassium.

Oregano Wild Rice

Yield: 6 servings | **Prep time:** 10 minutes | **Cook time:** 4 hours

- 2 cups wild rice
- 5 cups chicken stock
- 1 teaspoon dried oregano
- ½ teaspoon dried marjoram
- 1 tablespoon butter
- ½ teaspoon ground black pepper

1. Put the wild rice in the Crock Pot.
2. Add chicken stock, dried oregano, dried marjoram, and ground black pepper.
3. Close the lid and cook the rice on high for 4 hours.
4. Then add butter and stir the rice well.

per serving: 281 calories, 13g protein, 47.3g carbohydrates, 4.9g fat, 3.5g fiber, 11mg cholesterol, 304mg sodium, 445mg potassium.

Mushroom Rissoto

Yield: 4 servings | **Prep time:** 10 minutes | **Cook time:** 2.5 hours

- 1 cup cremini mushrooms, chopped
- 1 tablespoon cream cheese
- 1 cup basmati rice
- 1.5 cups chicken stock

1. Put basmati rice and chicken stock in the Crock Pot.
2. Add cremini mushrooms and close the lid.
3. Cook the risotto on High for 2 hours.
4. Then add cream cheese and stir the rice. Cook it on high for 30 minutes more.

per serving: 186 calories, 4.2g protein, 38.1g carbohydrates, 1.4g fat, 0.7g fiber, 3mg cholesterol, 297mg sodium, 142mg potassium

Chicken Pilaf

Yield: 3 servings | **Prep time:** 10 minutes | **Cook time:** 6 hours

- ½ cup basmati rice
- 2 cups of water
- 5 oz chicken fillet, chopped
- 1 teaspoon chili powder
- ½ teaspoon salt

1. Put the rice and chicken fillet in the Crock Pot.
2. Add chili powder, salt, and water. Carefully stir the ingredients and close the lid.
3. Cook the pilaf on Low for 6 hours.

per serving: 205 calories, 16g protein, 25.1g carbohydrates, 3.9g fat, 0.7g fiber, 42mg cholesterol, 443mg sodium, 169mg potassium.

Spinach Rice

Yield: 5 servings | **Prep time:** 10 minutes | **Cook time:** 3 hours 20 minutes

- 1 tablespoon sesame oil
- 1 teaspoon ground cumin
- 2 cups spinach, chopped
- ½ cup cream
- 1 cup long-grain rice
- 1 cup chicken stock

1. Mix spinach with cream, add ground cumin and transfer the mixture in the Crock Pot.
2. Cook it on high for 20 minutes.

3.   After this, add all remaining ingredients, carefully stir them and close the lid.
4.   Cook the meal on high for 3 hours.
per serving: 226 calories, 4.2g protein, 38.9g carbohydrates, 5.7g fat, 1g fiber, 6mg cholesterol, 216mg sodium, 161mg potassium.

Barley Pilaf
Yield: 4 servings | **Prep time:** 10 minutes | **Cook time:** 2.5 hours
- ¼ cup white rice
- ½ cup barley
- 3 cups vegetable stock
- 1 cup lima beans, cooked
- 1 tablespoon avocado oil
- 1 teaspoon salt
- 1 tablespoon tomato paste

1.   Mix vegetable stock and tomato paste and pour the liquid in the Crock Pot.
2.   Add barley and rice.
3.   Then add lima beans, avocado oil, and salt.
4.   Close the lid and cook the pilaf on High for 2.5 hours.
per serving: 183 calories, 6.6g protein, 36.5g carbohydrates, 2.9g fat, 6.4g fiber, 0mg cholesterol, 1132mg sodium, 351mg potassium.

Rice and Chorizo Bowl
Yield: 5 servings | **Prep time:** 15 minutes | **Cook time:** 3 hours
- 8 oz chorizo, sliced
- 2 oz green chiles, canned, chopped
- 1 garlic clove, diced
- ½ cup white rice
- 1.5 cup chicken stock
- 1 teaspoon avocado oil

1.   Put rice in the Crock Pot.
2.   Add chicken stock, garlic, chiles, and chicken stock.
3.   Close the lid and cook the rice on high for 3 hours.
4.   Meanwhile, heat the avocado oil in the skillet.
5.   Add chorizo and roast it for 2 minutes per side on medium heat.
6.   When the rice is cooked, transfer it in the bowls and top with roasted chorizo.
per serving: 283 calories, 12.5g protein, 16.9g carbohydrates, 17.8g fat, 0.3g fiber, 40mg cholesterol, 836mg sodium, 212mg potassium.

Farro Pilaf
Yield: 4 servings | **Prep time:** 15 minutes | **Cook time:** 7 hours
- ¼ onion, diced
- 1 tablespoon olive oil
- 1 cup farro
- 3 cups of water
- 1 teaspoon dried sage
- 4 oz beef sirloin, chopped

1.   Heat olive oil in the skillet.
2.   Add beef sirloin and roast it on medium heat for 3 minutes per side.
3.   Then transfer the meat in the Crock Pot.
4.   Add water, farro, sage, and onion.
5.   Close the lid and cook the pilaf on Low for 7 hours.
per serving: 246 calories,15.7g protein, 33.7g carbohydrates, 5.3g fat, 3.2g fiber, 25mg cholesterol, 54mg sodium, 128mg potassium.

Butter Pink Rice
Yield: 6 servings | **Prep time:** 5 minutes | **Cook time:** 5.5 hours
- 1 cup pink rice
- 1 cups chicken stock
- 1 teaspoon cream cheese
- 1 tablespoon butter

1.   Put all ingredients in the Crock Pot and stir gently.
2.   Close the lid and cook the meal on low for 5.5 hours.
per serving: 122 calories, 2.2g protein, 22.3g carbohydrates, 3g fat, 1g fiber, 6mg cholesterol, 143mg sodium, 52mg potassium.

Carrot Rice
Yield: 6 servings | **Prep time:** 10 minutes | **Cook time:** 4 hours
- 1 teaspoon sesame oil
- ½ cup carrot, grated
- 1 ½ cup risotto rice
- 4 cups chicken stock
- 1 teaspoon allspice
- 1 tablespoon butter

1.   Mix rice with sesame oil and transfer in the Crock Pot.
2.   Add carrot, chicken stock, and allspices.
3.   Close the lid and cook the rice on high for 4 hours.
4.   Then open the lid, add butter, and carefully mix the rice.
per serving: 204 calories, 3.9g protein, 38.6g carbohydrates, 3.4g fat, 0.9g fiber, 5mg cholesterol, 532mg sodium, 96mg potassium.

Cumin Rice
Yield: 6 servings | **Prep time:** 15 minutes | **Cook time:** 3.5 hours
- 2 cups long-grain rice
- 5 cups chicken stock
- 1 teaspoon cumin seeds
- 1 teaspoon olive oil
- 1 tablespoon cream cheese

1.   Heat the olive oil in the skillet.
2.   Add cumin seeds and roast them for 2-3 minutes.
3.   Then transfer the roasted cumin seeds in the Crock Pot.
4.   Add rice and chickens tock. Gently stir the ingredients.
5.   Close the lid and cook the rice on high for 3.5 hours.
6.   Then add cream cheese and stir the rice well.
per serving: 247 calories, 5.2g protein, 50.1g carbohydrates, 2.3g fat, 0.8g fiber, 2mg cholesterol, 645mg sodium, 91mg potassium.

Sweet Farro

Yield: 3 servings | **Prep time:** 10 minutes | **Cook time:** 6 hours

- ½ cup farro
- 2 cups of water
- ½ cup heavy cream
- 2 tablespoons dried cranberries
- 2 tablespoons sugar
1. Chop the cranberries and put in the Crock Pot.
2. Add water, heavy cream, sugar, and farro.
3. Mix the ingredients with the help of the spoon and close the lid.
4. Cook the farro on low for 6 hours.

per serving: 208 calories, 5.1g protein, 31g carbohydrates, 7.4g fat, 2.2g fiber, 27mg cholesterol, 32mg sodium, 24mg potassium.

Rice and Corn Bowl

Yield: 5 servings | **Prep time:** 10 minutes | **Cook time:** 3 hours

- 1 cup basmati rice
- 1.5 cup vegetable stock
- 1 cup corn kernels
- 1 teaspoon hot sauce
- 2 tablespoons butter
1. Put corn kernels and rice in the Crock Pot.
2. Add vegetable stock and cook the meal on high for 3 hours.
3. Then open the lid, add hot sauce and butter.
4. Carefully stir the meal and transfer in the bowls.

per serving: 205 calories, 3.7g protein, 36g carbohydrates, 5.8g fat, 1.3g fiber, 12mg cholesterol, 281mg sodium, 128mg potassium.

Wild Rice with Crumbled Cheese

Yield: 4 servings | **Prep time:** 15 minutes | **Cook time:** 4 hours

- 1 garlic clove, diced
- 1 teaspoon coconut oil
- ½ cup wild rice
- 1.5 cups chicken stock
- 4 oz goat cheese, crumbled
- 1 tablespoon butter
- ½ teaspoon dried oregano
1. Heat the skillet well.
2. Add coconut oil, dried oregano, and garlic. Roast the ingredients for 1 minute on high heat.
3. Then transfer them in the Crock Pot.
4. Add wild rice and chicken stock.
5. Close the lid and cook the mixture for 4 hours on High.
6. After this, add butter and carefully stir the ingredients.
7. Top the meal with crumbled goat cheese.

per serving: 253 calories, 10.7g protein, 19.8g carbohydrates, 14.5g fat, 0.4g fiber, 37mg cholesterol, 406mg sodium, 53mg potassium.

Basmati Rice with Artichoke Hearts

Yield: 5 servings | **Prep time:** 15 minutes | **Cook time:** 6 hours

- 4 artichoke hearts, canned, chopped
- 1 cup Arborio rice
- 1 tablespoon apple cider vinegar
- 2 cups of water
- ½ cup of coconut milk
- 1 teaspoon coconut oil
- 1 onion, sliced
- 1 oz Parmesan, grated
1. Put rice in the Crock Pot. Add coconut milk and water.
2. Close the lid and cook the mixture on low for 6 hours.
3. Meanwhile, melt the coconut oil.
4. Add onion and roast it for 2 minutes.
5. Then stir it well, add apple cider vinegar, and artichoke hearts.
6. Roast the ingredients for 3 minutes.
7. When the rice is cooked, transfer it in the plates and top with roasted artichoke mixture and Parmesan.

per serving: 289 calories, 9.4g protein, 47.5g carbohydrates, 8.3g fat, 9g fiber, 4mg cholesterol, 185mg sodium, 606mg potassium.

Creamy Polenta

Yield: 4 servings | **Prep time:** 10 minutes | **Cook time:** 2.5 hours

- 1 cup polenta
- 3 cups of water
- 1 cup heavy cream
- 1 teaspoon salt
1. Put all ingredients in the Crock Pot.
2. Close the lid and cook them on High for 2.5 hours.
3. When the polenta is cooked, stir it carefully and transfer it in the serving plates.

per serving: 242 calories, 3.5g protein, 31.3g carbohydrates, 11.4g fat, 1g fiber, 41mg cholesterol, 600mg sodium, 24mg potassium.

Butter Buckwheat

Yield: 4 servings | **Prep time:** 5 minutes | **Cook time:** 4 hours

- 2 tablespoons butter
- 1 cup buckwheat
- 2 cups chicken stock
- ½ teaspoon salt
1. Mix buckwheat with salt and transfer in the Crock Pot.
2. Add chicken stock and close the lid.
3. Cook the buckwheat on High for 4 hours.
4. Then add butter, carefully mixture the buckwheat, and transfer in the bowls.

per serving: 202 calories, 6g protein, 30.8g carbohydrates, 7.5g fat, 4.3g fiber, 15mg cholesterol, 714mg sodium, 205mg potassium.

Dumplings with Polenta

Yield: 6 servings | **Prep time:** 20 minutes | **Cook time:** 45 minutes

- 3 oz polenta
- 3 oz flour
- 2 oz Cheddar cheese, shredded
- ½ cup of coconut milk

- 1 egg, beaten
- 3 oz water, hot

1. Mix polenta and flour. Add egg and coconut milk. Mix the ingredients well.
2. Add cheddar cheese and knead the soft dough.
3. Cut the dough into 6 pieces and roll them into balls.
4. Pour water in the Crock Pot.
5. Add polenta balls and cook them for 45 minutes on HIGH. Drain the water and transfer the dumplings in the serving plates.

per serving: 198 calories, 6.3g protein, 23.5g carbohydrates, 8.9g fat, 1.2g fiber, 37mg cholesterol, 73mg sodium, 87mg potassium.

Apple Cups

Yield: 2 servings | **Prep time:** 15 minutes | **Cook time:** 6 hours

- 2 green apples
- 3 oz white rice
- 1 shallot, diced
- ¼ cup of water
- 1 tablespoon cream cheese

1. Scoop the flesh from the apples to make the apple cups.
2. Then mix the onion with rice, and curry paste.
3. Pour water in the Crock Pot.
4. Fill the apple cups with rice mixture and top with cream cheese,
5. Then combine the raisins, diced onion, white rice, salt, and curry. Cook the meal on Low for 6 hours.

per serving: 292 calories, 4.1g protein, 65.8g carbohydrates, 2.4g fat, 6g fiber, 6mg cholesterol, 20mg sodium, 310mg potassium.

Dinner Rice Casserole

Yield: 6 servings | **Prep time:** 10 minutes | **Cook time:** 8 hours

- 1 cup wild rice
- ½ cup broccoli, chopped
- ¼ cup red kidney beans, canned
- 1 cup plain yogurt
- 1 cup of water
- ¼ cup Mozzarella, shredded
- 1 teaspoon smoked paprika
- 1 teaspoon almond butter

1. Put the chopped broccoli in the Crock Pot.
2. Top it with red kidney beans.
3. Then add water and plain yogurt.
4. After this, add the layer of rice and sprinkle with smoked paprika.
5. Then add almond butter and Mozzarella.
6. Close the lid and cook the casserole on LOW for 8 hours.

per serving: 173 calories, 9.1g protein, 28.8g carbohydrates, 2.7g fat, 3.4g fiber, 3mg cholesterol, 42mg sodium, 366mg potassium.

Green Lentils Salad

Yield: 2 servings | **Prep time:** 10 minutes | **Cook time:** 4 hours

- ¼ cup green lentils

- 1 cup chicken stock
- ½ teaspoon ground cumin
- 2 cups lettuce, chopped
- ¼ cup Greek Yogurt

1. Mix green lentils with chicken stock and transfer in the Crock Pot.
2. Cook the ingredients on High for 4 hours.
3. Then cool the lentils and transfer them in the salad bowl.
4. Add ground cumin, lettuce, and Greek yogurt.
5. Mix the salad carefully.

per serving: 118 calories, 9.4g protein, 17.7g carbohydrates, 1.3g fat, 7.7g fiber, 1mg cholesterol, 395mg sodium, 359mg potassium.

Tomato Bulgur

Yield: 6 servings | **Prep time:** 15 minutes | **Cook time:** 6 hours

- 1 cup bulgur
- 2 cups of water
- 1 tablespoon tomato paste
- ¼ cup onion, diced
- ¼ cup bell pepper, diced
- 1 teaspoon cayenne pepper
- 1 tablespoon sesame oil

1. Heat sesame oil in the skillet.
2. Add onion and bell pepper and roast them for 5 minutes on medium heat.
3. Then transfer the roasted vegetables in the Crock Pot.
4. Add water and tomato paste. Stir the ingredients.
5. Then add bulgur and cayenne pepper.
6. Close the lid and cook the meal on Low for 6 hours.

per serving: 107 calories, 3.1g protein, 19.2g carbohydrates, 2.7g fat, 4.6g fiber, 0mg cholesterol, 9mg sodium, 146mg potassium.

Bacon Millet

Yield: 6 servings | **Prep time:** 10 minutes | **Cook time:** 6 hours

- 2 cups millet
- 4 cups of water
- 2 tablespoons butter
- ½ teaspoon salt
- 2 oz bacon, chopped, cooked

1. Put millet and salt in the Crock Pot.
2. Add water and cook the meal on low for 6 hours.
3. When the millet is cooked, carefully mix it with butter and transfer in the plates.
4. Add bacon.

per serving: 337 calories, 10.9g protein, 48.7g carbohydrates, 10.6g fat, 5.7g fiber, 21mg cholesterol, 447mg sodium, 186mg potassium.

Oregano Millet

Yield: 3 servings | **Prep time:** 5 minutes | **Cook time:** 3 hours

- ¼ cup heavy cream
- ½ cup millet
- 1 teaspoon dried oregano
- 1 cup of water

1. Put all ingredients from the list above in the Crock Pot.
2. Close the lid and cook on high for 3 hours.
per serving: 162 calories, 3.9g protein, 24.9g carbohydrates, 5.2g fat, 3g fiber, 14mg cholesterol, 6mg sodium, 81mg potassium.

Milky Semolina
Yield: 2 servings | **Prep time:** 15 minutes | **Cook time:** 1 hour

- ¼ cup semolina
- 1 ½ cup milk
- 1 teaspoon vanilla extract
- 1 teaspoon sugar
1. Put all ingredients in the Crock Pot.
2. Close the lid and cook the semolina on high for 1 hour.
3. When the meal is cooked, carefully stir it and cool it to room temperature.
per serving: 180 calories, 8.7g protein, 26.5g carbohydrates, 4g fat, 0.8g fiber, 15mg cholesterol, 87mg sodium, 147mg potassium.

Rice Boats
Yield: 4 servings | **Prep time:** 15 minutes | **Cook time:** 2.5 hours

- 2 medium eggplants
- ½ cup wild rice, cooked
- 1 teaspoon dried basil
- ¼ cup broccoli, shredded
- 1 teaspoon butter, melted
- ¼ teaspoon ground black pepper
- ¼ cup of water
1. Cut the eggplants into the halves and remove the flesh.
2. In the mixing bowl, mix rice with basil, broccoli, ground black pepper, and butter.
3. Then fill the eggplant halves with rice mixture and arrange them in the Crock Pot.
4. Add water and close the lid.
5. Cook the rice boats on High for 2.5 hours.
per serving: 151 calories, 5.8g protein, 31.6g carbohydrates, 1.7g fat, 11.1g fiber, 3mg cholesterol, 16mg sodium, 734mg potassium.

Tomato Dal
Yield: 6 servings | **Prep time:** 10 minutes | **Cook time:** 7 hours

- 1 teaspoon cumin seeds
- 1 cup red lentils
- ½ teaspoon fennel seeds
- 5 cups of water
- 1 cup tomatoes, chopped
- ¼ cup onion, diced
- ½ teaspoon ground ginger
- 1 cup of rice
1. Put ingredients from the list above in the Crock Pot.
2. Carefully stir the mixture and close the lid.
3. Cook the tomato dal on low for 7 hours.
per serving: 235 calories, 10.9g protein, 45.9g carbohydrates, 0.7g fat, 10.8g fiber, 0mg cholesterol, 12mg sodium, 432mg potassium.

Cherry Rice
Yield: 4 servings | **Prep time:** 10 minutes | **Cook time:** 3 hours

- 1 cup basmati rice
- 1 cup cherries, raw
- 3 cups of water
- 2 tablespoons of liquid honey
- 1 tablespoon butter, melted
1. Put cherries and rice in the Crock Pot.
2. Add water and cook the meal on high for 3 hours.
3. Meanwhile, mix liquid honey and butter.
4. When the rice is cooked, add liquid honey mixture and carefully stir.
per serving: 249 calories, 3.9g protein, 51.1g carbohydrates, 3.3g fat, 1.4g fiber, 8mg cholesterol, 29mg sodium, 136mg potassium.

Refried Red Kidney Beans
Yield: 4 servings | **Prep time:** 10 minutes | **Cook time:** 6 hours

- 2 cups red kidney beans, soaked
- 1 cayenne pepper, chopped
- ½ teaspoon garlic powder
- 1 teaspoon onion powder
- 8 cups of water
- 1 teaspoon coconut oil
1. Put all ingredients in the Crock Pot.
2. Cook the mixture for 6 hours on high.
3. Then transfer the cooked bean mixture in the blender and pulse for 15 seconds.
4. Transfer the meal in the bowls
per serving: 324 calories, 20.9g protein, 57.4g carbohydrates, 2.2g fat, 14.2g fiber, 0mg cholesterol, 26mg sodium, 1274mg potassium.

Black Beans Dip
Yield: 6 servings | **Prep time:** 10 minutes | **Cook time:** 7 hours

- 1 cup black beans, soaked
- ½ cup spinach, chopped
- 3 oz Monterey Jack cheese, shredded
- 1 cup tomatoes, chopped
- ½ cup of coconut milk
- 5 cups of water
1. Pour water in the Crock Pot.
2. Add black beans and cook them for 7 hours on low.
3. Then transfer the cooked, hot, drained black beans in the blender.
4. Add cheese, tomatoes, and coconut milk.
5. Blend the mixture until smooth and transfer it in the bowl.
per serving: 215 calories, 11.2g protein, 22.6g carbohydrates, 9.6g fat, 5.8g fiber, 13mg cholesterol, 90mg sodium, 631mg potassium.

Classic Huevos Rancheros
Yield: 6 servings | **Prep time:** 20 minutes | **Cook time:** 2 hours

- 6 eggs
- 2 oz chilies, canned, chopped

- 1 cup tomatoes, canned
- 1 onion, diced
- 1 tablespoon butter
- 1 teaspoon olive oil
- ½ cup bell pepper, chopped
- ½ cup of water
- 1 teaspoon smoked paprika
1. Mix chilies, tomatoes, onion, olive oil, bell pepper, water, and smoked paprika in the Crock Pot.
2. Close the lid and cook the mixture on high for 2 hours.
3. Meanwhile, melt the butter in the skillet.
4. Crack the eggs in the hot oil and roast them for 4 minutes or until the eggs are solid.
5. Then transfer the eggs in the plates.
6. Top them with cooked tomato mixture from the Crock Pot.
 per serving: 134 calories, 7.2g protein, 10.8g carbohydrates, 7.8g fat, 3.7g fiber, 169mg cholesterol, 87mg sodium, 361mg potassium.

Creamy Panade
Yield: 4 servings | **Prep time:** 10 minutes | **Cook time:** 2.5 hours
- 5 oz bread, toasted, chopped
- 1 teaspoon garlic powder
- ½ cup red kidney beans, canned
- ¼ cup Mozzarella, shredded
- 3 cups of water
- 6 oz sausages, chopped
1. Put chopped sausages in the Crock Pot.
2. Add water, cheese, red kidney beans, garlic powder, and bread.
3. Gently stir the mixture and close the lid.
4. Cook the panade on high for 2.5 hours.
 per serving: 323 calories,16.8g protein, 32.6g carbohydrates, 13.8g fat, 4.4g fiber, 37mg cholesterol, 579mg sodium, 483mg potassium.

Beef and Beans Saute
Yield: 6 servings | **Prep time:** 8 minutes | **Cook time:** 9 hours
- ½ cup white beans, soaked
- 1-pound beef sirloin, chopped
- 2 tablespoons tomato paste
- 1 teaspoon chili powder
- 5 cups of water
- ½ teaspoon salt
1. Put all ingredients in the Crock Pot.
2. Gently stir the mixture or until the tomato paste is dissolved.
3. Close the lid and cook the saute on Low for 9 hours.
 per serving: 202 calories, 27.1g protein, 11.4g carbohydrates, 5g fat, 2.9g fiber, 68mg cholesterol, 262mg sodium, 671mg potassium.

Beans and Peas Bowl
Yield: 4 servings | **Prep time:** 10 minutes | **Cook time:** 6 hours
- ½ cup black beans, soaked
- 1 cup green peas

- 4 cups of water
- 1 tablespoon tomato paste
- 1 teaspoon sriracha
1. Pour water in the Crock Pot.
2. Add black beans and cook them for 5 hours on High.
3. Then add green peas, tomato paste, and sriracha.
4. Stir the ingredients and cook the meal for 1 hour on High.
 per serving: 117 calories, 7.4g protein, 21.4g carbohydrates, 0.5g fat, 5.7g fiber, 0mg cholesterol, 23mg sodium, 491mg potassium.

Warm Bean Salad
Yield: 4 servings | **Prep time:** 10 minutes | **Cook time:** 5 hours
- ½ cup white beans, soaked
- 1 cup tomatoes, chopped
- ½ cup fresh parsley, chopped
- 4 oz chicken fillet, cut into strips
- 2 tablespoons sour cream
- ½ cup arugula, chopped
- 4 cups of water
1. Put chicken and white beans in the Crock Pot.
2. Cook the on high for 5 hours.
3. Then drain water and transfer the beans and chicken in the big salad bowl.
4. Add parsley, tomatoes, and arugula.
5. Then add sour cream and mix the salad.
 per serving: 162 calories, 15g protein, 17.8g carbohydrates, 3.7g fat, 4.7g fiber, 28mg cholesterol, 46mg sodium, 691mg potassium.

Red Beans Saute
Yield: 4 servings | **Prep time:** 10 minutes | **Cook time:** 7 hours
- 1 cup red beans, soaked
- 1 cup carrot, chopped
- 1 yellow onion, chopped
- 5 cups chicken stock
- 1 teaspoon Italian seasonings
- 1 teaspoon tomato paste
1. Mix chicken stock with tomato paste and pour the liquid in the Crock Pot.
2. Add Italian seasonings, onion, carrot, and soaked red beans.
3. Close the lid and cook the saute on Low for 7 hours.
 per serving: 194 calories, 11.8g protein, 34.8g carbohydrates, 1.6g fat, 8.3g fiber, 1mg cholesterol, 982mg sodium, 786mg potassium.

Turnip and Beans Casserole
Yield: 4 servings | **Prep time:** 10 minutes | **Cook time:** 6 hours
- ½ cup turnip, chopped
- 1 teaspoon chili powder
- ¼ cup of coconut milk
- 1 teaspoon coconut oil
- ¼ cup potato, chopped 1 carrot, diced
- 1 cup red kidney beans, canned
- ½ cup Cheddar cheese, shredded

1. Grease the Crock Pot bottom with coconut oil.
2. Then put the turnip and potato inside.
3. Sprinkle the vegetables with chili powder and coconut mil.
4. After this, top the with red kidney beans and Cheddar cheese.
5. Close the lid and cook the casserole on Low for 6 hours.
per serving: 266 calories, 14.5g protein, 31.4g carbohydrates, 10g fat, 7.9g fiber, 15mg cholesterol, 113mg sodium, 742mg potassium.

White Beans in Sauce
Yield: 4 servings | **Prep time:** 10 minutes | **Cook time:** 5 hours
- 1 cup white beans, soaked
- 1 cup BBQ sauce
- 1 cup chicken stock
- 3 cups of water
- 1 onion, diced
- 1 teaspoon dried sage
1. Mix BBQ sauce, chicken stock, and water in the Crock Pot.
2. Add onion, dried sage, and white beans.
3. Close the lid and cook the beans on High for 5 hours.
4. Serve the cooked beans with BBQ sauce gravy.
per serving: 278 calories, 13.1g protein, 56g carbohydrates, 0.7g fat, 8.7g fiber, 0mg cholesterol, 841mg sodium, 1080mg potassium.

Garlic Bean Dip
Yield: 8 servings | **Prep time:** 10 minutes | **Cook time:** 5 hours
- 1 cup red kidney beans, canned
- 1 tablespoon tomato paste
- 1 teaspoon minced garlic
- 1 teaspoon dried cilantro
- 1 teaspoon ground paprika
- ½ cup of water
1. Mix water with tomato paste and pour the liquid in the Crock Pot.
2. Add red kidney beans, ground paprika, minced garlic, and cilantro.
3. Close the lid and cook the mixture on low for 5 hours.
4. Then blend the mixture gently with the help of the blender.
per serving: 80 calories, 5.3g protein, 14.7g carbohydrates, 0.3g fat, 3.7g fiber, 0mg cholesterol, 5mg sodium, 341mg potassium.

Chicken Dip
Yield: 4 servings | **Prep time:** 10 minutes | **Cook time:** 3.5 hours
- ½ cup white beans, canned, drained
- ½ cup ground chicken
- 1 teaspoon dried parsley
- ¼ cup BBQ sauce
- 1 teaspoon cayenne pepper
- ½ cup of water
1. Blend the canned beans and transfer them in the Crock Pot.

2. Add ground chicken, dried parsley, BBQ sauce, cayenne pepper, and water.
3. Stir the ingredients and close the lid.
4. Cook the dip on High for 3.5 hours.
per serving: 142 calories, 11g protein, 21.2g carbohydrates, 1.6g fat, 4.1g fiber, 16mg cholesterol, 195mg sodium, 539mg potassium.

Salted Caramel Rice Pudding
Yield: 2 servings | **Prep time:** 10 minutes | **Cook time:** 3 hours
- 2 teaspoons salted caramel
- ½ cup basmati rice
- 1.5 cup milk
- 1 teaspoon vanilla extract
1. Pour milk in the Crock Pot.
2. Add vanilla extract and basmati rice. Cook the rice on high or 3 hours.
3. Then add salted caramel and carefully mix the pudding.
4. Cool it to the room temperature and transfer in the bowls.
per serving: 284 calories, 9.8g protein, 48.9g carbohydrates, 4.7g fat, 0.8g fiber, 16mg cholesterol, 99mg sodium, 161mg potassium.

Chocolate Rice
Yield: 5 servings | **Prep time:** 10 minutes | **Cook time:** 7 hours
- 1 teaspoon vanilla extract
- 1 teaspoon ground cinnamon
- 1 cup of rice
- 2 cups of coconut milk
- 1 tablespoon cocoa powder
- 1 tablespoon sugar
1. Mix coconut milk and cocoa powder and whisk until smooth.
2. Pour the liquid in the Crock Pot.
3. Add sugar, rice, ground cinnamon, and vanilla extract.
4. Close the lid and cook the meal on Low for 7 hours.
per serving: 371 calories, 5.1g protein, 38.4g carbohydrates, 23.3g fat, 3.2g fiber, 0mg cholesterol, 17mg sodium, 325mg potassium.

Barley Saute
Yield: 2 servings | **Prep time:** 10 minutes | **Cook time:** 8 hours
- ¼ cup barley
- ½ cup ground pork
- 1 teaspoon dried thyme
- ½ cup tomatoes, chopped
- 1 jalapeno pepper, diced
- 3 cups of water
1. Put barley, ground pork, and tomatoes in the Crock Pot.
2. Sprinkle the ingredients with dried thyme and jalapeno pepper.
3. Add water and close the lid.
4. Cook the saute for 8 hours on low.

per serving: 325 calories, 23.5g protein, 19.4g carbohydrates, 7g fat, 4.9g fiber, 74mg cholesterol, 73mg sodium, 517mg potassium.

Oatmeal Lunch Bars
Yield: 4 servings | **Prep time:** 10 minutes | **Cook time:** 6 hours

- 1 cup oatmeal
- 2 dried apricots, chopped
- 1 tablespoon whole-grain flour
- 1 tablespoon raisins, chopped
- 1 egg, beaten
- 1 tablespoon sunflower seeds
- 1 teaspoon coconut oil

1. In the bowl mix oatmeal, apricots, flour, raisins, egg, sunflower seeds, and coconut oil.
2. Stir the mixture until smooth.
3. Knead the dough.
4. Line the Crock Pot bowl with baking paper.
5. Arrange the oatmeal dough inside and flatten it.
6. Cut the dough into bars and close the lid.
7. Cook the meal on Low for 6 hours.

per serving: 129 calories, 4.8g protein, 19.1g carbohydrates, 4.1g fat, 2.8g fiber, 41mg cholesterol, 17mg sodium, 163mg potassium.

Pasta Fritters
Yield: 4 servings | **Prep time:** 15 minutes | **Cook time:** 5 hours

- 5 oz whole-grain pasta, cooked
- 1 egg, beaten
- ½ cup Cheddar cheese
- 1 teaspoon ground turmeric
- 1 tablespoon whole-grain flour
- 1 teaspoon sesame oil

1. Chop the pasta into small pieces and mix with egg, ground turmeric, and flour.
2. Then shred the cheese and add it in the pasta mixture.
3. Make the small fritters from the mixture.
4. After this, brush the Crock Pot bowl with sesame oil.
5. Put the fritters inside and cook them on low for 5 hours.

per serving: 144 calories, 7g protein, 12.4g carbohydrates, 7.4g fat, 1.6g fiber, 56mg cholesterol, 103mg sodium, 103g potassium.

Vegetable Pasta
Yield: 2 servings | **Prep time:** 10 minutes | **Cook time:** 6 hours

- 4 oz whole-grain penne pasta
- 1 tomato, chopped
- 2 bell pepper, chopped
- 1 cup chicken stock
- 1 teaspoon dried dill
- 1 teaspoon butter

1. Pour chicken stock in the Crock Pot.
2. Add penne pasta, tomato, bell peppers, chicken stock, and dried dill.
3. Then add butter and cook the meal on Low for 6 hours.
4. Carefully mix the pasta before serving.

per serving: 193 calories, 7.3g protein, 34.3g carbohydrates, 3.8g fat, 6.2g fiber, 5mg cholesterol, 407mg sodium, 322mg potassium.

Sweet Popcorn
Yield: 4 servings | **Prep time:** 10 minutes | **Cook time:** 20 minutes

- 2 cups popped popcorn
- 2 tablespoons butter
- 2 tablespoons brown sugar
- ½ teaspoon ground cinnamon

1. Put butter and sugar in the Crock Pot.
2. Add ground cinnamon and cook the mixture on High or 15 minutes.
3. Then open the lid, stir the mixture, and add popped popcorn.
4. Carefully mix the ingredients with the help of the spatula and cook on high for 5 minutes more.

per serving: 84 calories, 0.6g protein, 7.8g carbohydrates, 5.9g fat, 0.7g fiber, 15mg cholesterol, 43mg sodium, 22mg potassium.

Dinner Millet Bowl
Yield: 5 servings | **Prep time:** 15 minutes | **Cook time:** 8 hours

- 2 cups whole-grain millet
- 2 cups chicken stock
- 3 cups of water
- 1 teaspoon butter
- 1 teaspoon salt
- ¼ cup pomegranate seeds
- 1 cup sauerkraut

1. Mix water with chicken stock and pour the liquid in the Crock Pot.
2. Add salt and millet and cook the ingredients on low for 8 hours.
3. Then mix the cooked millet with butter and pomegranate seeds.
4. Transfer the millet in the bowls and top with sauerkraut.

per serving: 323 calories, 9.4g protein, 61g carbohydrates, 4.4g fat, 7.7g fiber, 2mg cholesterol, 972mg sodium, 212mg potassium.

Coconut Millet with Apples
Yield: 4 servings | **Prep time:** 10 minutes | **Cook time:** 4 hours

- 1 cup millet
- 1 cup of coconut milk
- 3 cups of water
- ½ cup apples, diced
- 4 teaspoons cream cheese
- 1 tablespoon sugar

1. Mix water with coconut milk, and millet, and transfer the mixture in the Crock Pot.
2. Add sugar and apples, and cook it for 4 hours on High.
3. Then add cream cheese and carefully mix the meal.

per serving: 364 calories, 7.2g protein, 46.7g carbohydrates, 17.6g fat, 6.3g fiber, 4mg cholesterol, 27mg sodium, 291mg potassium.

Cinnamon Buckwheat

Yield: 5 servings | **Prep time:** 10 minutes | **Cook time:** 4.5 hours

- 1 cup buckwheat
- 1 teaspoon ground cinnamon
- ½ cup raisins, chopped
- 4 cups of milk
- 4 pecans, chopped
- 1 tablespoon honey

1. Mix milk and buckwheat in the Crock Pot.
2. Add ground cinnamon and close the lid.
3. Cook the buckwheat on High for 4.5 hours.
4. Then mix the cooked buckwheat with chopped pecans and raisins.
5. Transfer the meal in the bowls and top with a small amount of honey.

per serving: 349 calories, 12.6g protein, 50.8g carbohydrates, 13.2g fat, 5.4g fiber, 16mg cholesterol, 94mg sodium, 428mg potassium.

Barley Risotto
Yield: 6 servings | **Prep time:** 15 minutes | **Cook time:** 8.5 hours

- 1 cup pearl barley
- 2 cups chicken stock
- 1 cup white mushrooms, chopped
- 1 carrot, grated
- 1 onion, diced
- 2 tablespoons coconut oil
- 1 teaspoon Italian seasonings
- ½ cup cream

1. Pour chicken stock in the Crock Pot.
2. Add barley.
3. Then melt the coconut oil in the skillet.
4. Add carrot, mushrooms, and onion.
5. Sprinkle the vegetables with Italian seasonings and roast for 10 minutes on low heat.
6. Add the vegetables in the barley and close the lid.
7. Cook the meal on Low for 8 hours.
8. Then add cream and carefully mix the cooked risotto. Cook it on High or 30 minutes.

per serving: 189 calories, 4.3g protein, 29.9g carbohydrates, 6.5g fat, 6g fiber, 4mg cholesterol, 273mg sodium, 202mg potassium.

3-Grain Porridge
Yield: 6 servings | **Prep time:** 10 minutes | **Cook time:** 8 hours

- ½ cup of wheat berries
- ½ cup pearl barley
- ¼ wild rice
- 3 oz goat cheese, crumbled
- 2 tablespoons butter
- 1 teaspoon salt
- 5 cups of water

1. Pour water in the Crock Pot.
2. Add wheat berries, pearl barley, and wild rice.
3. Then add salt and cook the mixture on low for 8 hours.
4. When the grains are cooked, add goat cheese and butter.
5. Carefully mix the meal and transfer in the serving plates.

per serving: 198 calories, 7.7g protein, 22.1g carbohydrates, 9.3g fat, 3.1g fiber, 25mg cholesterol, 473mg sodium, 100mg potassium.

Wild Rice Medley
Yield: 4 servings | **Prep time:** 10 minutes | **Cook time:** 6 hours

- 1/3 cup wild rice
- 1 cup carrot, chopped
- 1 onion, chopped
- 1 oz pine nuts
- 1 teaspoon butter
- 1.5 cup vegetable stock

1. Mix wild rice with vegetable stock and transfer in the Crock Pot.
2. Add carrot and onion.
3. Cook the mixture on low for 6 hours.
4. Then add butter and stir the medley.
5. Top it with pine nuts.

per serving: 128 calories, 3.6g protein, 16.5g carbohydrates, 6g fat, 2.6g fiber, 3mg cholesterol, 47mg sodium, 228mg potassium.

Spring Pilaf
Yield: 5 servings | **Prep time:** 10 minutes | **Cook time:** 4 hours

- ½ cup carrot, diced
- ½ cup green peas, frozen
- 1 cup long-grain rice
- 2 oz chives, chopped
- 1 tablespoon olive oil
- 2.5 cups chicken stock
- ½ cup fresh parsley, chopped

1. Mix rice with olive oil and put it in the Crock Pot.
2. Add chicken stock and all remaining ingredients.
3. Close the lid and cook the pilaf on High for 4 hours.

per serving: 186 calories, 4.4g protein, 34g carbohydrates, 3.5g fat, 2g fiber, 0mg cholesterol, 396mg sodium, 187mg potassium.

Multi-Grain Cereal Bowl
Yield: 4 servings | **Prep time:** 10 minutes | **Cook time:** 6 hours

- ¼ cup quinoa
- ½ cup of wheat berries
- ½ cup steel cut oats
- 4 cups of water
- 2 oz Parmesan, grated
- 1 teaspoon butter

1. Put quinoa, wheat berries, and steel-cut oats in the Crock Pot.
2. Add water and cook the mixture for 6 hours on low.
3. Then add butter and carefully mix.
4. Transfer the meal in the bowls and top with Parmesan.

per serving: 159 calories, 8.4g protein, 20g carbohydrates, 5.5g fat, 1.9g fiber, 13mg cholesterol, 149mg sodium, 122mg potassium.

Spiced Bulgur

Yield: 3 servings | **Prep time:** 15 minutes | **Cook time:** 6 hours

- 1 cup bulgur
- 1.5 cup chicken stock
- ½ cup of water
- ½ teaspoon cayenne pepper
- ½ teaspoon ground nutmeg
- ½ teaspoon ground cardamom
- 1 tablespoon coconut oil

1. Melt the coconut oil in the skillet, add bulgur and roast for 2-3 minutes on high heat.
2. Then transfer the bulgur in the Crock Pot.
3. Add chicken stock and all remaining ingredients.
4. Close the lid and cook the meal on low for 6 hours.

per serving: 207 calories, 6.2g protein, 36.4g carbohydrates, 5.6g fat, 8.8g fiber, 0mg cholesterol, 390mg sodium, 210mg potassium.

Ginger Bulgur

Yield: 4 servings | **Prep time:** 15 minutes | **Cook time:** 4 hours

- 1 garlic clove, diced
- 1 teaspoon fresh ginger, grated
- 1 tablespoon olive oil
- 2 cups of water
- 1 cup bulgur
- 1 tablespoon sour cream

1. Heat olive oil in the skillet, add ginger and garlic and roast the vegetable for 2-3 minutes. Stir them from time to time to avoid burning.
2. Then transfer them in the Crock Pot.
3. Add water, bulgur, and close the lid.
4. Cook the bulgur on high for 4 hours.
5. Add sour cream and mix the cooked meal.

per serving: 159 calories, 4.5g protein, 27.3g carbohydrates, 4.6g fat, 6.5g fiber, 1mg cholesterol, 11mg sodium, 159mg potassium.

Pesto Freekeh

Yield: 4 servings | **Prep time:** 10 minutes | **Cook time:** 2 hours

- 2 tablespoons pesto sauce
- 1 tablespoon sesame oil
- 1 oz raisins
- 1 cup freekeh
- 3 cups chicken stock

1. Pour the chicken stock in the Crock Pot.
2. Add freekeh and raisins and cook the ingredients on High for 2 hours. The cooked freekeh should be tender.
3. Then transfer the freekeh mixture in the bowl.
4. Add sesame oil and pesto sauce.
5. Carefully mix the meal.

per serving: 125 calories, 3.5g protein, 13.2g carbohydrates, 7.4g fat, 1.4g fiber, 2mg cholesterol, 621mg sodium, 64mg potassium.

Poultry

Chicken Pockets

Yield: 4 servings | **Prep time:** 10 minutes | **Cook time:** 4 hours

- 4 tablespoons plain yogurt
- 1 oz fresh cilantro, chopped
- ½ teaspoon dried thyme
- 1-pound chicken fillet, sliced
- 2 tablespoons cream cheese
- 1 red onion, sliced
- 1/3 cup water
- 4 pita bread

1. Mix plain yogurt with chicken, water, dried thyme, and transfer in the Crock Pot.
2. Cook the chicken for 4 hours on High.
3. Then fill the pita bread with cream cheese, onion, cilantro, and chicken.

per serving: 422 calories, 40g protein, 37.5g carbohydrates, 11.1g fat, 2.2g fiber, 107mg cholesterol, 450mg sodium, 468mg potassium.

Jerk Chicken

Yield: 4 servings | **Prep time:** 15 minutes | **Cook time:** 7 hours

- 1 lemon
- 1-pound chicken breast, skinless, boneless
- 1 tablespoon taco seasoning
- 1 teaspoon garlic powder
- 1 teaspoon ground black pepper
- ½ teaspoon minced ginger
- 1 tablespoon soy sauce
- 1 cup of water

1. Chop the lemon and put it in the blender.
2. Add taco seasoning, garlic powder, ground black pepper, minced ginger, and soy sauce.
3. Blend the mixture until smooth.
4. After this, cut the chicken breast into the servings and rub with the lemon mixture carefully.
5. Transfer the chicken in the Crock Pot, add water, and cook on Low for 7 hours.

per serving: 150 calories, 24.7g protein, 4.7g carbohydrates, 2.9g fat, 0.7g fiber, 73mg cholesterol, 496mg sodium, 466mg potassium.

Lemon Chicken Thighs

Yield: 4 servings | **Prep time:** 10 minutes | **Cook time:** 7 hours

- 4 chicken thighs, skinless, boneless
- 1 lemon, sliced
- 1 teaspoon ground black pepper
- ½ teaspoon ground nutmeg
- 1 teaspoon olive oil
- 1 cup of water

1. Rub the chicken thighs with ground black pepper, nutmeg, and olive oil.
2. Then transfer the chicken in the Crock Pot.
3. Add lemon and water.
4. Close the lid and cook the meal on LOW for 7 hours.

per serving: 294 calories, 42.5g protein, 1.8g carbohydrates, 12.2g fat, 0.6g fiber, 130mg cholesterol, 128mg sodium, 383mg potassium.

Chicken Bowl

Yield: 6 servings | **Prep time:** 15 minutes | **Cook time:** 4 hours

- 1-pound chicken breast, skinless, boneless, chopped
- 1 cup sweet corn, frozen
- 1 teaspoon ground paprika
- 1 teaspoon onion powder
- 1 cup tomatoes, chopped
- 1 cup of water
- 1 teaspoon olive oil

1. Mix chopped chicken breast with ground paprika and onion powder. Transfer it in the Crock Pot.
2. Add water and sweet corn. Cook the mixture on High for 4 hours.
3. Then drain the liquid and transfer the mixture in the bowl.
4. Add tomatoes and olive oil. Mix the meal.

per serving: 122 calories, 17.2g protein, 6.3g carbohydrates, 3g fat, 1.1g fiber, 48mg cholesterol, 45mg sodium, 424mg potassium.

Asian Style Chicken

Yield: 4 servings | **Prep time:** 10 minutes | **Cook time:** 8 hours

- 1 teaspoon hot sauce
- ¼ cup of soy sauce
- 1 teaspoon sesame oil
- 2 oz scallions, chopped
- ½ cup of orange juice
- 1 teaspoon ground coriander
- 1-pound chicken breast, skinless, boneless, roughly chopped

1. Put all ingredients in the Crock Pot.
2. Close the lid and cook the meal on Low for 8 hours.
3. Then transfer the chicken and little amount of the chicken liquid in the bowls.

per serving: 166 calories, 25.5g protein, 5.5g carbohydrates, 4.1g fat, 0.6g fiber, 73mg cholesterol, 991mg sodium, 557mg potassium.

Oregano Chicken Breast

Yield: 4 servings | **Prep time:** 10 minutes | **Cook time:** 4 hours

- 1-pound chicken breast, skinless, boneless, roughly chopped
- 1 tablespoon dried oregano
- 1 bay leaf
- 1 teaspoon peppercorns
- 1 teaspoon salt
- 2 cups of water

1. Pour water in the Crock Pot and add peppercorns and bay leaf.
2. Then sprinkle the chicken with the dried oregano and transfer in the Crock Pot.
3. Close the lid and cook the meal on High for 4 hours.

per serving: 135 calories, 24.2g protein, 1.3g carbohydrates, 3g fat, 0.3g fiber, 73mg cholesterol, 643mg sodium, 448mg potassium.

Thai Chicken

Yield: 4 servings | **Prep time:** 15 minutes | **Cook time:** 4 hours

- 12 oz chicken fillet, sliced
- ½ cup of coconut milk
- 1 teaspoon dried lemongrass
- 1 teaspoon chili powder
- 1 teaspoon tomato paste
- 1 teaspoon ground cardamom
- 1 cup of water

1. Rub the chicken with chili powder, tomato paste, ground cardamom, and dried lemongrass. Transfer it in the Crock Pot.
2. Add water and coconut milk.
3. Close the lid and cook the meal on High for 4 hours.

per serving: 236 calories, 25.5g protein, 2.7g carbohydrates, 13.6g fat, 1.1g fiber, 76mg cholesterol, 87mg sodium, 321mg potassium.

Chicken Teriyaki

Yield: 4 servings | **Prep time:** 10 minutes | **Cook time:** 4 hours

- 1-pound chicken wings
- ½ cup teriyaki sauce
- ½ cup of water
- 1 carrot, chopped
- 1 onion, chopped
- 1 teaspoon butter

1. Toss butter in the pan and melt it.
2. Add onion and carrot and roast the vegetables for 5 minutes on medium heat.
3. Then transfer them in the Crock Pot.
4. Add chicken wings, teriyaki sauce, and water.
5. Close the lid and cook the meal for 4 hours on High.

per serving: 273 calories, 35.4g protein, 9.7g carbohydrates, 9.4g fat, 1g fiber, 103mg cholesterol, 1497mg sodium, 446mg potassium.

Stuffed Chicken Breast

Yield: 4 servings | **Prep time:** 15 minutes | **Cook time:** 6 hours

- 1-pound chicken breast, skinless, boneless
- 1 tomato, sliced
- 2 oz mozzarella, sliced
- 1 teaspoon fresh basil
- 1 teaspoon olive oil
- 1 teaspoon salt
- 1 cup of water

1. Make the horizontal cut in the chicken breast in the shape of the pocket.
2. Then fill it with sliced mozzarella, tomato, and basil.
3. Secure the cut with the help of the toothpicks and sprinkle the chicken with olive oil and salt.
4. Place it in the Crock Pot and add water.
5. Cook the chicken on low for 6 hours.

per serving: 182 calories, 28.2g protein, 1.1g carbohydrates, 6.5g fat, 0.2g fiber, 80mg cholesterol, 727mg sodium, 458mg potassium.

Chicken Pate

Yield: 6 servings | **Prep time:** 15 minutes | **Cook time:** 8 hours

- 1 carrot, peeled
- 1 teaspoon salt
- 1-pound chicken liver
- 2 cups of water
- 2 tablespoons coconut oil

1. Chop the carrot roughly and put it in the Crock Pot.
2. Add chicken liver and water.
3. Cook the mixture for 8 hours on Low.
4. Then drain water and transfer the mixture in the blender.
5. Add coconut oil and salt.
6. Blend the mixture until smooth.
7. Store the pate in the fridge for up to 7 days.

per serving: 169 calories, 18.6g protein, 1.7g carbohydrates, 9.5g fat, 0.3g fiber, 426mg cholesterol, 454mg sodium, 232mg potassium.

Chicken Masala

Yield: 4 servings | **Prep time:** 15 / minutes | **Cook time:** 4 hours

- 1 teaspoon garam masala
- 1 teaspoon ground ginger
- 1 cup of coconut milk
- 1-pound chicken fillet, sliced
- 1 teaspoon olive oil

1. Mix coconut milk with ground ginger, garam masala, and olive oil.
2. Add chicken fillet and mix the ingredients.
3. Then transfer them in the Crock Pot and cook on High for 4 hours.

per serving: 365 calories, 34.2g protein, 3.6g carbohydrates, 23.9g fat, 1.4g fiber, 101mg cholesterol, 108mg sodium, 439mg potassium.

Chicken Minestrone

Yield: 4 servings | **Prep time:** 10 minutes | **Cook time:** 3.5 hours

- 10 oz chicken fillet, sliced
- 2 cup of water
- 1 cup tomatoes, chopped 1 teaspoon chili powder
- 1 teaspoon ground paprika
- 1 teaspoon ground cumin
- 1 cup swiss chard, chopped
- ¼ cup red kidney beans, canned

1. Sprinkle the chicken fillet with chili powder, ground paprika, and ground cumin.
2. Transfer it in the Crock Pot.
3. Add tomatoes, water, swiss chard, and red kidney beans.
4. Close the lid and cook the meal on High for 3.5 hours.

per serving: 189 calories, 23.9g protein, 10g carbohydrates, 5.8g fat, 2.9g fiber, 63mg cholesterol, 95mg sodium, 505mg potassium.

French-Style Chicken

Yield: 4 servings | **Prep time:** 10 minutes | **Cook time:** 7 hours

- 1 can onion soup
- 4 chicken drumsticks
- ½ cup celery stalk, chopped
- 1 teaspoon dried tarragon
- ¼ cup white wine

1. Put ingredients in the Crock Pot and carefully mix them.
2. Then close the lid and cook the chicken on low for 7 hours.

per serving: 127 calories, 15.1g protein, 5.8g carbohydrates, 3.7g fat, 0.7g fiber, 40mg cholesterol, 688mg sodium, 185mg potassium.

Paella

Yield: 6 servings | **Prep time:** 10 minutes | **Cook time:** 4 hours

- 12 oz chicken fillet, chopped
- 4 oz chorizo, chopped
- ½ cup white rice
- 1 teaspoon garlic, diced
- 2 cups chicken stock
- 1 teaspoon dried cilantro
- 1 teaspoon chili flakes
- Cooking spray

1. Spray the skillet with cooking spray and put the chorizo inside.
2. Roast the chorizo for 2 minutes per side and transfer in the Crock Pot.
3. Then put rice in the Crock Pot.
4. Then add all remaining ingredients and carefully stir the paella mixture.
5. Cook it on High for 4 hours.

per serving: 254 calories, 22.3g protein, 13.1g carbohydrates, 11.7g fat, 0.2g fiber, 67mg cholesterol, 538mg sodium, 238mg potassium.

Sweet Chicken Breast

Yield: 4 servings | **Prep time:** 20 minutes | **Cook time:** 4 hours

- 2 red onions
- 2 tablespoons of liquid honey
- 1 tablespoon butter
- ½ cup of water
- 1-pound chicken breast, skinless, boneless
- 1 teaspoon curry paste

1. Rub the chicken breast with curry paste and transfer in the Crock Pot.
2. Slice the onion and add it to the cooker too.
3. Then add water and close the lid.
4. Cook the chicken breast on High for 4 hours.
5. After this, toss the butter in the skillet.
6. Melt it and add chicken.
7. Sprinkle the chicken with liquid honey and roast for 1 minute per side.
8. Slice the chicken breast.

per serving: 217 calories, 24.8g protein, 14.1g carbohydrates, 6.5g fat, 1.2g fiber, 80mg cholesterol, 82mg sodium, 506mg potassium.

Basil Chicken

Yield: 4 servings | **Prep time:** 15 minutes | **Cook time:** 7 hours

- 2 tablespoons balsamic vinegar
- 1 cup of water
- 1 teaspoon dried basil
- 1 teaspoon dried oregano
- 1-pound chicken fillet, sliced
- 1 teaspoon mustard

1. Mix chicken fillet with mustard and balsamic vinegar.
2. Add dried basil, oregano, and transfer in the Crock Pot.
3. Add water and close the lid.
4. Cook the chicken on low for 7 hours.

per serving: 222 calories, 33.1g protein, 0.6g carbohydrates, 8.7g fat, 0.3g fiber, 101mg cholesterol, 100mg sodium, 294mg potassium.

BBQ Chicken

Yield: 2 servings | **Prep time:** 15 minutes | **Cook time:** 7 hours

- 1 teaspoon minced garlic
- ½ cup BBQ sauce
- 1 tablespoon avocado oil
- 3 tablespoons lemon juice
- ½ cup of water
- 7 oz chicken fillet, sliced

1. In the bowl BBQ sauce, minced garlic, avocado oil, and lemon juice.
2. Add chicken fillet and mix the mixture.
3. After this, transfer it to the Crock Pot. Add water and close the lid.
4. Cook the chicken on low for 7 hours.

per serving: 299 calories, 29.1g protein, 24g carbohydrates, 8.6g fat, 0.8g fiber, 88mg cholesterol, 792mg sodium, 428mg potassium.

Sugar Chicken

Yield: 6 servings | **Prep time:** 10 minutes | **Cook time:** 6 hours

- 1 teaspoon chili flakes
- 6 chicken drumsticks
- 2 tablespoons brown sugar
- 1 tablespoon butter, melted
- 1 tablespoon lemon juice
- 1 teaspoon ground black pepper
- ¼ cup milk

1. In the bowl mix chili flakes, brown sugar, butter, lemon juice, and ground black pepper.
2. Then brush every chicken drumstick with the sweet mixture and transfer in the Crock Pot.
3. Add milk and close the lid. Cook the meal on Low for 6 hours.

per serving: 113 calories, 13.1g protein, 3.7g carbohydrates, 4.8g fat, 0.1g fiber, 46mg cholesterol, 57mg sodium, 110mg potassium.

Chili Chicken

Yield: 4 servings | **Prep time:** 15 minutes | **Cook time:** 7 hours

- 1 teaspoon chili powder

- 1 tablespoon hot sauce
- 1 tablespoon coconut oil, melted
- ½ teaspoon ground turmeric
- 1 teaspoon garlic, minced
- ½ cup of water
- 1-pound chicken wings

1. Rub the chicken wings with hot sauce, chili powder, ground turmeric, garlic, and coconut oil.
2. Then pour water in the Crock Pot and add prepared chicken wings.
3. Cook the chicken on low for 7 hours.

per serving: 249 calories, 33g protein, 0.8g carbohydrates, 12g fat, 0.3g fiber, 101mg cholesterol, 200mg sodium, 303mg potassium.

Orange Chicken

Yield: 4 servings | **Prep time:** 10 minutes | **Cook time:** 8 hours

- 1 orange, chopped
- 1 teaspoon ground turmeric
- 1 teaspoon peppercorn
- 1 teaspoon olive oil
- 1 teaspoon salt
- 1 cup of water
- 1-pound chicken breast, skinless, boneless, sliced

1. Put all ingredients in the Crock Pot and gently mix them.
2. Close the lid and cook the meal on Low for 8 hours.
3. When the time is finished, transfer the chicken in the serving bowls and top with orange liquid from the Crock Pot.

per serving: 164 calories, 24.6g protein, 6.1g carbohydrates, 4.1g fat, 1.g4 fiber, 73mg cholesterol, 641mg sodium, 524mg potassium.

Bacon Chicken

Yield: 4 servings | **Prep time:** 10 minutes | **Cook time:** 7 hours

- 4 bacon slices, cooked
- 4 chicken drumsticks
- ½ cup of water
- ¼ tomato juice
- 1 teaspoon salt
- ½ teaspoon ground black pepper

1. Sprinkle the chicken drumsticks with the salt and ground black pepper.
2. Then wrap every chicken drumstick in the bacon and arrange it in the Crock Pot.
3. Add water and tomato juice. Cook the meal on Low for 7 hours.

per serving: 184 calories, 19.8g protein, 1.1g carbohydrates, 10.6g fat, 0.1g fiber, 61mg cholesterol, 1099mg sodium, 237mg potassium.

Bourbon Chicken Cubes

Yield: 4 servings | **Prep time:** 10 minutes | **Cook time:** 4 hours

- ½ cup bourbon
- 1 teaspoon liquid honey
- 1 tablespoon BBQ sauce

- 1 white onion, diced
- 1 teaspoon garlic powder
- 1-pound chicken fillet, cubed

1. Put all ingredients in the Crock Pot.
2. Mix the mixture until liquid honey is dissolved.
3. Then close the lid and cook the meal on high for 4 hours.

per serving: 304 calories, 33.2g protein, 5.9g carbohydrates, 8.5g fat, 0.7g fiber, 101mg cholesterol, 143mg sodium, 333mg potassium.

Mexican Chicken

Yield: 2 servings | **Prep time:** 10 minutes | **Cook time:** 6 hours

- ½ cup sweet pepper, sliced
- 1 teaspoon cayenne pepper
- 2 chicken thighs, skinless, boneless
- 1 red onion, sliced
- ½ cup salsa verde
- 1 cup of water

1. Pour water in the Crock Pot.
2. Add salsa verde and onion.
3. Then add cayenne pepper and chicken thighs.
4. Cook the mixture on High for 3 hours.
5. After this, add sweet pepper and cook the meal on Low for 3 hours.

per serving: 327 calories, 44g protein, 10.5g carbohydrates, 11.3g fat, 2.1g fiber, 130mg cholesterol, 477mg sodium, 510mg potassium.

Curry Chicken Wings

Yield: 4 servings | **Prep time:** 15 minutes | **Cook time:** 7 hours

- 1-pound chicken wings
- 1 teaspoon curry paste
- ½ cup heavy cream
- 1 teaspoon minced garlic
- ½ teaspoon ground nutmeg
- ½ cup of water

1. In the bowl mix curry paste, heavy cream, minced garlic, and ground nutmeg.
2. Add chicken wings and stir.
3. Then pour water in the Crock Pot.
4. Add chicken wings with all remaining curry paste mixture and close the lid.
5. Cook the chicken wings on Low for 7 hours.

per serving: 278 calories, 33.2g protein, 1.1g carbohydrates, 14.8g fat, 0.1g fiber, 121mg cholesterol, 104mg sodium, 291mg potassium.

Thyme Whole Chicken

Yield: 6 servings | **Prep time:** 15 minutes | **Cook time:** 9 hours

- 1.5-pound whole chicken
- 1 tablespoon dried thyme
- 1 tablespoon olive oil
- 1 teaspoon salt
- 1 cup of water

1. Chop the whole chicken roughly and sprinkle with dried thyme, olive oil, and salt.
2. Then transfer it in the Crock Pot, add water.
3. Cook the chicken on low for 9 hours.

per serving: 237 calories, 32.9g protein, 0.3g carbohydrates, 10.8g fat, 0.2g fiber, 101mg cholesterol, 487mg sodium, 280mg potassium.

Fennel and Chicken Saute

Yield: 4 servings | **Prep time:** 10 minutes | **Cook time:** 7 hours

- 1 cup fennel, peeled, chopped
- 10 oz chicken fillet, chopped
- 1 tablespoon tomato paste
- 1 cup of water
- 1 teaspoon ground black pepper
- 1 teaspoon olive oil
- ½ teaspoon fennel seeds

1. Heat the olive oil in the skillet.
2. Add fennel seeds and roast them until you get saturated fennel smell.
3. Transfer the seeds in the Crock Pot.
4. Add fennel, chicken fillet, tomato paste, water, and ground black pepper.
5. Close the lid and cook the meal on Low for 7 hours.

per serving: 157 calories, 28.1g protein, 2.8g carbohydrates, 6.5g fat, 1.1g fiber, 63mg cholesterol, 78mg sodium, 314mg potassium.

Russian Chicken

Yield: 4 servings | **Prep time:** 10 minutes | **Cook time:** 4 hours

- 2 tablespoons mayonnaise
- 4 chicken thighs, skinless, boneless
- 1 teaspoon minced garlic
- 1 teaspoon ground black pepper
- 1 teaspoon sunflower oil
- 1 teaspoon salt
- ½ cup of water

1. In the bowl mix mayonnaise, minced garlic, ground black pepper, salt, and oil.
2. Then add chicken thighs and mix the ingredients well.
3. After this, pour water in the Crock Pot. Add chicken thighs mixture.
4. Cook the meal on High for 4 hours.

per serving: 319 calories, 42.4g protein, 2.3g carbohydrates, 14.5g fat, 0.2g fiber, 132mg cholesterol, 760mg sodium, 365mg potassium.

Cocoa Chicken

Yield: 8 servings | **Prep time:** 10 minutes | **Cook time:** 8 hours

- 2 tablespoons cocoa powder
- 1 cup of water
- 2-pound chicken breast, skinless, boneless
- 1 tablespoon tomato paste
- 1 teaspoon hot sauce
- ½ cup cream

1. Whisk cocoa powder with cream until smooth and pour the liquid in the Crock Pot.
2. Mix chicken breast with tomato paste and hot sauce and put in the Crock Pot.
3. Then add water and close the lid.
4. Cook the chicken on low for 8 hours.

5. Then shred the chicken and serve it with cocoa gravy.

per serving: 144 calories, 24.5g protein, 1.6g carbohydrates, 3.9g fat, 0.5g fiber, 75mg cholesterol, 82mg sodium, 480mg potassium.

Easy Chicken Adobo

Yield: 4 servings | **Prep time:** 10 minutes | **Cook time:** 4 hours

- 1 teaspoon minced garlic
- 1 cup onion, chopped
- ½ teaspoon ground ginger
- 4 chicken thighs, skinless, boneless
- 1 tablespoon balsamic vinegar
- 1 tablespoon soy sauce
- ½ teaspoon ground black pepper
- ½ cup of water

1. Put the onion in the Crock Pot.
2. Then mix soy sauce with balsamic vinegar and minced garlic.
3. Rub the chicken with garlic mixture and put it in the Crock Pot.
4. Then add ground black pepper, ginger, and water.
5. Cook the meal on High for 4 hours.

per serving: 294 calories, 42.9g protein, 3.6g carbohydrates, 10.9g fat, 0.8g fiber, 130g cholesterol, 354mg sodium, 418mg potassium.

Stuffed Whole Chicken

Yield: 10 servings | **Prep time:** 15 minutes | **Cook time:** 6 hours

- 3-pound whole chicken
- 1 tablespoon taco seasonings
- 1 cup apples, chopped
- 1 tablespoon olive oil
- 2 cups of water

1. Fill the chicken with apples.
2. Then rub the chicken with taco seasonings and brush with olive oil.
3. Place it in the Crock Pot. Add water.
4. Cook the chicken on High for 6 hours.
5. When the chicken is cooked, chop it into servings and serve with cooked apples.

per serving: 285 calories, 39.4g protein, 3.7g carbohydrates, 11.5g fat, 0.5g fiber, 121mg cholesterol, 182mg sodium, 355mg potassium.

Lime Chicken

Yield: 4 servings | **Prep time:** 10 minutes | **Cook time:** 6 hours

- 3 tablespoons lime juice
- 1 teaspoon lime zest
- 1 teaspoon olive oil
- ½ teaspoon ground black pepper
- 1-pound chicken fillet
- ½ cup of coconut milk

1. Cut the chicken fillet into servings.
2. In the shallow bowl mix lime zest, lime juice, olive oil, and ground black pepper.
3. Mix chickens servings with lime mixture and put in the Crock Pot.

4. Add coconut milk and cook the meal on Low for 6 hours.
 per serving: 297 calories, 33.6g protein, 2.4g carbohydrates, 16.8g fat, 0.8g fiber, 101mg cholesterol, 103mg sodium, 364mg potassium.

Sesame Chicken Drumsticks
Yield: 4 servings | **Prep time:** 15 minutes | **Cook time:** 7 hours
- 1-pound chicken drumsticks
- 1 teaspoon salt
- 1 teaspoon ground turmeric
- 1 teaspoon chili powder
- 1 tablespoon sesame seeds
- 1 tablespoon olive oil
- 1 cup of water

1. Sprinkle the chicken drumsticks with salt, ground turmeric, chili powder, and sesame oil. Mix the chicken well.
2. Then heat olive oil well and add the chicken drumsticks.
3. Roast them on high heat for 2 minutes per side.
4. Transfer the roasted chicken drumsticks in the Crock Pot, add water, and close the lid.
5. Cook the chicken drumsticks on Low for 7 hours.
 per serving: 239 calories, 31.7g protein, 1.3g carbohydrates, 11.3g fat, 0.6g fiber, 100mg cholesterol, 681mg sodium, 263mg potassium.

Algerian Chicken
Yield: 2 servings | **Prep time:** 15 minutes | **Cook time:** 4 hours
- 6 oz chicken breast, skinless, boneless, sliced
- 1 teaspoon peanut oil
- 1 teaspoon harissa
- 1 teaspoon tomato paste
- 1 tablespoon sesame oil
- 1 cup tomatoes, canned
- ¼ cup of water

1. Mix tomato paste with harissa, peanut oil, and sesame oil. Whisk the mixture and mix it with sliced chicken breast.
2. After this, transfer the chicken in the Crock Pot in one layer.
3. Add water and close the lid.
4. Cook the chicken on High for 4 hours.
 per serving: 204 calories, 19.1 protein, 5g carbohydrates, 11.8g fat, 1.2g fiber, 55mg cholesterol, 81mg sodium, 555mg potassium.

Butter Chicken
Yield: 4 servings | **Prep time:** 10 minutes | **Cook time:** 4 hours
- 12 oz chicken fillet
- ½ cup butter
- 1 teaspoon garlic powder
- 1 teaspoon salt

1. Put all ingredients in the Crock Pot.
2. Cook them on High for 4 hours.
3. Then shred the chicken and transfer in the plates.

4. Sprinkle the chicken with fragrant butter from the Crock Pot.
 per serving: 367 calories, 25g protein, 0.5g carbohydrates, 29.3g fat, 0.1g fiber, 137mg cholesterol, 818mg sodium, 221mg potassium.

Chicken in Sweet Soy Sauce
Yield: 6 servings | **Prep time:** 15 minutes | **Cook time:** 6 hours
- ½ cup of soy sauce
- 2 teaspoons maple syrup
- ½ teaspoon ground cinnamon
- 6 chicken thighs, skinless, boneless
- ¼ cup of water

1. Pour water and soy sauce in the Crock Pot.
2. Add chicken thighs, ground cinnamon, and maple syrup.
3. Close the lid and cook the meal on Low for 6 hours.
 per serving: 295 calories, 43.6g protein, 3.3g carbohydrates, 10.8g fat, 0.3g fiber, 130mg cholesterol, 1324mg sodium, 406mg potassium.

Jamaican Chicken
Yield: 3 servings | **Prep time:** 10 minutes | **Cook time:** 4 hours
- 12 oz chicken fillet
- ½ teaspoon ground coriander
- ½ teaspoon dried cilantro
- ½ teaspoon lemon zest
- 1 jalapeno, sliced
- 1 teaspoon olive oil
- 1 cup tomato juice

1. Rub the chicken fillet with ground coriander, cilantro, lemon zest, and olive oil.
2. Put the chicken in the Crock Pot.
3. Add tomato juice and jalapeno.
4. Cook the meal on High for 4 hours.
 per serving: 244 calories, 33.5g protein, 3.8g carbohydrates, 10g fat, 0.5g fiber, 101mg cholesterol, 316mg sodium, 472mg potassium.

Turkey in Pomegranate Juice
Yield: 4 servings | **Prep time:** 10 minutes | **Cook time:** 7 hours
- 1-pound turkey fillet, sliced
- ½ cup pomegranate juice
- 1 tablespoon maple syrup
- 1 teaspoon cornstarch
- 1 teaspoon dried thyme
- 1 teaspoon butter
- ¼ cup of water

1. Pour water and pomegranate juice in the Crock Pot.
2. Add cornstarch and whisk the mixture until smooth.
3. Then add all remaining ingredients and close the lid.
4. Cook the meal on Low for 7 hours.
 per serving: 150 calories, 23.6g protein, 8.8g carbohydrates, 1.5g fat, 0.1g fiber, 61mg cholesterol, 266mg sodium, 88mg potassium.

Tender Duck Fillets

Yield: 3 servings | **Prep time:** 15 minutes | **Cook time:** 8 hours

- 1 tablespoon butter
- 1 teaspoon dried rosemary
- 1 teaspoon ground nutmeg
- 9 oz duck fillet
- 1 cup of water
1. Slice the fillet.
2. Then melt the butter in the skillet.
3. Add sliced duck fillet and roast it for 2-3 minutes per side on medium heat.
4. Transfer the roasted duck fillet and butter in the Crock Pot.
5. Add dried rosemary, ground nutmeg, and water.
6. Close the lid and cook the meal on Low for 8 hours.

per serving: 145 calories, 25.2g protein, 0.6g carbohydrates, 4.7g fat, 0.3g fiber, 10mg cholesterol, 158mg sodium, 61mg potassium.

Chicken Mole

Yield: 4 servings | **Prep time:** 10 minutes | **Cook time:** 4.5 hours

- 1 onion, minced
- 1 tablespoon raisins
- 1 tablespoon chipotle, chopped
- 1 tablespoon adobo sauce
- 1 teaspoon of cocoa powder
- 1 cup of water
- 1-pound chicken breast, skinless, boneless, chopped
1. Pour water in the Crock Pot. Add cocoa powder and whisk the mixture until smooth.
2. Add raisins, chipotle, adobo sauce, and chicken breast.
3. Close the lid and cook the mole on High for 4.5 hours.

per serving: 175 calories, 24.5g protein, 5.9g carbohydrates, 5.3g fat, 0.8g fiber, 74mg cholesterol, 212mg sodium, 489mg potassium.

Curry Chicken Strips

Yield: 6 servings | **Prep time:** 15 minutes | **Cook time:** 3.5 hours

- 1 tablespoon curry paste
- 1-pound chicken fillet, cut into strips
- 1 teaspoon liquid honey
- 1 teaspoon olive oil
- 1 tablespoon cream cheese
- 1/3 cup water
1. Mix curry paste with honey, olive oil, and cream cheese,
2. Then mix the curry mixture with chicken strips and carefully mix.
3. Put the chicken strips in the Crock Pot, add water, and close the lid.
4. Cook the meal in High for 3.5 hours.

per serving: 176 calories, 22.1g protein, 1.7g carbohydrates, 8.4g fat, 0g fiber, 69mg cholesterol, 70mg sodium, 186mg potassium.

Easy Chicken Continental

Yield: 2 servings | **Prep time:** 15 minutes | **Cook time:** 7 hours

- 2 oz dried beef
- 8 oz chicken breast, skinless, boneless, chopped
- ½ cup cream
- ½ can onion soup
- 1 tablespoon cornstarch
1. Put 1 oz of the dried beef in the Crock Pot in one layer.
2. Then add chicken breast and top it with remaining dried beef.
3. After this, mix cream cheese, onion, and cornstarch. Whisk the mixture and pour it over the chicken and dried beef.
4. Cook the meal on Low for 7 hours.

per serving: 270 calories, 35.4g protein, 10.5g carbohydrates, 9g fat, 0.6g fiber, 109mg cholesterol, 737mg sodium, 598mg potassium.

Pineapple Chicken

Yield: 4 servings | **Prep time:** 15 minutes | **Cook time:** 8 hours

- 12 oz chicken fillet
- 1 cup pineapple, canned, chopped
- ½ cup Cheddar cheese, shredded
- 1 tablespoon butter, softened
- 1 teaspoon ground black pepper
- ¼ cup of water
1. Grease the Crock Pot bowl bottom with softened butter.
2. Then cut the chicken fillet into servings and put in the Crock Pot in one layer.
3. After this, top the chicken with ground black pepper, water, pineapple, and Cheddar cheese.
4. Close the lid and cook the meal on Low for 8 hours.

per serving: 266 calories, 28.4g protein, 5.9g carbohydrates, 13.9g fat, 0.7g fiber, 98mg cholesterol, 183mg sodium, 273mg potassium.

Cinnamon Turkey

Yield: 5 servings | **Prep time:** 10 minutes | **Cook time:** 6 hours

- 1 teaspoon ground cinnamon
- 1-pound turkey fillet, chopped
- ½ teaspoon dried thyme
- 1 teaspoon salt
- ½ cup cream
1. Mix turkey with cinnamon, salt, and thyme.
2. Transfer it in the Crock Pot.
3. Add cream and cook the meal on Low for 6 hours.

per serving: 102 calories, 19g protein, 1.1g carbohydrates, 1.8g fat, 0.2g fiber, 52mg cholesterol, 678mg sodium, 11mg potassium.

BBQ Pulled Chicken

Yield: 3 servings | **Prep time:** 15 minutes | **Cook time:** 8 hours

- 12 oz chicken breast, skinless, boneless
- ½ cup BBQ sauce

- 1 teaspoon dried rosemary
- 1 cup of water
1.   Pour water in the Crock Pot.
2.   Add chicken breast and dried rosemary. Cook the chicken on High for 5 hours.
3.   Then drain the water and shred the chicken with the help of the fork.
4.   Add BBQ sauce, carefully mix the chicken and cook it on Low for 3 hours.
 per serving: 193 calories, 24.1g protein, 15.4g carbohydrates, 3g fat, 0.4g fiber, 73mg cholesterol, 527mg sodium, 511mg potassium.

Basil Chicken Saute
Yield: 4 servings | **Prep time:** 10 minutes | **Cook time:** 7 hours
- 1 cup bell pepper
- 2 tomatoes, chopped
- 1 jalapeno pepper, chopped
- ½ cup of water
- 10 oz chicken fillet, chopped
- 1 teaspoon dried basil
1.   Pour water in the Crock Pot.
2.   Add all remaining ingredients and close the lid.
3.   Cook the chicken saute on Low for 7 hours.
 per serving: 156 calories, 21.4g protein, 4.9g carbohydrates, 5.5g fat, 1.2g fiber, 63mg cholesterol, 66mg sodium, 382mg potassium.

Chicken Mix
Yield: 4 servings | **Prep time:** 10 minutes | **Cook time:** 8 hours
- 1 cup carrot, chopped
- 1-pound chicken wings
- 1 cup of water
- ½ cup tomato juice
- 1 teaspoon salt
- 1 teaspoon dried rosemary
1.   Put chicken wings in the Crock Pot.
2.   Add carrot, tomato juice, water, salt, and dried rosemary.
3.   Close the lid and cook the meal on low for 8 hours.
 per serving: 233 calories, 33.3g protein, 4.2g carbohydrates, 8.g 5fat, 0.9g fiber, 101mg cholesterol, 781mg sodium, 437mg potassium.

Chicken Parm
Yield: 3 servings | **Prep time:** 10 minutes | **Cook time:** 4 hours
- 9 oz chicken fillet
- 1/3 cup cream
- 3 oz Parmesan, grated
- 1 teaspoon olive oil
1.   Brush the Crock Pot bowl with olive oil from inside.
2.   Then slice the chicken fillet and place it in the Crock Pot.
3.   Top it with Parmesan and cream.
4.   Close the lid and cook the meal on High for 4 hours.

 per serving: 283 calories, 33.9g protein, 1.8g carbohydrates, 15.4g fat, 0g fiber, 101mg cholesterol, 345mg sodium, 216mg potassium.

Chicken Cacciatore
Yield: 2 servings | **Prep time:** 10 minutes | **Cook time:** 7 hours
- 1 teaspoon sesame oil
- 2 chicken thighs, skinless, boneless
- 1 teaspoon tomato paste
- 1 carrot, sliced
- ½ cup mushrooms, sliced
- 1 cup of water
- 1 teaspoon Italian seasonings
- ¼ cup green beans, canned
1.   Put all ingredients in the Crock Pot and gently stir them.
2.   Then close the lid and cook the meal on Low for 7 hours.
 per serving: 327 calories, 43.4g protein, 5.3g carbohydrates, 13.9g fat, 1.5g fiber, 132mg cholesterol, 155mg sodium, 566mg potassium.

Fanta Chicken
Yield: 4 servings | **Prep time:** 10 minutes | **Cook time:** 4.5 hours
- 1 cup Fanta
- 1-pound chicken breast, skinless, boneless, chopped
- 1 teaspoon ground cumin
- 1 teaspoon ground nutmeg
1.   Mix chicken breast with cumin and ground nutmeg and transfer in the Crock Pot.
2.   Add Fanta and close the lid.
3.   Cook the meal on high for 4.5 hours.
 per serving: 162 calories, 24.2g protein, 9.3g carbohydrates, 3.2g fat, 0.2g fiber, 73mg cholesterol, 68mg sodium, 431mg potassium.

Horseradish Chicken Wings
Yield: 4 servings | **Prep time:** 10 minutes | **Cook time:** 6 hours
- 3 tablespoons horseradish, grated
- 1 teaspoon ketchup
- 1 tablespoon mayonnaise
- ½ cup of water
- 1-pound chicken wings
1.   Mix chicken wings with ketchup, horseradish, and mayonnaise,
2.   Put them in the Crock Pot and add water.
3.   Cook the meal on Low for 6 hours.
 per serving: 236 calories, 33g protein, 2.5g carbohydrates, 9.7g fat, 0.4g fiber, 102mg cholesterol, 174mg sodium, 309mg potassium.

Mustard Chicken
Yield: 4 servings | **Prep time:** 10 minutes | **Cook time:** 6 hours
- 1 tablespoon avocado oil
- 1-pound chicken breast, skinless, boneless and roughly cubed
- ½ cup of water

- 1 tablespoon mustard
- 1 teaspoon chili flakes
- 2 tablespoons apple cider vinegar
- 1 garlic clove, peeled

1.   Mix avocado oil with mustard, chili flakes, and apple cider vinegar.
2.   Mix the chicken with mustard mixture and transfer it in the Crock Pot.
3.   Add water and garlic clove.
4.   Cook the chicken on low for 6 hours.

per serving: 150 calories, 24.8g protein, 1.5g carbohydrates, 4.1g fat, 0.6g fiber, 73mg cholesterol, 60mg sodium, 459mg potassium.

Spinach Chicken
Yield: 4 servings | **Prep time:** 15 minutes | **Cook time:** 8 hours

- 1-pound chicken breasts, skinless, boneless, chopped
- 1 cup baby spinach
- 1 teaspoon ground black pepper
- ½ teaspoon salt
- 1 cup of water
- 1 jalapeno pepper

1.   Chop the jalapeno pepper and put it in the Crock Pot.
2.   Add baby spinach, chicken breast, salt, ground black pepper, and water.
3.   Close the lid and cook the chicken on low for 8 hours.

per serving: 220 calories, 33.1g protein, 0.8g carbohydrates, 8.5g fat, 0.4g fiber, 101mg cholesterol, 396mg sodium, 332mg potassium.

Greece Style Chicken
Yield: 6 servings | **Prep time:** 10 minutes | **Cook time:** 8 hours

- 12 oz chicken fillet, chopped
- 1 cup green olives, chopped
- 1 cup of water
- 1 tablespoon cream cheese
- ½ teaspoon dried thyme

1.   Put all ingredients in the Crock Pot.
2.   Close the lid and cook the meal on Low for 8 hours.
3.   Then transfer the cooked chicken in the bowls and top with olives and hot liquid from the Crock Pot.

per serving: 124 calories, 16.7g protein, 0.8g carbohydrates, 5.7g fat, 0.3g fiber, 52mg cholesterol, 167mg sodium, 142mg potassium.

Turkey with Plums
Yield: 5 servings | **Prep time:** 10 minutes | **Cook time:** 8 hours

- 1-pound turkey fillet, chopped
- 1 cup plums, pitted, halved
- 1 teaspoon ground cinnamon
- 1 cup of water
- 1 teaspoon ground black pepper

1.   Mix the turkey with ground cinnamon and ground black pepper.
2.   Then transfer it in the Crock Pot.

3.   Add water and plums.
4.   Close the lid and cook the meal on Low for 8 hours.

per serving: 94 calories, 19g protein, 2.2g carbohydrates, 0.5g fat, 0.5g fiber, 47mg cholesterol, 207mg sodium, 29mg potassium.

Chicken with Vegetables
Yield: 4 servings | **Prep time:** 10 minutes | **Cook time:** 4 hours

- 1-pound chicken fillet, cut into slices
- 1 cup broccoli, chopped
- ½ cup green peas, frozen
- ½ cup corn kernels, frozen
- 1 cup of water
- 1 teaspoon dried rosemary
- ½ teaspoon peppercorns

1.   Put all ingredients in the Crock Pot.
2.   Close the lid and cook the meal on High for 4 hours.

per serving: 256 calories, 35.1g protein, 8.1g carbohydrates, 8.8g fat, 2.2g fiber, 101mg cholesterol, 111mg sodium, 451mg potassium.

Cyprus Chicken
Yield: 4 servings | **Prep time:** 10 minutes | **Cook time:** 4.5 hours

- 1-pound chicken breast, skinless, boneless
- 1 tablespoon sesame seeds
- ½ cup black olives, pitted and halved
- ½ cup pearl onions, peeled
- 1 teaspoon cumin seeds
- 1 cup of water

1.   Chop the chicken breast roughly and put it in the Crock Pot.
2.   Add sesame seeds, black olives, onions, cumin seeds, and water.
3.   Close the lid and cook the meal on high for 4.5 hours.

per serving: 169 calories, 24.8g protein, 3.2g carbohydrates, 5.9g fat, 1.2g fiber, 73mg cholesterol, 208mg sodium, 463mg potassium.

Duck Saute
Yield: 3 servings | **Prep time:** 10 minutes | **Cook time:** 5 hours

- 8 oz duck fillet, sliced
- 1 cup of water
- 1 cup mushrooms, sliced
- 1 teaspoon salt
- 1 teaspoon ground black pepper
- 1 tablespoon olive oil

1.   Heat the olive oil in the skillet well.
2.   Add mushrooms and roast them for 3-5 minutes on medium heat.
3.   Transfer the roasted mushrooms in the Crock Pot.
4.   Add duck fillet, and all remaining ingredients.
5.   Close the lid and cook saute for 5 hours on High.

per serving: 141 calories, 23.1g protein, 1.2g carbohydrates, 5.2g fat, 0.4g fiber, 0mg cholesterol, 893mg sodium, 131mg potassium.

Chicken Drumsticks with Zucchini

Yield: 4 servings | **Prep time:** 10 minutes | **Cook time:** 7 hours

- 4 chicken drumsticks
- 1 teaspoon ground black pepper
- ½ teaspoon salt
- ½ teaspoon ground turmeric
- 1 cup of water
- 1 large zucchini, chopped
1.   Put all ingredients in the Crock Pot.
2.   Close the lid and cook the meal on Low for 7 hours.

per serving: 93 calories, 13.7g protein, 3.2g carbohydrates, 2.8g fat, 1.1g fiber, 40mg cholesterol, 338mg sodium, 318mg potassium.

Garlic Duck

Yield: 4 servings | **Prep time:** 10 minutes | **Cook time:** 5 hours

- 1-pound duck fillet
- 1 tablespoon minced garlic
- 1 tablespoon butter, softened
- 1 teaspoon dried thyme
- 1/3 cup coconut cream
1.   Mix minced garlic with butter, and dried thyme.
2.   Then rub the suck fillet with garlic mixture and place it in the Crock Pot.
3.   Add coconut cream and cook the duck on High for 5 hours.
4.   Then slice the cooked duck fillet and sprinkle it with hot garlic coconut milk.

per serving: 216 calories, 34.1g protein, 2g carbohydrates, 8.4g fat, 0.6g fiber, 8mg cholesterol, 194mg sodium, 135mg potassium.

Chicken and Cabbage Bowl

Yield: 4 servings | **Prep time:** 10 minutes | **Cook time:** 7 hours

- 1-pound chicken fillet, sliced
- 1 cup white cabbage, shredded
- 1 tablespoon tomato paste
- 1 teaspoon dried rosemary
- 1 teaspoon salt
- 1 teaspoon dried dill
- 2 cups of water
1.   Mix water with tomato paste and whisk until smooth.
2.   Pour the liquid in the Crock Pot.
3.   Add cabbage, chicken fillet, and all remaining ingredients.
4.   Close the lid and cook the meal on Low for 7 hours.
5.   When the meal is cooked, transfer it in the serving bowls.

per serving: 225 calories, 33.3g protein, 2.1g carbohydrates, 8.5g fat, 0.8g fiber, 101mg cholesterol, 690mg sodium, 358mg potassium.

Garlic Pulled Chicken

Yield: 4 servings | **Prep time:** 10 minutes | **Cook time:** 4 hours

- 1-pound chicken breast, skinless, boneless
- 1 tablespoon minced garlic
- 2 cups of water
- ½ cup plain yogurt
1.   Put the chicken breast in the Crock Pot.
2.   Add minced garlic and water.
3.   Close the lid and cook the chicken on High for 4 hours.
4.   Then drain water and shred the chicken breast.
5.   Add plain yogurt and stir the pulled chicken well.

per serving: 154 calories, 25.9g protein, 2.9g carbohydrates, 3.2g fat, 0g fiber, 74mg cholesterol, 83mg sodium, 501mg potassium.

Orange Chicken

Yield: 4 servings | **Prep time:** 10 minutes | **Cook time:** 7 hours

- 1-pound chicken fillet, roughly chopped
- 4 oranges, peeled, chopped
- 1 cup of water
- 1 teaspoon peppercorns
- 1 onion, diced
1.   Put chicken and oranges in the Crock Pot.
2.   Add water, peppercorns, and onion.
3.   Close the lid and cook the meal on Low for 7 hours.

per serving: 314 calories, 34.9g protein, 24.5g carbohydrates, 8.7g fat, 5.2g fiber, 101mg cholesterol, 101mg sodium, 656mg potassium.

Pepper Whole Chicken

Yield: 4 servings | **Prep time:** 15 minutes | **Cook time:** 8 hours

- 16 oz whole chicken
- 1 tablespoon ground black pepper
- 1 teaspoon salt
- 1 cup bell pepper, chopped
- 2 cup of water
- 1 tablespoon butter, softened
1.   Rub the chicken with butter, salt, and ground black pepper.
2.   Then fill it with bell pepper and put it in the Crock Pot.
3.   Add water and close the lid.
4.   Cook the chicken on low for 8 hours.

per serving: 254 calories, 33.3g protein, 3.3g carbohydrates, 11.4g fat, 0.8g fiber, 109mg cholesterol, 704mg sodium, 354mg potassium.

Italian Style Tenders

Yield: 4 servings | **Prep time:** 20 minutes | **Cook time:** 3 hours

- 12 oz chicken fillet
- 1 tablespoon Italian seasonings
- ½ cup of water
- 1 tablespoon olive oil
- 1 teaspoon salt

1. Cut the chicken into tenders and sprinkle with salt and Italian seasonings.
2. Then heat the oil in the skillet.
3. Add chicken tenders and cook them on high heat for 1 minute per side.
4. Then put the chicken tenders in the Crock Pot.
5. Add water and close the lid.
6. Cook the chicken for 3 hours on High.

per serving: 202 calories, 24.6g protein, 0.4g carbohydrates, 10.8g fat, 0g fiber, 75mg cholesterol, 657mg sodium, 209mg potassium.

Tarragon Chicken
Yield: 4 servings | **Prep time:** 20 minutes | **Cook time:** 3.5 hours

- 1-pound chicken breast, skinless
- 1 teaspoon dried tarragon
- 3 tablespoons lemon juice
- 1 tablespoon plain yogurt
- 1 tablespoon olive oil
- ½ cup of water

1. Mix olive oil with plain yogurt, lemon juice, and tarragon.
2. Then brush the chicken breast with tarragon mixture and leave for 10-15 minutes to marinate.
3. After this, pour water in the Crock Pot. Add chicken breast and close the lid.
4. Cook the chicken on High for 3.5 hours.

per serving: 165 calories, 24.4g protein, 0.6g carbohydrates, 6.5g fat, 0.1g fiber, 73mg cholesterol, 64mg sodium, 448mg potassium.

Salsa Chicken Wings
Yield: 5 servings | **Prep time:** 10 minutes | **Cook time:** 6 hours

- 2-pounds chicken wings
- 2 cups salsa
- ½ cup of water

1. Put all ingredients in the Crock Pot.
2. Carefully mix the mixture and close the lid.
3. Cook the chicken wings on low for 6 hours.

per serving: 373 calories, 54.1g protein, 6.5g carbohydrates, 13.6g fat, 1.7g fiber, 161mg cholesterol, 781mg sodium, 750mg potassium.

Bali Style Chicken
Yield: 4 servings | **Prep time:** 30 minutes | **Cook time:** 4 hours

- 4 chicken drumsticks
- 1 teaspoon chili powder
- 1 teaspoon allspices
- 1 teaspoon minced garlic
- 2 tablespoons olive oil
- ½ cup tomato juice
- 1 jalapeno pepper, chopped

1. Mix chili powder, allspices, minced garlic, olive oil, jalapeno pepper, and tomato juice in the bowl.
2. Add chicken drumsticks and mix the mixture. Marinate the chicken for 30 minutes.
3. Then transfer the chicken with tomato juice mixture in the Crock Pot and close the lid.
4. Cook the chicken on High for 4 hours.

per serving: 148 calories, 13.1g protein, 2.4g carbohydrates, 9.8g fat, 0.6g fiber, 40mg cholesterol, 126mg sodium, 189mg potassium.

Cannellini Chicken
Yield: 4 servings | **Prep time:** 10 minutes | **Cook time:** 3 hours

- 1 cup cannellini beans, canned
- 12 oz chicken fillet, chopped
- 1 teaspoon lemon zest, grated
- 1 teaspoon dried oregano
- 1 teaspoon salt
- 1 cup of water
- 1 tablespoon butter
- 1 garlic clove, chopped

1. Put the chopped chicken in the Crock Pot.
2. Add lemon zest, salt, water, butter, and garlic.
3. Close the lid and cook the chicken on high for 2 hours.
4. Then add cannellini beans and stir the chicken well.
5. Close the lid and cook the chicken on High for 1 hour.

per serving: 343 calories, 35.6g protein, 28.2g carbohydrates, 9.6g fat, 11.7g fiber, 83mg cholesterol, 688mg sodium, 866mg potassium.

Honey Turkey Breast
Yield: 4 servings | **Prep time:** 15 minutes | **Cook time:** 3.5 hours

- 1-pound turkey breast, skinless, boneless
- 3 tablespoons of liquid honey
- 1 teaspoon chili powder
- 1 teaspoon smoked paprika
- ½ teaspoon salt
- 1 cup of water
- 3 tablespoons butter

1. Sprinkle the turkey breast with salt, smoked paprika, and chili powder.
2. Put the turkey in the Crock Pot, add water, and close the lid.
3. Cook the meal on High for 3 hours.
4. Then drain water and sprinkle the turkey breast with butter and liquid honey. Carefully mix the turkey breast and cook it on High for 30 minutes.

per serving: 246 calories, 19.7g protein, 18.4g carbohydrates, 10.7g fat, 1g fiber, 72mg cholesterol, 1512mg sodium, 379mg potassium.

Chicken with Figs
Yield: 4 servings | **Prep time:** 10 minutes | **Cook time:** 7 hours

- 5 oz fresh figs, chopped
- 14 oz chicken fillet, chopped
- 1 cup of water
- 1 teaspoon peppercorns
- 1 tablespoon dried dill

1. Put all ingredients in the Crock Pot.
2. Close the lid and cook the meal on Low for 7 hours.

per serving: 280 calories, 30.1g protein, 23.4g carbohydrates, 7.7g fat, 3.7g fiber, 88mg cholesterol, 93mg sodium, 515mg potassium.

Ground Turkey Bowl

Yield: 4 servings | **Prep time:** 10 minutes | **Cook time:** 2.5 hours

- 2 tomatoes, chopped
- 10 oz ground turkey
- 1 cup Monterey Jack cheese, shredded
- ½ cup cream
- 1 teaspoon ground black pepper

1. Put ground turkey in the Crock Pot.
2. Add cheese, cream, and ground black pepper.
3. Close the lid and cook the meal on High for 2.5 hours.
4. Then carefully mix the mixture and transfer in the serving bowls.
5. Top the ground turkey with chopped tomatoes.

per serving: 275 calories, 27.2g protein, 3.9g carbohydrates, 18.1g fat, 0.9g fiber, 103mg cholesterol, 240mg sodium, 378mg potassium.

Tomato Chicken Sausages

Yield: 4 servings | **Prep time:** 15 minutes | **Cook time:** 2 hours

- 1-pound chicken sausages
- 1 cup tomato juice
- 1 tablespoon dried sage
- 1 teaspoon salt
- 1 teaspoon olive oil

1. Heat the olive oil in the skillet well.
2. Add chicken sausages and roast them for 1 minute per side on high heat.
3. Then transfer the chicken sausages in the Crock Pot.
4. Add all remaining ingredients and close the lid.
5. Cook the chicken sausages on High for 2 hours.

per serving: 236 calories, 15.3g protein, 10.5g carbohydrates, 13.7g fat, 1.1g fiber, 0mg cholesterol, 1198mg sodium, 145mg potassium.

Chili Sausages

Yield: 4 servings | **Prep time:** 15 minutes | **Cook time:** 3 hours

- 1-pound chicken sausages, roughly chopped
- ½ cup of water
- 1 tablespoon chili powder
- 1 teaspoon tomato paste

1. Sprinkle the chicken sausages with chili powder and transfer in the Crock Pot.
2. Then mix water and tomato paste and pour the liquid over the chicken sausages.
3. Close the lid and cook the meal on High for 3 hours.

per serving: 221 calories, 15g protein, 8.9g carbohydrates, 12.8g fat, 1.4g fiber, 0mg cholesterol, 475mg sodium, 50mg potassium.

Cinnamon and Cumin Chicken Drumsticks

Yield: 4 servings | **Prep time:** 10 minutes | **Cook time:** 6 hours

- 8 chicken drumsticks
- 1 teaspoon cumin seeds
- 1 teaspoon ground cinnamon
- 1 onion, peeled, chopped
- 1 teaspoon salt
- 2 cups of water

1. Put all ingredients in the Crock Pot and carefully mix.
2. Close the lid and cook the chicken on low for 6 hours.

per serving: 170 calories, 25.g protein, 3.3g carbohydrates, 5.4g fat, 1g fiber, 81mg cholesterol, 661mg sodium, 237mg potassium.

Stuffed Chicken Fillets

Yield: 6 servings | **Prep time:** 20 minutes | **Cook time:** 4 hours

- ½ cup green peas, cooked
- ½ cup long-grain rice, cooked
- 16 oz chicken fillets
- 1 cup of water
- 1 teaspoon Italian seasonings

1. Make the horizontal cuts in chicken fillets.
2. After this, mix Italian seasonings with rice and green peas.
3. Fill the chicken fillet with rice mixture and secure them with toothpicks.
4. Put the chicken fillets in the Crock Pot.
5. Add water and close the lid.
6. Cook the chicken on high for 4 hours.

per serving: 212 calories, 23.6g protein, 14.2g carbohydrates, 6g fat, 0.8g fiber, 68mg cholesterol, 68mg sodium, 232mg potassium.

Vinegar Chicken Wings

Yield: 8 servings | **Prep time:** 10 minutes | **Cook time:** 3 hours

- ½ cup apple cider vinegar
- 1 teaspoon garlic powder
- 1 teaspoon smoked paprika
- ½ cup plain yogurt
- 3-pounds chicken wings

1. Mix plain yogurt with smoked paprika, garlic powder, and apple cider vinegar.
2. Pour the liquid in the Crock Pot.
3. Add chicken wings and close the lid.
4. Cook the meal on High for 3 hours.

per serving: 339 calories, 50.2g protein, 1.6g carbohydrates, 12.8g fat, 0.1g fiber, 152mg cholesterol, 158mg sodium, 470mg potassium.

Zucchini Chicken

Yield: 4 servings | **Prep time:** 10 minutes | **Cook time:** hours

- 4 chicken drumsticks
- 3 large zucchinis, chopped
- 1 cup of water
- 1 teaspoon white pepper
- 1 carrot, grated
- 1 teaspoon salt

1. Put all ingredients in the Crock Pot.
2. Carefully mix the mixture and close the lid.
3. Cook the meal on Low for 6 hours.
4. When the time is finished, gently transfer the meal in the plates.

per serving: 124 calories, 15.8g protein, 10g carbohydrates, 3.1g fat, 3.2g fiber, 40mg cholesterol, 655mg sodium, 782mg potassium.

Rosemary Chicken in Yogurt
Yield: 4 servings | **Prep time:** 10 minutes | **Cook time:** 6 hours

- 1 cup plain yogurt
- 1 tablespoon dried rosemary
- 2 tablespoons olive oil
- 1 teaspoon onion powder
- 1-pound chicken breast, skinless, boneless, chopped

1. Rub the chicken breast with onion powder, dried rosemary, and olive oil.
2. Transfer the chicken in the Crock Pot.
3. Add plain yogurt and close the lid.
4. Cook the chicken on low for 6 hours.
5. When the meal is cooked, transfer it in the plates and top with hot yogurt mixture from the Crock Pot.

per serving: 238 calories, 27.6g protein, 5.3g carbohydrates, 10.7g fat, 0.4g fiber, 76mg cholesterol, 101mg sodium, 577mg potassium.

Mexican Style Chicken Wings
Yield: 4 servings | **Prep time:** 20 minutes | **Cook time:** 3 hours

- 1-pound chicken wings, boneless, skinless
- 1 tablespoon Mexican seasonings
- 2 tablespoon sesame oil
- 1 tablespoon mayonnaise
- 1 teaspoon tomato paste
- ½ cup of water

1. Mix sesame oil with mayonnaise, tomato paste, and Mexican seasonings.
2. Rub the chicken wings with Mexican seasonings mixture and leave for 10-15 minutes to marinate.
3. Transfer the marinated chicken wings and all remaining Mexican seasonings mixture in the Crock Pot.
4. Add water and close the lid.
5. Cook the chicken wings on High for 3 hours.

per serving: 297 calories, 33.1g protein, 2.3g carbohydrates, 16.4g fat, 0.1g fiber, 102mg cholesterol, 242mg sodium, 290mg potassium.

Cream Chicken with Spices
Yield: 4 servings | **Prep time:** 10 minutes | **Cook time:** 7 hours

- 1 cup cream
- 1-pound chicken fillet, chopped
- 1 teaspoon dried sage
- 1 teaspoon dried lemongrass
- 1 teaspoon coriander seeds
- 1 teaspoon salt
- 1 tablespoon dried cilantro

1. Pour cream in the Crock Pot.
2. Add dried sage, dried lemongrass, coriander, seeds, salt, and dried cilantro.
3. Then add chicken and close the lid.
4. Cook the meal on Low for 7 hours.

5. Serve the chicken with fragrant cream gravy.

per serving: 255 calories, 33.3g protein, 2.1g carbohydrates, 11.8g fat, 0.1g fiber, 112mg cholesterol, 698mg sodium, 303mg potassium.

Chicken in Apricots
Yield: 4 servings | **Prep time:** 10 minutes | **Cook time:** 5 hours

- 4 chicken drumsticks
- 1 cup of water
- 1 teaspoon white pepper
- 1 teaspoon smoked paprika
- 1 teaspoon chili pepper
- 1 cup apricots, pitted, halved
- 1 teaspoon butter

1. Put all ingredients in the Crock Pot and gently stir them.
2. Close the lid and cook the chicken on low for 5 hours.

per serving: 108 calories, 13.3g protein, 5g carbohydrates, 3.9g fat, 1.1g fiber, 43mg cholesterol, 46mg sodium, 215mg potassium.

Bacon Chicken Wings
Yield: 4 servings | **Prep time:** 10 minutes | **Cook time:** 3 hours

- 4 chicken wings, boneless
- 4 bacon slices
- 1 tablespoon maple syrup
- ½ teaspoon ground black pepper
- ½ cup of water

1. Sprinkle the chicken wings with ground black pepper and maple syrup.
2. Then wrap every chicken wing in the bacon and place it in the Crock Pot.
3. Add water and close the lid.
4. Cook the chicken wings in High for 3 hours.

per serving: 367 calories, 16.1g protein, 25.8g carbohydrates, 22g fat, 1.1g fiber, 41mg cholesterol, 840mg sodium, 121mg potassium.

Chicken in Onion Rings
Yield: 4 servings | **Prep time:** 15 minutes | **Cook time:** 3.5 hours

- 1-pound chicken fillet, roughly chopped
- 3 white onions, sliced into rings
- 2 tablespoons butter
- 1 oz Parmesan, grated
- 1 cup of water
- 1 teaspoon sugar

1. Put butter in the Crock Pot.
2. Then make the layer of the onion rings and sprinkle them with sugar.
3. After this, add chicken fillet and Parmesan.
4. Add water and close the lid.
5. Cook the meal on high for 3.5 hours.

per serving: 326 calories, 36.1g protein, 9g carbohydrates, 15.8g fat, 1.8g fiber, 121mg cholesterol, 209mg sodium, 398mg potassium.

Chicken Sausages in Jam
Yield: 4 servings | **Prep time:** 10 minutes | **Cook time:** 6 hours

- ½ cup of strawberry jam
- ½ cup of water
- 1-pound chicken breast, skinless, boneless, chopped
- 1 teaspoon white pepper
1. Sprinkle the chicken meat with white pepper and put it in the Crock Pot.
2. Then mix jam with water and pour the liquid over the chicken.
3. Close the lid and cook it on Low for 6 hours.
 per serving: 282 calories, 24.1g protein, 37.5g carbohydrates, 2.9g fat, 0.1g fiber, 73mg cholesterol, 59mg sodium, 427mg potassium.

Curry Drumsticks
Yield: 4 servings | **Prep time:** 10 minutes | **Cook time:** 3 hours
- 8 chicken drumsticks
- 1 cup cream
- 1 teaspoon curry paste
- 1 teaspoon olive oil
1. Mix the curry paste with cream and pour the liquid in the Crock Pot.
2. Add olive oil and chicken drumsticks.
3. Close the lid and cook the chicken on High for 3 hours.
 per serving: 212 calories, 25.8g protein, 2.2g carbohydrates, 10.5g fat, 0g fiber, 92mg cholesterol, 93mg sodium, 205mg potassium.

Sichuan Chicken
Yield: 4 servings | **Prep time:** 10 minutes | **Cook time:** 4 hours
- 1 chili pepper, chopped
- 1 oz fresh ginger, chopped
- 1 onion, chopped
- 1-pound chicken fillet, chopped
- 3 oz scallions, chopped
- 1 garlic clove, chopped
- 2 tablespoons mustard
- 1 cup of water
1. Mix mustard with chicken and leave for 10 minutes to marinate.
2. Meanwhile, put all remaining ingredients in the Crock Pot.
3. Add marinated chicken and close the lid.
4. Cook the chicken on High for 4 hours.
 per serving: 286 calories, 36.5g protein, 11.5g carbohydrates, 10.5g fat, 2.9g fiber, 101mg cholesterol, 107mg sodium, 514mg potassium.

Gung Bao Chicken
Yield: 4 servings | **Prep time:** 10 minutes | **Cook time:** 7 hours
- ¼ cup of soy sauce
- ¼ cup apple cider vinegar
- 1 teaspoon brown sugar
- 1 teaspoon chili powder
- 1 tablespoon olive oil
- 2 oz scallions, chopped
- ½ cup of water
- 1 teaspoon cayenne pepper

- 1-pound chicken breast, skinless, boneless, chopped
1. Put all ingredients in the Crock Pot and carefully mix.
2. Close the lid and cook the chicken on Low doe 7 hours.
 per serving: 182 calories, 25.g protein, 3.7g carbohydrates, 6.6g fat, 0.8g fiber, 73mg cholesterol, 967mg sodium, 527mg potassium.

Cardamom Chicken in Coconut Milk
Yield: 4 servings | **Prep time:** 15 minutes | **Cook time:** 3 hours
- 12 oz chicken fillet, chopped
- 1 onion, diced
- 1 teaspoon ground cardamom
- 1 cup of coconut milk
- 1 teaspoon chili pepper
- 1 teaspoon ground ginger
- 3 garlic cloves, diced
- 1 tablespoon coconut oil
1. Melt the coconut oil in the skillet.
2. Add diced onion, ground cardamom, chili pepper, ground ginger, and garlic.
3. Roast the mixture for 1 minute.
4. Then transfer it in the Crock Pot.
5. Add chicken fillet and coconut milk. Stir the mixture and close the lid.
6. Cook the chicken on high for 3 hours.
 per serving: 347 calories, 26.5g protein, 7.4g carbohydrates, 24.1g fat, 2.2g fiber, 76mg cholesterol, 84mg sodium, 429mg potassium.

Braised Chicken with Bay Leaf
Yield: 4 servings | **Prep time:** 10 minutes | **Cook time:** 8 hours
- 1-pound chicken breast, skinless
- 1 teaspoon salt
- 4 bay leaves
- 1 teaspoon garlic powder
- 3 cups of water
1. Put all ingredients in the Crock Pot and close the lid.
2. Cook the chicken on low for 8 hours.
3. Then chop the chicken and transfer in the bowls.
4. Add chicken liquid from the Crock Pot.
 per serving: 135 calories, 24.2g protein, 1.3g carbohydrates, 2.9g fat, 0.3g fiber, 73mg cholesterol, 645mg sodium, 434mg potassium.

Buffalo Chicken Tenders
Yield: 4 servings | **Prep time:** 10 minutes | **Cook time:** 3.5 hours
- 12 oz chicken fillet
- 3 tablespoons buffalo sauce
- ½ cup of coconut milk
- 1 jalapeno pepper, chopped
1. Cut the chicken fillet into tenders and sprinkle the buffalo sauce.
2. Put the chicken tenders in the Crock Pot.
3. Add coconut milk and jalapeno pepper.

4.	Close the lid and cook the meal on high for 3.5 hours.
per serving: 235 calories, 25.3g protein, 2.4g carbohydrates, 13.5g fat, 1g fiber, 76mg cholesterol, 318mg sodium, 293mg potassium.

Chicken Casserole
Yield: 4 servings | **Prep time:** 15 minutes | **Cook time:** 4 hours
- 4 jalapeno pepper, chopped
- 1 onion, chopped
- 10 oz ground chicken
- 1 cup Cheddar cheese, shredded
- 1 cup of water
- 1 teaspoon olive oil
- ½ teaspoon salt
1.	Brush the Crock Pot bottom with olive oil.
2.	Then mix ground chicken with salt and jalapeno pepper.
3.	Put the mixture in the Crock Pot in one layer.
4.	After this, top the ground chicken with chopped onion and Cheddar cheese.
5.	Add water and close the lid.
6.	Cook the casserole on High for 4 hours.
per serving: 274 calories, 28g protein, 3.g carbohydrates, 15.9g fat, 1g fiber, 93mg cholesterol, 530mg sodium, 271mg potassium.

Wine Chicken
Yield: 4 servings | **Prep time:** 15 minutes | **Cook time:** 3 hours
- 1 cup red wine
- 1-pound chicken breast, skinless, boneless, chopped
- 1 anise star
- 1 teaspoon cayenne pepper
- 2 garlic cloves, crushed
1.	Pour red wine in the Crock Pot.
2.	Add anise star, cayenne pepper, and garlic cloves.
3.	Then add chopped chicken and close the lid.
4.	Cook the meal on High for 3 hours.
5.	Serve the chicken with hot wine sauce.
per serving: 182 calories, 24.2g protein, 2.4g carbohydrates, 2.9g fat, 0.2g fiber, 73mg cholesterol, 61mg sodium, 493mg potassium.

Turmeric Meatballs
Yield: 4 servings | **Prep time:** 15 minutes | **Cook time:** 2.5 hours
- 1-pound ground chicken
- 1 tablespoon ground turmeric
- ½ teaspoon ground ginger
- 1 teaspoon salt
- 1 tablespoon corn starch
- ½ cup cream
1.	Mix ground chicken with ground turmeric, ginger, salt, and corn starch.
2.	Then make the medium-size meatballs.
3.	Preheat the skillet well.
4.	Put the meatballs in the hot skillet and cook them for 30 seconds per side.

5.	Then transfer the meatballs in the Crock Pot, add cream, and close the lid.
6.	Cook the meatballs on High for 2.5 hours.
per serving: 250 calories, 33.2g protein, 4.5g carbohydrates, 10.3g fat, 0.4g fiber, 107mg cholesterol, 689mg sodium, 333mg potassium.

Carrot Meatballs
Yield: 6 servings | **Prep time:** 20 minutes | **Cook time:** 6 hours
- 1 cup carrot, shredded
- 14 oz ground chicken
- 1 teaspoon cayenne pepper
- ½ cup of water
- 1 tablespoon butter
- 1 teaspoon salt
- 1 teaspoon ground cumin
1.	Mix carrot with ground chicken
2.	Then add cayenne pepper, salt, and ground cumin.
3.	After this, make the small meatballs and put them in the Crock Pot.
4.	Add water and butter.
5.	Close the lid and cook the meatballs on low for 6 hours.
per serving: 152 calories, 19.4g protein, 2.1g carbohydrates, 7g fat, 0.6g fiber, 64mg cholesterol, 472mg sodium, 232mg potassium.

Chicken and Lentils Meatballs
Yield: 4 servings | **Prep time:** 20 minutes | **Cook time:** 2.5 hours
- ½ cup red lentils, cooked
- 10 oz ground chicken
- 1 teaspoon ground black pepper
- ½ teaspoon salt
- 2 tablespoons flour
- 1 teaspoon sesame oil
- ½ cup chicken stock
1.	Mix lentils with ground chicken.
2.	Add ground black pepper, salt, and flour.
3.	Make the meatballs and put them in the hot skillet.
4.	Add sesame oil and roast the meatballs for 1 minute per side on high heat.
5.	Pour chicken stock in the Crock Pot.
6.	Add meatballs and cook them on High for 2.5 hours.
per serving: 246 calories, 27.2g protein, 17.8g carbohydrates, 6.8g fat, 7.6g fiber, 63mg cholesterol, 449mg sodium, 414mg potassium.

Bulgur Meatballs
Yield: 4 servings | **Prep time:** 15 minutes | **Cook time:** 3 hours
- ½ teaspoon ground turmeric
- 1 teaspoon ground paprika
- 1 teaspoon onion powder
- ½ cup bulgur, grinded
- 8 oz ground chicken
- 1 tablespoon coconut oil
- ½ cup of water

- ½ cup hot water
1. Mix hot water with grinded bulgur and leave for 5 minutes.
2. Then mix cooked bulgur with ground paprika, ground turmeric, onion powder, and ground chicken.
3. Make the meatballs and put them in the Crock Pot.
4. Add coconut oil and cook the meatballs on High for 30 minutes.
5. Then add water and close the lid.
6. Cook the meal on High for 2.5 hours.

per serving: 201 calories, 18.7g protein, 14.2g carbohydrates, 7.9g fat, 3.5g fiber, 50mg cholesterol, 53mg sodium, 235mg potassium.

Broccoli Meatballs
Yield: 4 servings | **Prep time:** 20 minutes | **Cook time:** 3 hours

- 1 teaspoon garam masala
- 1 cup broccoli, shredded
- 14 oz ground chicken
- 1 tablespoon avocado oil
- 1 teaspoon dried dill
- ½ cup of water
1. Mix shredded broccoli with garam masala and ground chicken.
2. Then add dill and make balls from the chicken mixture.
3. After this, pour the avocado oil in the skillet.
4. Preheat it well.
5. Add the chicken balls and roast them for 1.5 minutes per side on high heat or until you get the light crunchy crust.
6. Transfer the balls in the Crock Pot, add water, and close the lid.
7. Cook the meatballs on High for 3 hours.

per serving: 202 calories, 29.4g protein, 1.9g carbohydrates, 7.9g fat, 0.8g fiber, 88mg cholesterol, 95mg sodium, 333mg potassium.

Chopped Balls
Yield: 4 servings | **Prep time:** 25 minutes | **Cook time:** 2.5 hours

- 1-pound chicken fillet, diced
- 2 tablespoon corn starch
- 1 tablespoon flour
- 1 teaspoon cayenne pepper
- ½ teaspoon salt
- 2 eggs, beaten
- 1 tablespoon coconut oil
- ½ cup of water
1. Mix diced chicken fillet with corn starch, flour, cayenne pepper, salt, and eggs.
2. Then preheat the coconut oil in the skillet well.
3. With the help of the spoon make the chicken balls and put them in the hot skillet.
4. Roast them on high heat for 30 seconds per side.
5. Transfer the chicken balls in the Crock Pot, add water, and close the lid.
6. Cook the meal on High for 2.5 hours.

per serving: 302 calories, 35.8g protein, 6.4g carbohydrates, 14.1g fat, 0.2g fiber, 183mg cholesterol, 420mg sodium, 317mg potassium.

Chicken Pancake
Yield: 4 servings | **Prep time:** 10 minutes | **Cook time:** 3 hours

- 16 oz ground chicken
- 2 tablespoons flour
- 1 teaspoon ground black pepper
- 3 eggs, beaten
- 1 teaspoon olive oil
- 1 teaspoon dried oregano
1. Brush the Crock Pot bottom with olive oil.
2. Then mix ground chicken with flour, ground black pepper, oregano, and eggs.
3. When the mixture is homogenous, transfer it in the Crock Pot and flatten the surface.
4. Close the lid and cook the pancake on high for 3 hours.
5. Then cool the cooked meal little and cut into 4 servings.

per serving: 289 calories, 37.5g protein, 3.8g carbohydrates, 13g fat, 0.4g fiber, 224mg cholesterol, 144mg sodium, 337mg potassium.

Beer Chicken
Yield: 4 servings | **Prep time:** 20 minutes | **Cook time:** 6 hours

- 4 chicken thighs, skinless, boneless
- 1 cup beer
- 1 tablespoon garlic, diced
- 1 teaspoon coriander seeds
- 1 teaspoon chili flakes
- 1 tablespoon soy sauce
1. Mix beer with garlic, coriander seeds, chili flakes, and soy sauce.
2. Put the chicken thighs in the beer mixture and leave for 10-15 minutes to marinate.
3. After this, transfer the mixture in the Crock Pot.
4. Cook the chicken on low for 6 hours.

per serving: 308 calories, 42.9g protein, 3.1g carbohydrates, 10.8g fat, 0.1g fiber, 130mg cholesterol, 354mg sodium, 389mg potassium.

Banana Chicken
Yield: 6 servings | **Prep time:** 15 minutes | **Cook time:** 9 hours

- 2 bananas, chopped
- 2-pound whole chicken
- 1 tablespoon taco seasonings
- 1 tablespoon olive oil
- ½ cup of soy sauce
- ½ cup of water
1. Fill the chicken with bananas and secure the whole.
2. Then rub the chicken with taco seasonings and brush with olive oil.
3. After this, pour water and soy sauce in the Crock Pot.
4. Add chicken and close the lid.
5. Cook it on Low for 9 hours.

per serving: 360 calories, 45.5g protein, 11.9g carbohydrates, 13.7g fat, 1.2g fiber, 135mg cholesterol, 1469mg sodium, 555mg potassium.

Chicken Cordon Bleu

Yield: 4 servings | **Prep time:** 20 minutes | **Cook time:** 3.5 hours

- 4 ham slices
- 1-pound chicken fillet
- 4 Cheddar cheese slices
- 1 egg, beaten
- 1 teaspoon salt
- 1 teaspoon ground black pepper
- ½ cup of water
- 1 tablespoon olive oil

1. Cut the chicken fillet into 4 servings.
2. Then beat every chicken fillet and sprinkle with salt and ground black pepper.
3. Put the ham and cheese on the fillets and roll them.
4. Secure the chicken fillets with toothpicks and sprinkle with olive oil.
5. Place the chicken fillets in the Crock Pot.
6. Add water and close the lid.
7. Cook the meal on High for 3.5 hours.

per serving: 421 calories, 45.9g protein, 1.9g carbohydrates, 24.7g fat, 0.5g fiber, 187mg cholesterol, 1234mg sodium, 405mg potassium.

Chicken Pasta Casserole

Yield: 6 servings | **Prep time:** 15 minutes | **Cook time:** 7 hours

- 1 cup pasta, cooked, chopped
- 1 cup cream
- 1 teaspoon cayenne pepper
- 1 teaspoon salt
- ½ cup Mozzarella, shredded
- 12 oz ground chicken
- 1 teaspoon avocado oil

1. Pour the avocado oil in the Crock Pot.
2. Then mix ground chicken with salt and cayenne pepper.
3. Put the ground chicken in the Crock Pot and flatten it gently.
4. After this, add pasta and shredded Mozzarella.
5. Add cream and close the lid.
6. Cook the casserole on Low for 7 hours.

per serving: 167 calories, 18.4g protein, 6.3g carbohydrates, 7.2g fat, 0.1g fiber, 66mg cholesterol, 465mg sodium, 166mg potassium.

Chicken Soufflé

Yield: 6 servings | **Prep time:** 15 minutes | **Cook time:** 3.5 hours

- 1-pound ground chicken
- 1 teaspoon dried oregano
- 1 teaspoon dried sage
- 1 teaspoon butter, softened
- 1 teaspoon salt
- ½ cup cream
- 4 eggs, beaten
- 2 oz provolone cheese, shredded

1. Mix ground chicken with dried oregano, sage, butter, and salt.
2. Then mix the ground mixture with eggs and transfer in the ramekins.
3. Add cream and cheese.
4. Cover the ramekins with foil and transfer in the Crock Pot.
5. Cook the soufflé on High for 3.5 hours.

per serving: 238 calories, 28.2g protein, 1.3g carbohydrates, 12.8g fat, 0.2g fiber, 188mg cholesterol, 587mg sodium, 249mg potassium.

Halved Chicken

Yield: 4 servings | **Prep time:** 15 minutes | **Cook time:** 5 hours

- 2-pounds whole chicken, halved
- 1 tablespoon salt
- 1 teaspoon ground black pepper
- 2 tablespoons mayonnaise
- ½ cup of water

1. Mix the ground black pepper with salt and mayonnaise.
2. Then rub the chicken halves with mayonnaise mixture and transfer in the Crock Pot.
3. Add water and close the lid.
4. Cook the chicken on High for 5 hours.

per serving: 461 calories, 65.7g protein, 2.1g carbohydrates, 19.3g fat, 1.2g fiber, 0.1mg cholesterol, 1993mg sodium, 559mg potassium.

Chili Chicken Liver

Yield: 6 servings | **Prep time:** 10 minutes | **Cook time:** 2.5 hours

- 1-pound chicken liver, diced
- 1 teaspoon chili powder
- ½ cup of water
- 1 onion, diced
- 1 teaspoon butter
- 1 teaspoon salt

1. Pour water in the Crock Pot.
2. Add salt, butter, diced onion, chili powder, and diced chicken liver.
3. Close the lid and cook the meal on High for 2.5 hours.

per serving: 141 calories, 18.8g protein, 2.6g carbohydrates, 5.6g fat, 0.5g fiber, 427mg cholesterol, 455mg sodium, 234mg potassium.

Chopped Chicken Liver Balls

Yield: 6 servings | **Prep time:** 15 minutes | **Cook time:** 4 hours

- 1 egg, beaten
- 3 tablespoon semolina
- 1 teaspoon Italian seasonings
- 1 tablespoon flour
- ½ teaspoon salt
- 1-pound liver, minced
- 1/3 cup water

1. Mix egg with semolina, Italian seasonings, flour, salt, and minced liver.
2. When the mixture is homogenous, make the medium size balls and put them in the Crock Pot.
3. Add water and close the lid.

4. Cook the liver balls on High for 4 hours.
per serving: 169 calories, 21.8g protein, 8.8g carbohydrates, 4.6g fat, 0.2g fiber, 316mg cholesterol, 263mg sodium, 287mg potassium.

Chicken Stuffed with Plums
Yield: 6 servings | **Prep time:** 15 minutes | **Cook time:** 4 hours

- 6 chicken fillets
- 1 cup plums, pitted, sliced
- 1 cup of water
- 1 teaspoon salt
- 1 teaspoon white pepper

1. Beat the chicken fillets gently and rub with salt and white pepper.
2. Then put the sliced plums on the chicken fillets and roll them.
3. Secure the chicken rolls with toothpicks and put in the Crock Pot.
4. Add water and close the lid.
5. Cook the meal on High for 4 hours.
6. Then remove the chicken from the Crock Pot, remove the toothpicks and transfer in the serving plates.
per serving: 283 calories, 42.4g protein, 1.6g carbohydrates, 10.9g fat, 0.2g fiber, 130mg cholesterol, 514mg sodium, 377mg potassium.

Chickpea and Chicken Bowl
Yield: 7 servings | **Prep time:** 15 minutes | **Cook time:** 3 hours

- 2 cups chickpeas, cooked
- 1-pound chicken fillet, sliced
- 1 teaspoon taco seasonings
- 1 cup fresh cilantro, chopped
- ½ cup plain yogurt
- ½ cup of water

1. Mix chicken slices with taco seasonings and transfer in the Crock Pot.
2. Add water and close the lid.
3. Cook the chicken on High for 3 hours.
4. Then drain water and transfer the chicken in the bowls.
5. Add chickpeas and top with fresh cilantro and plain yogurt.
per serving: 347 calories, 30.8g protein, 36.5g carbohydrates, 8.5g fat, 10g fiber, 59mg cholesterol, 143mg sodium, 710mg potassium.

Stuffed Pasta
Yield: 6 servings | **Prep time:** 20 minutes | **Cook time:** 4 hours

- 12 oz cannelloni
- 9 oz ground chicken
- 1 teaspoon Italian seasonings
- 2 oz Parmesan, grated
- ½ cup tomato juice
- ½ cup of water

1. Mix the ground chicken with Italian seasonings and fill the cannelloni.
2. Put the stuffed cannelloni in the Crock Pot.
3. Add all remaining ingredients and close the lid.
4. Cook the meal on High for 4 hours.

per serving: 250 calories, 21.5g protein, 14g carbohydrates, 12.1g fat, 0.8g fiber, 62mg cholesterol, 373mg sodium, 150mg potassium.

Grape Chicken Saute
Yield: 6 servings | **Prep time:** 10 minutes | **Cook time:** 7 hours

- 1-pound chicken
- 1 cup tomato, chopped
- 2 cups green grapes, chopped
- 1 cup of water
- 1 teaspoon cayenne pepper
- ½ teaspoon dried sage
- 1 teaspoon butter

1. Put all ingredients in the Crock Pot.
2. Close the lid and cook the saute on Low for 7 hours.
per serving: 147 calories, 22.4g protein, 6.6g carbohydrates, 3.2g fat, 0.7g fiber, 60mg cholesterol, 55mg sodium, 278mg potassium.

Lemongrass Chicken Thighs
Yield: 6 servings | **Prep time:** 15 minutes | **Cook time:** 4 hours

- 6 chicken thighs
- 1 tablespoon dried sage
- 1 teaspoon salt
- 1 teaspoon ground paprika
- 2 tablespoons sesame oil
- 1 cup of water

1. Mix dried sage with salt, and ground paprika.
2. Then rub the chicken thighs with the sage mixture and transfer in the Crock Pot.
3. Sprinkle the chicken with sesame oil and water.
4. Close the chicken on High for 4 hours.
per serving: 320 calories, 42.3g protein, 0.4g carbohydrates, 15.4g fat, 0.3g fiber, 130mg cholesterol, 514mg sodium, 367mg potassium.

Cauliflower Chicken
Yield: 6 servings | **Prep time:** 10 minutes | **Cook time:** 7 hours

- 2 cups cauliflower, chopped
- 1-pound ground chicken
- 1 teaspoon chili powder
- 1 teaspoon ground turmeric
- 1 teaspoon salt
- 1 cup of water
- 3 tablespoons plain yogurt

1. Mix ground chicken with chili powder, ground turmeric, and salt.
2. Then mix the chicken mixture with cauliflower and transfer in the Crock Pot.
3. Add plain yogurt and water.
4. Close the lid and cook the meal on Low for 7 hours.
per serving: 160 calories, 23.1g protein, 2.8g carbohydrates, 5.8g fat, 1.1g fiber, 68mg cholesterol, 473mg sodium, 320mg potassium.

Breadcrumbs Mini Balls
Yield: 6 servings | **Prep time:** 15 minutes | **Cook time:** 3 hours

- 1-pound ground chicken
- 1 teaspoon cayenne pepper
- 1 teaspoon salt
- ½ cup bread crumbs
- ½ cup of water
1. Mix ground chicken with cayenne pepper, salt, and bread crumbs.
2. Then make the small balls and put them in the Crock Pot.
3. Add water and close the lid.
4. Cook the mini balls on High for 3 hours.
 per serving: 180 calories, 23.1g protein, 6.7g carbohydrates, 6.1g fat, 0.5g fiber, 67mg cholesterol, 519mg sodium, 208mg potassium.

Jalapeno Chicken Wings
Yield: 6 servings | **Prep time:** 15 minutes | **Cook time:** 3 hours
- 5 jalapenos, minced
- ½ cup tomato juice
- 2-pounds chicken wings, skinless
- 1 teaspoon salt
- ¼ cup of water
1. Mix minced jalapenos with tomato juice, salt, and water.
2. Pour the liquid in the Crock Pot.
3. Add chicken wings and close the lid.
4. Cook the meal on High for 3 hours.
 per serving: 294 calories, 44.1g protein, 1.6g carbohydrates, 11.3g fat, 0.4g fiber, 135mg cholesterol, 573mg sodium, 439mg potassium.

Avocado Chicken Salad
Yield: 6 servings | **Prep time:** 15 minutes | **Cook time:** 3.5 hours
- 1-pound chicken fillet, chopped
- 1 teaspoon salt
- 1 teaspoon ground black pepper
- ½ cup of water
- 1 avocado, pitted, peeled, chopped
- 1 tomato, chopped
- 2 tablespoons plain yogurt
- 1 tablespoon lemon juice
1. Mix chicken fillet with salt and ground black pepper.
2. Put the chicken in the Crock Pot, add water, and cook on High for 3.5 hours.
3. Meanwhile, mix avocado with tomato in the salad bowl.
4. In the shallow bowl mix lemon juice and plain yogurt.
5. When the chicken is cooked, add it in the salad and mix well.
6. Sprinkle the meal with plain yogurt mixture.
 per serving: 219 calories, 23g protein, 3.9g carbohydrates, 12.2g fat, 2.5g fiber, 68mg cholesterol, 460mg sodium, 390mg potassium.

Lettuce and Chicken Salad
Yield: 6 servings | **Prep time:** 15 minutes | **Cook time:** 7 hours
- ½ cup of soy sauce
- 2 oz scallions, chopped
- 2 cups lettuce, chopped
- 2 oz Mozzarella, chopped
- 1 tablespoon olive oil
- 8 oz chicken fillet, chopped
1. Pour soy sauce in the Crock Pot.
2. Add chicken and close the lid.
3. Cook the chicken on low for 7 hours.
4. Drain soy sauce and transfer the chicken in the salad bowl.
5. Add all remaining ingredients and stir the salad well.
 per serving: 135 calories, 15.2g protein, 3.2g carbohydrates, 6.9g fat, 0.5g fiber, 39mg cholesterol, 1290mg sodium, 190mg potassium.

Chicken Pocket
Yield: 4 servings | **Prep time:** 20 minutes | **Cook time:** 4 hours
- 1-pound chicken fillet, skinless, boneless
- 3 oz prunes, chopped
- 1 teaspoon dried cilantro
- 1 tablespoon olive oil
- 1 teaspoon salt
- ½ cup of water
1. Make the horizontal cut in the chicken fillet and fill it with prunes.
2. Then secure the cut and rub the chicken fillet with dried cilantro and salt.
3. Sprinkle the chicken with olive oil and transfer in the Crock Pot.
4. Add water and close the lid.
5. Cook the chicken on High for 4 hours.
6. Drain water and remove the toothpicks.
7. Cut the cooked meal into 4 servings.
 per serving: 297 calories, 33.3g protein, 13.6g carbohydrates, 12g fat, 1.5g fiber, 101mg cholesterol, 680mg sodium, 432mg potassium.

Sweet Chicken Mash
Yield: 6 servings | **Prep time:** 10 minutes | **Cook time:** 7 hours
- 3 tablespoons maple syrup
- 1-pound ground chicken
- 1 teaspoon dried dill
- 1 cup Cheddar cheese, shredded
- 1 cup of water
1. Put all ingredients in the Crock Pot and carefully mix.
2. Close the lid and cook the mash on Low for 7 hours.
 per serving: 246 calories, 26.6g protein, 7g carbohydrates, 11.9g fat, 0g fiber, 87mg cholesterol, 184mg sodium, 229mg potassium.

Okra Chicken Saute
Yield: 6 servings | **Prep time:** 10 minutes | **Cook time:** 8 hours
- 1 cup bell pepper, chopped
- 1 cup tomatoes, chopped
- 2 cups okra, chopped
- 1-pound chicken fillet, chopped
- 1 teaspoon salt
- 1 teaspoon ground black pepper

- 2 cups of water
1. Put all ingredients in the Crock Pot.
2. Close the lid and cook the saute on Low for 8 hours.

per serving: 170 calories, 23g protein, 5.4g carbohydrates, 5.8g fat, 1.8g fiber, 67mg cholesterol, 459mg sodium, 397mg potassium.

Chicken Wings in Vodka Sauce
Yield: 4 servings | **Prep time:** 10 minutes | **Cook time:** 6 hours

- 1-pound chicken wings
- ½ cup vodka sauce
- 1 tablespoon olive oil

1. Put all ingredients in the Crock Pot and mix well.
2. Close the lid and cook the meal on Low for 6 hours.

per serving: 273 calories, 34.1g protein, 2.8g carbohydrates, 13.2g fat, 0g fiber, 102mg cholesterol, 208mg sodium, 276mg potassium.

Green Chicken Salad
Yield: 4 servings | **Prep time:** 15 minutes | **Cook time:** 3.5 hours

- 1 cup celery stalk, chopped
- 10 oz chicken fillet
- 1 teaspoon salt
- 1 teaspoon ground black pepper
- 1 cup of water
- 1 tablespoon mustard
- 1 tablespoon mayonnaise
- 1 teaspoon lemon juice
- 1 cup arugula, chopped
- 1 cup of green grapes

1. Put the chicken in the Crock Pot.
2. Add salt and ground black pepper. Add water.
3. Cook the chicken in high for 3.5 hours.
4. Meanwhile, put green grapes, arugula, and celery stalk in the bowl.
5. Then chopped the cooked chicken and add it in the arugula mixture.
6. In the shallow bowl, mix mustard with lemon juice, and mayonnaise.
7. Add the mixture in the salad and shake it well.

per serving: 184 calories, 21.7g protein, 7.1g carbohydrates, 7.5g fat, 1.3g fiber, 64mg cholesterol, 693mg sodium, 329mg potassium.

Chicken Burger Meat
Yield: 4 servings | **Prep time:** 15 minutes | **Cook time:** 2 hours

- 1-pound ground chicken
- 1 teaspoon dried cilantro
- 1 teaspoon salt
- 1 teaspoon chili powder
- 1 teaspoon olive oil
- ¼ cup of water

1. Mix ground chicken with dried cilantro, salt, and chili powder.
2. Make the meatballs and press them gently.
3. Pour olive oil in the skillet and heat it well.

4. Add the meatballs and roast them for 2 minutes per side.
5. Then transfer them in the Crock Pot, add water, and close the lid.
6. Cook the burgers on High for 2 hours.

per serving: 228 calories, 32.9g protein, 0.4g carbohydrates, 9.7g fat, 0.2g fiber, 101mg cholesterol, 686mg sodium, 289mg potassium.

Party Chicken Wings
Yield: 4 servings | **Prep time:** 15 minutes | **Cook time:** 4 hours

- 1-pound chicken wings
- 3 tablespoons hot sauce
- 2 tablespoons butter
- ¼ cup of soy sauce

1. Put all ingredients in the Crock Pot and close the lid.
2. Cook the chicken wings on High for 4 hours.
3. Then transfer the chicken wings in the big bowl and sprinkle with hot sauce gravy from the Crock Pot.

per serving: 276 calories, 33.9g protein, 1.4g carbohydrates, 14.2g fat, 0.2g fiber, 116mg cholesterol, 1322mg sodium, 327mg potassium.

Sheriff Chicken Wings
Yield: 4 servings | **Prep time:** 15 minutes | **Cook time:** 3 hours

- 1-pound chicken wings
- 1 cup plain yogurt
- ¼ cup pickled cucumbers, grated
- 1 tablespoon lemon juice
- 1 teaspoon white pepper
- 1 teaspoon salt
- 1 teaspoon cayenne pepper
- 1 cup of water

1. Put chicken wings in the Crock Pot.
2. Add cayenne pepper and salt.
3. Then add water and cook the chicken on High for 3 hours.
4. Meanwhile, mix plain yogurt with grated pickled cucumbers, and white pepper.
5. When the chicken wings are cooked, transfer them in the serving plates and top with plain yogurt sauce.

per serving: 264 calories, 36.5g protein, 5.2g carbohydrates, 9.3g fat, 0.3g fiber, 105mg cholesterol, 725mg sodium, 450mg potassium.

Asparagus Chicken Salad
Yield: 4 servings | **Prep time:** 15 minutes | **Cook time:** 4 hours

- 12 oz chicken fillet
- 7 oz asparagus, chopped, boiled
- 2 tablespoons mayonnaise
- 1 tablespoon lemon juice
- 1 teaspoon cayenne pepper
- 1 cup of water

1. Put the chicken in the Crock Pot. Add water and close the lid.
2. Cook the chicken on high for 4 hours.
3. Then shred it and mix with chopped asparagus.

4.   Add lemon juice, cayenne pepper, and mayonnaise.
5.   Mix the salad.
per serving: 203 calories, 25.8g protein, 4g carbohydrates, 8.9g fat, 1.2g fiber, 78mg cholesterol, 127mg sodium, 321mg potassium.

Scallions and Chicken Salad

Yield: 4 servings | **Prep time:** 15 minutes | **Cook time:** 3 hours

- 4 oz scallions, chopped
- 2 eggs, hard-boiled, cooked, chopped
- 2 tablespoons mayonnaise
- 1 tablespoon plain yogurt
- 5 oz chicken fillet
- 1 cup of water
- 1 teaspoon ground black pepper

1.   Put the chicken in the Crock Pot. Add water.
2.   Close the lid and cook the chicken on high for 3 hours.
3.   Then shred the chicken and add all remaining ingredients from the list above.
4.   Carefully mix the salad.
per serving: 141 calories, 13.9g protein, 4.6g carbohydrates, 7.4g fat, 0.9g fiber, 116mg cholesterol, 123mg sodium, 211mg potassium.

Corn and Chicken Saute

Yield: 4 servings | **Prep time:** 10 minutes | **Cook time:** 8 hours

- 1 cup carrot, chopped
- 2 corn on cobs, roughly chopped
- 1 cup of water
- 1-pound chicken fillet, chopped
- 1 teaspoon Italian seasonings
- 1 teaspoon salt

1.   Put all ingredients from the list above in the Crock Pot.
2.   Close the lid and cook the meal on Low for 8 hours.
per serving: 308 calories, 35.3g protein, 18.8g carbohydrates, 10.5g fat, 0.7g fiber, 105mg cholesterol, 714mg sodium, 544mg potassium.

Beef

Beef and Zucchini Saute

Yield: 4 servings | **Prep time:** 10 minutes | **Cook time:** 5 hours

- 1-pound beef sirloins, chopped
- 1 cup zucchini, chopped
- 1 teaspoon ground black pepper
- 1 cup bell pepper, chopped
- 2 cup of water
- 1 teaspoon salt

1. Mix beef sirloin with ground black pepper and salt.
2. Transfer the meat in the Crock Pot.
3. Top it with zucchini and bell pepper.
4. Add water and close the lid.
5. Cook the beef on high for 5 hours.

per serving: 226 calories, 35.1g protein, 3.5g carbohydrates, 7.2g fat, 0.9g fiber, 101mg cholesterol, 663mg sodium, 595mg potassium.

Beef in Sauce

Yield: 4 servings | **Prep time:** 10 minutes | **Cook time:** 9 hours

- 1-pound beef stew meat, chopped
- 1 teaspoon garam masala
- 1 cup of water
- 1 tablespoon flour
- 1 teaspoon garlic powder
- 1 onion, diced

1. Whisk flour with water until smooth and pour the liquid in the Crock Pot.
2. Add garam masala and beef stew meat.
3. After this, add onion and garlic powder.
4. Close the lid and cook the meat on low for 9 hours.
5. Serve the cooked beef with thick gravy from the Crock Pot.

per serving: 231 calories, 35g protein, 4.6g carbohydrates, 7.1g fat, 0.7g fiber, 101mg cholesterol, 79mg sodium, 507mg potassium

Beef with Greens

Yield: 3 servings | **Prep time:** 15 minutes | **Cook time:** 8 hours

- 1 cup fresh spinach, chopped
- 9 oz beef stew meat, cubed
- 1 cup swiss chard, chopped
- 2 cups of water 1 teaspoon olive oil
- 1 teaspoon dried rosemary

1. Heat olive oil in the skillet.
2. Add beef and roast it for 1 minute per side.
3. Then transfer the meat in the Crock Pot.
4. Add swiss chard, spinach, water, and rosemary.
5. Close the lid and cook the meal on Low for 8 hours.

per serving: 177 calories, 26.3g protein, 1.1g carbohydrates, 7g fat, 0.6g fiber, 76mg cholesterol, 95mg sodium, 449mg potassium.

Beef and Scallions Bowl

Yield: 4 servings | **Prep time:** 10 minutes | **Cook time:** 5 hours

- 1 teaspoon chili powder
- 2 oz scallions, chopped
- 1-pound beef stew meat, cubed
- 1 cup corn kernels, frozen
- 1 cup of water
- 2 tablespoons tomato paste
- 1 teaspoon minced garlic

1. Mix water with tomato paste and pour the liquid in the Crock Pot.
2. Add chili powder, beef, corn kernels, and minced garlic.
3. Close the lid and cook the meal on high for 5 hours.
4. When the meal is cooked, transfer the mixture in the bowls and top with scallions.

per serving: 258 calories, 36.4g protein, 10.4g carbohydrates, 7.7g fat, 2g fiber, 101mg cholesterol, 99mg sodium, 697mg potassium.

Balsamic Beef

Yield: 4 servings | **Prep time:** 15 minutes | **Cook time:** 9 hours

- 1 pound beef stew meat, cubed
- 1 teaspoon cayenne pepper
- 4 tablespoons balsamic vinegar
- ½ cup of water
- 2 tablespoons butter

1. Toss the butter in the skillet and melt it.
2. Then add meat and roast it for 2 minutes per side on medium heat.
3. Transfer the meat with butter in the Crock Pot.
4. Add balsamic vinegar, cayenne pepper, and water.
5. Close the lid and cook the meal on Low for 9 hours.

per serving: 266 calories, 34.5g protein, 0.4g carbohydrates, 12.9g fat, 0.1g fiber, 117mg cholesterol, 117mg sodium, 479mg potassium.

Onion Beef

Yield: 14 servings | **Prep time:** 10 minutes | **Cook time:** 5.5 hours

- 4-pounds beef sirloin, sliced
- 2 cups white onion, chopped
- 3 cups of water
- ½ cup butter
- 1 teaspoon ground black pepper
- 1 teaspoon salt
- 1 bay leaf

1. Mix beef sirloin with salt and ground black pepper and transfer in the Crock Pot.
2. Add butter, water, onion, and bay leaf.
3. Close the lid and cook the meat on High for 5.5 hours.

per serving: 306 calories, 39.6g protein, 1.7g carbohydrates, 14.7g fat, 0.4g fiber, 133mg cholesterol, 301mg sodium, 551mg potassium.

Cilantro Beef

Yield: 4 servings | **Prep time:** 10 minutes | **Cook time:** 4.5 hours

- 1-pound beef loin, roughly chopped
- ¼ cup apple cider vinegar
- 1 tablespoon dried cilantro
- ½ teaspoon dried basil
- 1 cup of water
- 1 teaspoon tomato paste

1. Mix meat with tomato paste, dried cilantro, and basil.
2. Then transfer it in the Crock Pot.
3. Add apple cider vinegar and water.
4. Cook the cilantro beef for 4.5 hours on High.

per serving: 211 calories, 30.4g protein, 0.4g carbohydrates, 9.5g fat, 0.1g fiber, 81mg cholesterol, 66mg sodium, 412mg potassium.

Beef and Artichokes Bowls

Yield: 2 servings | **Prep time:** 10 minutes | **Cook time:** 7 hours

- 6 oz beef sirloin, chopped
- ½ teaspoon cayenne pepper
- ½ teaspoon white pepper
- 4 artichoke hearts, chopped
- 1 cup of water
- 1 teaspoon salt

1. Mix meat with white pepper and cayenne pepper. Transfer it in the Crock Pot bowl.
2. Add salt, artichoke hearts, and water.
3. Close the lid and cook the meal on Low for 7 hours.

per serving: 313 calories, 36.5g protein, 34.6g carbohydrates, 5.9g fat, 17.8g fiber, 76mg cholesterol, 1527mg sodium, 1559mg potassium.

Mustard Beef

Yield: 4 servings | **Prep time:** 10 minutes | **Cook time:** 8 hours

- 1-pound beef sirloin, chopped
- 1 tablespoon capers, drained
- 1 cup of water
- 2 tablespoons mustard
- 1 tablespoon coconut oil

1. Mix meat with mustard and leave for 10 minutes to marinate.
2. Then melt the coconut oil in the skillet.
3. Add meat and roast it for 1 minute per side on high heat.
4. After this, transfer the meat in the Crock Pot.
5. Add water and capers.
6. Cook the meal on Low for 8 hours.

per serving: 267 calories, 35.9g protein, 2.1g carbohydrates, 12.1g fat, 0.9g fiber, 101mg cholesterol, 140mg sodium, 496mg potassium.

Beef Masala

Yield: 6 servings | **Prep time:** 15 minutes | **Cook time:** 9 hours

- 1-pound beef sirloin, sliced
- 1 teaspoon garam masala
- 2 tablespoons lemon juice
- 1 teaspoon ground paprika
- ½ cup of coconut milk
- 1 teaspoon dried mint

1. In the bowl mix coconut milk with dried mint, ground paprika, lemon juice, and garam masala.
2. Then add beef sirloin and mix the mixture. Leave it for at least 10 minutes to marinate.
3. Then transfer the mixture in the Crock Pot.
4. Cook it on Low for 9 hours.

per serving: 283 calories, 35.3g protein, 2.2g carbohydrates, 14.4g fat, 0.9g fiber, 101mg cholesterol, 82mg sodium, 560mg potassium.

Beef Saute with Endives

Yield: 4 servings | **Prep time:** 10 minutes | **Cook time:** 8 hours

- 1-pound beef sirloin, chopped
- 3 oz endives, roughly chopped
- 1 teaspoon peppercorns
- 1 carrot, diced
- 1 onion, sliced
- 1 cup of water
- ½ cup tomato juice

1. Mix beef with onion, carrot, and peppercorns.
2. Place the mixture in the Crock Pot.
3. Add water and tomato juice.
4. Then close the lid and cook it on High for 5 hours.
5. After this, add endives and cook the meal for 3 hours on Low.

per serving: 238 calories, 35.4g protein, 6.4g carbohydrates, 7.2g fat, 1.9g fiber, 101mg cholesterol, 175mg sodium, 689mg potassium.

Turkish Meat Saute

Yield: 4 servings | **Prep time:** 10 minutes | **Cook time:** 10 hours

- 1 cup green peas
- 1 cup potatoes, chopped
- 2 cups of water
- 10 oz beef sirloin, chopped
- 1 teaspoon ground black pepper
- 1 teaspoon salt
- 1 tablespoon tomato paste

1. Put all ingredients in the Crock Pot and carefully mix.
2. Then close the lid.
3. Cook the saute on Low for 10 hours.

per serving: 192 calories, 24.3g protein, 12.2g carbohydrates, 4.7g fat, 3.1g fiber, 63mg cholesterol, 640mg sodium, 575mg potassium.

Sweet Beef

Yield: 4 servings | **Prep time:** 10 minutes | **Cook time:** 5 hours

- 1-pound beef roast, sliced
- 1 tablespoon maple syrup
- 2 tablespoons lemon juice
- 1 teaspoon dried oregano
- 1 cup of water

1. Mix water with maple syrup, lemon juice, and dried oregano.
2. Then pour the liquid in the Crock Pot.
3. Add beef roast and close the lid.
4. Cook the meal on High for 5 hours.

per serving: 227 calories, 34.5g protein, 3.8g carbohydrates, 7.2g fat, 0.2g fiber, 101mg cholesterol, 78mg sodium, 483mg potassium.

Thyme Beef

Yield: 2 servings | **Prep time:** 15 minutes | **Cook time:** 5 hours

- 8 oz beef sirloin, chopped
- 1 tablespoon dried thyme
- 1 tablespoon olive oil
- ½ cup of water
- 1 teaspoon salt
1.   Preheat the skillet well.
2.   Then mix beef with dried thyme and olive oil.
3.   Put the meat in the hot skillet and roast for 2 minutes per side on high heat.
4.   Then transfer the meat in the Crock Pot.
5.   Add salt and water.
6.   Cook the meal on High for 5 hours.

per serving: 274 calories, 34.5g protein, 0.9g carbohydrates, 14.2g fat, 0.5g fiber, 101mg cholesterol, 1240mg sodium, 469mg potassium.

Hot Beef

Yield: 4 servings | **Prep time:** 15 minutes | **Cook time:** 8 hours

- 1-pound beef sirloin, chopped
- 2 tablespoons hot sauce
- 1 tablespoon olive oil
- ½ cup of water
1.   In the shallow bowl mix hot sauce with olive oil.
2.   Then mix beef sirloin with hot sauce mixture and leave for 10 minutes to marinate.
3.   Put the marinated beef in the Crock Pot.
4.   Add water and close the lid.
5.   Cook the meal on Low for 8 hours.

per serving: 241 calories, 34.4g protein, 0.1g carbohydrates, 10.6g fat, 0g fiber, 101mg cholesterol, 266mg sodium, 467mg potassium.

Beef Chops with Sprouts

Yield: 5 servings | **Prep time:** 10 minutes | **Cook time:** 7 hours

- 1-pound beef loin
- ½ cup bean sprouts
- 1 cup of water
- 1 tablespoon tomato paste
- 1 teaspoon chili powder
- 1 teaspoon salt
1.   Cut the beef loin into 5 beef chops and sprinkle the beef chops with chili powder and salt.
2.   Then place them in the Crock Pot.
3.   Add water and tomato paste. Cook the meat on low for 7 hours.
4.   Then transfer the cooked beef chops in the plates, sprinkle with tomato gravy from the Crock Pot, and top with bean sprouts.

per serving: 175 calories, 25.2g protein, 1.6g carbohydrates, 7.8g fat, 0.3g fiber, 64mg cholesterol, 526mg sodium, 386mg potassium.

Beef Ragout with Beans

Yield: 5 servings | **Prep time:** 10 minutes | **Cook time:** 5 hours

- 1 tablespoon tomato paste
- 1 cup mung beans, canned
- 1 carrot, grated
- 1-pound beef stew meat, chopped
- 1 teaspoon ground black pepper
- 2 cup of water
1.   Pour water in the Crock Pot.
2.   Add meat, ground black pepper, and carrot.
3.   Cook the mixture on High for 4 hours.
4.   Then add tomato paste and mung beans. Stir the meal and cook it on high for 1 hour more.

per serving: 321 calories, 37.7g protein, 28g carbohydrates, 6.2g fat, 7.3g fiber, 81mg cholesterol, 81mg sodium, 959mg potassium.

Braised Beef

Yield: 2 servings | **Prep time:** 8 minutes | **Cook time:** 9 hours

- 8 oz beef tenderloin, chopped
- 1 garlic clove, peeled
- 1 teaspoon peppercorn
- 1 teaspoon salt
- 1 tablespoon dried basil
- 2 cups of water
1.   Put all ingredients from the list above in the Crock Pot.
2.   Gently stir the mixture and close the lid.
3.   Cook the beef on low for 9 hours.

per serving: 239 calories, 33.1g protein, 1.2g carbohydrates, 10.4g fat, 0.3g fiber, 104mg cholesterol, 1238mg sodium, 431mg potassium.

Coconut Beef

Yield: 5 servings | **Prep time:** 10 minutes | **Cook time:** 8 hours

- 1 cup baby spinach, chopped
- 1 cup of coconut milk
- 1-pound beef tenderloin, chopped
- 1 teaspoon avocado oil
- 1 teaspoon dried rosemary
- 1 teaspoon garlic powder
1.   Roast meat in the avocado oil for 1 minute per side on high heat.
2.   Ten transfer the meat in the Crock Pot.
3.   Add garlic powder, dried rosemary, coconut milk, and baby spinach.
4.   Close the lid and cook the meal on Low for 8 hours.

per serving: 303 calories, 27.6g protein, 3.5g carbohydrates, 19.9g fat, 1.4g fiber, 83mg cholesterol, 66mg sodium, 495mg potassium.

Beef Roast

Yield: 5 servings | **Prep time:** 10 minutes | **Cook time:** 6 hours

- 1-pound beef chuck roast
- 1 tablespoon ketchup
- 1 tablespoon mayonnaise
- 1 teaspoon chili powder
- 1 teaspoon olive oil

- 1 teaspoon lemon juice
- ½ cup of water

1. In the bowl mix ketchup, mayonnaise, chili powder, olive oil, and lemon juice.
2. Then sprinkle the beef chuck roast with ketchup mixture.
3. Pour the water in the Crock Pot.
4. Add beef chuck roast and close the lid.
5. Cook the meat on High for 6 hours.

per serving: 354 calories, 23.9g protein, 1.8g carbohydrates, 27.3g fat, 0.2g fiber, 94mg cholesterol, 119mg sodium, 230mg potassium.

Lunch Beef

Yield: 2 servings | **Prep time:** 10 minutes | **Cook time:** 8 hours

- ½ white onion, sliced
- 1 teaspoon brown sugar
- 1 teaspoon chili powder
- 1 teaspoon hot sauce
- ½ cup okra, chopped
- 1 cup of water
- 7 oz beef loin, chopped

1. Mix the beef loin with hot sauce, chili powder, and brown sugar.
2. Transfer the meat in the Crock Pot.
3. Add water, okra, and onion.
4. Cook the meal on Low for 8 hours.

per serving: 179 calories, 19.3g protein, 7.8g carbohydrates, 7.4g fat, 1.8g fiber, 53mg cholesterol, 520mg sodium, 146mg potassium.

Braised Beef Strips

Yield: 4 servings | **Prep time:** 10 minutes | **Cook time:** 5 hours

- ½ cup mushroom, sliced
- 1 onion, sliced
- 1 cup of water
- 1 tablespoon coconut oil
- 1 teaspoon salt
- 1 teaspoon white pepper
- 10 oz beef loin, cut into strips

1. Melt the coconut oil in the skillet.
2. Add mushrooms and roast them for 5 minutes on medium heat.
3. Then transfer the mushrooms in the Crock Pot.
4. Add all remaining ingredients and close the lid.
5. Cook the meal on High for 5 hours

per serving: 173 calories, 19.6g protein, 3.2g carbohydrates, 9.4g fat, 0.8g fiber, 50mg cholesterol, 624mg sodium, 316mg potassium.

Beef Dip

Yield: 6 servings | **Prep time:** 10 minutes | **Cook time:** 10 hours

- ½ cup heavy cream
- 1 onion, diced
- 1 teaspoon cream cheese
- ½ cup Cheddar cheese, shredded
- 1 teaspoon garlic powder
- 4 oz dried beef, chopped
- ½ cup of water

1. Put all ingredients in the Crock Pot.
2. Gently stir the ingredients and close the lid.
3. Cook the dip on Low for 10 hours.

per serving: 118 calories, 8.6g protein, 2.5g carbohydrates, 8.2g fat, 0.4g fiber, 41mg cholesterol, 78mg sodium, 126mg potassium.

Beef and Sauerkraut Bowl

Yield: 4 servings | **Prep time:** 10 minutes | **Cook time:** 5 hours

- 1 cup sauerkraut
- 1-pound corned beef, chopped
- ¼ cup apple cider vinegar
- 1 cup of water

1. Pour water and apple cider vinegar in the Crock Pot.
2. Add corned beef and cook it on High for 5 hours.
3. Then chop the meat roughly and put in the serving bowls.
4. Top the meat with sauerkraut.

per serving: 202 calories, 15.5g protein, 1.7g carbohydrates, 14.2g fat, 1g fiber, 71mg cholesterol, 1240mg sodium, 236mg potassium.

Cilantro Meatballs

Yield: 6 servings | **Prep time:** 20 minutes | **Cook time:** 4 hours

- 1-pound minced beef
- 1 teaspoon minced garlic
- 1 egg, beaten
- 1 teaspoon chili flakes
- 2 teaspoons dried cilantro
- 1 tablespoon semolina
- ½ cup of water
- 1 tablespoon sesame oil

1. In the bowl mix minced beef, garlic, egg, chili flakes, cilantro, and semolina.
2. Then make the meatballs.
3. After this, heat the sesame oil in the skillet.
4. Cook the meatballs in the hot oil on high heat for 1 minute per side.
5. Transfer the roasted meatballs in the Crock Pot, add water, and close the lid.
6. Cook the meatballs on High for 4 hours.

per serving: 178 calories, 24.1g protein, 1.5g carbohydrates, 7.7g fat, 0.1g fiber, 95mg cholesterol, 61mg sodium, 321mg potassium.

Stuffed Jalapenos

Yield: 3 servings | **Prep time:** 10 minutes | **Cook time:** 4.5 hours

- 6 jalapenos, deseed
- 4 oz minced beef
- 1 teaspoon garlic powder
- ½ cup of water

1. Mix the minced beef with garlic powder.
2. Then fill the jalapenos with minced meat and arrange it in the Crock Pot.
3. Add water and cook the jalapenos on High for 4.5 hours.

per serving: 55 calories, 7.5g protein, 2.3g carbohydrates, 1.9g fat, 0.9g fiber, 0mg cholesterol, 2mg sodium, 71mg potassium.

Burgers

Yield: 4 servings | **Prep time:** 10 minutes | **Cook time:** 4 hours

- 10 oz ground beef
- 1 tablespoon minced onion
- 1 teaspoon dried dill
- 2 tablespoons water
- 1 teaspoon ground black pepper
- 1/3 cup chicken stock

1. Mix the minced beef with onion, dill, water, and ground black pepper.
2. Make 4 burgers and arrange them in the Crock Pot bowl.
3. Add chicken stock and close the lid.
4. Cook the burgers on high for 4 hours.

per serving: 135 calories, 21.7g protein, 0.8g carbohydrates, 4.5g fat, 0.2g fiber, 63mg cholesterol, 111mg sodium, 305mg potassium.

BBQ Beef Short Ribs

Yield: 4 servings | **Prep time:** 10 minutes | **Cook time:** 5 hours

- 1-pound beef short ribs
- ¼ cup of water
- 1/3 cup BBQ sauce
- 1 teaspoon chili powder

1. Rub the beef short ribs with chili powder and put in the Crock Pot.
2. Mix water with BBQ sauce and pour the liquid in the Crock Pot.
3. Cook the meat on High for 5 hours.

per serving: 266 calories, 32.8g protein, 7.9g carbohydrates, 10.4g fat, 0.3g fiber, 103mg cholesterol, 308mg sodium, 468mg potassium.

Spiced Beef

Yield: 4 servings | **Prep time:** 10 minutes | **Cook time:** 9 hours

- 1-pound beef loin
- 1 teaspoon allspice
- 1 teaspoon olive oil
- 1 tablespoon minced onion
- 1 cup of water

1. Rub the beef loin with allspice, olive oil, and minced onion.
2. Put the meat in the Crock Pot.
3. Add water and close the lid.
4. Cook the beef on Low for 9 hours.
5. When the meat is cooked, slice it into servings.

per serving: 219 calories, 30.4g protein, 0.6g carbohydrates, 10.7g fat, 0.2g fiber, 81mg cholesterol, 65mg sodium, 395mg potassium.

Ginger Beef

Yield: 2 servings | **Prep time:** 10 minutes | **Cook time:** 4.5 hours

- 10 oz beef brisket, sliced
- 1 teaspoon minced ginger
- 1 teaspoon ground coriander
- 1 tablespoon olive oil
- 1 tablespoon lemon juice
- 1 cup of water

1. In the bowl mix lemon juice and olive oil.
2. Then mix beef brisket with ground coriander and minced ginger.
3. Sprinkle the meat with oil mixture and transfer in the Crock Pot.
4. Add water and cook the meal on High for 4.5 hours.

per serving: 328 calories, 43.1g protein, 0.8g carbohydrates, 15.9g fat, 0.1g fiber, 127mg cholesterol, 99mg sodium, 595mg potassium.

Turmeric Beef Brisket

Yield: 5 servings | **Prep time:** 10 minutes | **Cook time:** 5 hours

- 12 oz beef brisket, chopped
- 1 tablespoon ground turmeric
- 1 teaspoon chili powder
- ½ teaspoon garlic powder
- 1 cup of water
- 1 tablespoon coconut oil

1. Toss the coconut oil in the skillet and melt it.
2. Meanwhile, mix the meat with ground turmeric, chili powder, and garlic powder.
3. Put the meat in the hot oil and roast it for 2 minutes per side on high heat.
4. After this, pour water in the Crock Pot.
5. Add roasted meat and close the lid.
6. Cook the meal on High for 5 hours.

per serving: 157 calories, 20.9g protein, 1.4g carbohydrates, 7.2g fat, 0.5g fiber, 61mg cholesterol, 52mg sodium, 322mg potassium.

Aromatic Meatloaf

Yield: 6 servings | **Prep time:** 10 minutes | **Cook time:** 6 hours

- 1 potato, grated
- 1 teaspoon garlic powder
- 1 onion, minced
- 10 oz minced beef
- 1 egg, beaten
- 1 teaspoon avocado oil
- 1 cup of water

1. In the mixing bowl, mix grated potato, garlic powder, minced onion, minced beef, and egg.
2. Then brush the meatloaf mold with avocado oil.
3. Place the minced beef mixture inside and flatten it.
4. Then pour the water in the Crock Pot.
5. Place the mold with meatloaf in water.
6. Close the lid and cook the meal on High for 6 hours.

per serving: 130 calories, 16.1g protein, 7.1g carbohydrates, 3.8g fat, 1.1g fiber, 69mg cholesterol, 45mg sodium, 354mg potassium.

Beef Casserole

Yield: 5 servings | **Prep time:** 10 minutes | **Cook time:** 7 hours

- 7 oz ground beef
- 1 cup Cheddar cheese, shredded
- ½ cup cream
- 1 teaspoon Italian seasonings
- ½ cup broccoli, chopped

1. Mix ground beef with Italian seasonings and put in the Crock Pot.
2. Top the meat with broccoli and Cheddar cheese.
3. Then pour the cream over the casserole mixture and close the lid.
4. Cook the casserole on Low for 7 hours.

per serving: 186 calories, 18.1g protein, 1.7g carbohydrates, 11.6g fat, 0.2g fiber, 64mg cholesterol, 178mg sodium, 220mg potassium.

Bacon Beef Strips

Yield: 4 servings | **Prep time:** 15 minutes | **Cook time:** 5 hours

- 1-pound beef tenderloin, cut into strips
- 4 oz bacon, sliced
- 1 teaspoon salt
- ½ teaspoon ground black pepper
- ½ cup of water

1. Mix beef with salt and ground black pepper.
2. Then wrap every beef strip with sliced bacon and arrange it in the Crock Pot.
3. Add water and close the lid.
4. Cook the meal on High for 5 hours.

per serving: 258 calories,28.9g protein, 0.4g carbohydrates, 14.8g fat, 0.1g fiber, 90mg cholesterol, 869mg sodium, 379mg potassium.

Beef Curry

Yield: 3 servings | **Prep time:** 10 minutes | **Cook time:** 8 hours

- 7 oz beef tenderloin, chopped
- 1 teaspoon curry powder
- 1 cup of coconut milk
- ¼ cup of water
- ½ cup potatoes, chopped
- 1 onion, sliced

1. Mix coconut milk with curry powder and pour the liquid in the Crock Pot.
2. Add beef, potatoes, and sliced onion.
3. Then add water and close the lid.
4. Cook the meal on low for 8 hours.

per serving: 354 calories, 21.9g protein, 12.2g carbohydrates, 25.3g fat, 3.4g fiber, 61mg cholesterol, 55mg sodium, 612mg potassium.

Aromatic Tomato Beef

Yield: 5 servings | **Prep time:** 10 minutes | **Cook time:** 5 hours

- 1-pound beef brisket, roughly chopped
- 1 cup tomatoes, chopped
- 1 tablespoon tomato paste
- 1 tablespoon fennel seeds
- 1 teaspoon cardamom
- 1 cup of water

1. Preheat the skillet until hot.
2. Put the cardamom and fennel seeds inside and roast them for 2-3 minutes or until they start to smell.
3. Then transfer the spices in the Crock Pot.
4. Add water, tomato paste, tomatoes, and beef brisket.
5. Close the lid and cook the meal on High for 5 hours.

per serving: 183 calories, 28.2g protein, 2.9g carbohydrates, 5.9g fat, 1.1g fiber, 81mg cholesterol, 67mg sodium, 508mg potassium.

Pesto Beef

Yield: 4 servings | **Prep time:** 10 minutes | **Cook time:** 8 hours

- 4 beef chops
- 4 teaspoons pesto sauce
- 1/3 cup beef broth

1. Rub every beef chop with pesto sauce and arrange in the Crock Pot in one layer.
2. Then add beef broth and close the lid.
3. Cook the meal on Low for 8 hours.

per serving: 246 calories, 17.9g protein, 0.4g carbohydrates, 18.3g fat, 0.1g fiber, 46mg cholesterol, 415mg sodium, 17mg potassium.

Chili Beef Sausages

Yield: 5 servings | **Prep time:** 10 minutes | **Cook time:** 4 hours

- 1-pound beef sausages
- 1 tablespoon olive oil
- ¼ cup of water
- 1 teaspoon chili powder

1. Pour olive oil in the Crock Pot.
2. Then sprinkle the beef sausages with chili powder and put in the Crock Pot.
3. Add water and close the lid.
4. Cook the beef sausages on high for 4 hours.

per serving: 385 calories, 12.6g protein, 2.7g carbohydrates, 35.8g fat, 0.2g fiber, 64mg cholesterol, 736mg sodium, 182mg potassium.

Beef Pate

Yield: 4 servings | **Prep time:** 15 minutes | **Cook time:** 4 hours

- 10 oz beef liver
- 1 onion
- 2 cups of water
- 2 tablespoons butter
- 1 teaspoon salt
- 1 teaspoon olive oil

1. Dice the onion and roast it with olive oil in the skillet until light brown.
2. Then pour water in the Crock Pot.
3. Add liver and cook it on High for 4 hours.
4. After this, chop the cooked liver and transfer it in the food processor.
5. Blend it until smooth.
6. Add butter and roasted onion.
7. Stir the pate and store it in the fridge for up to 3 days.

per serving: 196 calories, 19.2g protein, 6.2g carbohydrates, 10.3g fat, 0.6g fiber, 285mg cholesterol, 682mg sodium, 292mg potassium.

Chili Beef Ribs

Yield: 4 servings | **Prep time:** 15 minutes | **Cook time:** 5 hours

- 10 oz beef ribs, chopped
- 1 teaspoon hot sauce
- 1 teaspoon chili powder

- 1 tablespoon sesame oil
- ½ cup of water
1. Mix the beef ribs with chili powder.
2. Then heat the sesame oil in the skillet until hot.
3. Add beef ribs and roast them for 2-3 minutes per side or until they are light brown.
4. After this, transfer the beef ribs in the Crock Pot.
5. Add water and hot sauce.
6. Close the lid and cook them on High for 5 hours.
 per serving: 164 calories, 21.6g protein, 0.4g carbohydrates, 7.9g fat, 0.2g fiber, 63mg cholesterol, 86mg sodium, 300mg potassium.

Basil Beef
Yield: 4 servings | **Prep time:** 15 minutes | **Cook time:** 4 hours
- 1-pound beef loin, chopped
- 2 tablespoons dried basil
- 2 tablespoons butter
- ½ cup of water
- 1 teaspoon salt
1. Toss the butter in the skillet and melt it.
2. Then mix the beef loin with dried basil and put in the hot butter.
3. Roast the meat for 2 minutes per side and transfer in the Crock Pot.
4. Add salt and water.
5. Close the lid and cook the beef on high for 4 hours.
 per serving: 220 calories, 21g protein, 1.4g carbohydrates, 13.9g fat, 0g fiber, 76mg cholesterol, 1123mg sodium, 6mg potassium.

5-Ingredients Chili
Yield: 4 servings | **Prep time:** 10 minutes | **Cook time:** 5 hours
- 8 oz ground beef
- ½ cup Cheddar cheese, shredded
- 2 cup tomatoes, chopped
- 1 teaspoon chili seasonings
- ½ cup of water
1. Mix the ground beef with chili seasonings and transfer in the Crock Pot.
2. Add tomatoes and water.
3. Close the lid and cook the chili on high for 3 hours.
4. After this, open the lid and mix the chili well. Top it with cheddar cheese and close the lid.
5. Cook the chili on low for 2 hours more.
 per serving: 180 calories, 21.6g protein, 4g carbohydrates, 8.4g fat, 1.1g fiber, 66mg cholesterol, 150mg sodium, 456mg potassium.

Beef and Parsnip Saute
Yield: 2 servings | **Prep time:** 10 minutes | **Cook time:** 7 hours
- 1 cup parsnip, peeled, chopped
- 6 oz beef tenderloin, chopped
- 1 tablespoon tomato paste
- 1 teaspoon dried dill
- 1 teaspoon salt
- 1 teaspoon chili powder

- 2 cup of water
1. Put all ingredients in the Crock Pot and carefully mix with the help of the spoon.
2. Close the lid and cook the saute on Low for 7 hours.
 per serving: 237 calories, 26g protein, 14.5g carbohydrates, 8.3g fat, 4.1g fiber, 78mg cholesterol, 1249mg sodium, 678mg potassium.

Lemon Beef Chuck Roast
Yield: 4 servings | **Prep time:** 15 minutes | **Cook time:** 4.5 hours
- 1-pound beef chuck roast
- 1 lemon, sliced
- 1 teaspoon dried thyme
- 1 teaspoon salt
- 1 apple, chopped
- 3 cups of water
1. Rub the beef chuck roast with thyme and salt and transfer in the Crock Pot.
2. Add water, apple, and lemon.
3. Close the lid and cook the meal on high for 4.5 hours.
 per serving: 446 calories, 30g protein, 9.2g carbohydrates, 31.7g fat, 1.9g fiber, 117mg cholesterol, 660mg sodium, 342mg potassium.

Cauliflower and Beef Ragout
Yield: 4 servings | **Prep time:** 15 minutes | **Cook time:** 4 hours
- 2 cups cauliflower florets, chopped
- 2 tablespoons tomato paste
- 1 onion, sliced
- 1 teaspoon ground black pepper
- 2 cups of water
- 7 oz beef loin, chopped
- 1 tablespoon avocado oil
1. Mix the beef loin with ground black pepper and put it in the skillet.
2. Add avocado oil and roast the beef for 3 minutes per side.
3. Transfer the meat in the Crock Pot.
4. Add all remaining ingredients and close the lid.
5. Cook the ragout on High for 4 hours.
 per serving: 110 calories, 10.9g protein, 7.9g carbohydrates, 4.1g fat, 2.5g fiber, 27mg cholesterol, 246mg sodium, 292mg potassium.

Beef with Yams
Yield: 4 servings | **Prep time:** 10 minutes | **Cook time:** 8 hours
- 2 cups yams, chopped
- 4 beef chops
- 1 cup of water
- 2 tablespoons butter
- 1 teaspoon salt
- 1 teaspoon peppercorns
1. Pour water in the Crock Pot.
2. Add peppercorns, salt, butter, and beef chops.
3. Then add yams and close the lid.
4. Cook the meal on Low for 8 hours.

per serving: 351 calories, 18.1g protein, 19g carbohydrates, 21.9g fat, 2.8g fiber, 60mg cholesterol, 950mg sodium, 465mg potassium.

Beef Brisket in Orange Juice
Yield: 4 servings | **Prep time:** 15 minutes | **Cook time:** 5 hours

- 1 cup of orange juice
- 2 cups of water
- 2 tablespoons butter
- 12 oz beef brisket
- ½ teaspoon salt

1. Toss butter in the skillet and melt.
2. Put the beef brisket in the melted butter and roast on high heat for 3 minutes per side.
3. Then sprinkle the meat with salt and transfer in the Crock Pot.
4. Add orange juice and water.
5. Close the lid and cook the meat on High for 5 hours.

per serving: 237 calories, 26.3g protein, 6.5g carbohydrates, 11.2g fat, 0.1g fiber, 91mg cholesterol, 392mg sodium, 470mg potassium.

Tomato Beef Chowder
Yield: 4 servings | **Prep time:** 10 minutes | **Cook time:** 7 hours

- 1 cup potatoes, peeled, chopped
- 1 cup tomato juice
- 3 cups of water
- 1 onion, chopped
- 12 oz beef sirloin, chopped
- 1 teaspoon fresh parsley, chopped
- 1 teaspoon salt

1. Put all ingredients in the Crock Pot.
2. Gently stir the mixture and close the lid.
3. Cook the chowder on Low for 7 hours.

per serving: 205 calories, 27.2g protein, 11.1g carbohydrates, 5.4g fat, 1.7g fiber, 76mg cholesterol, 810mg sodium, 678mg potassium.

Beef Sausages in Maple Syrup
Yield: 4 servings | **Prep time:** 15 minutes | **Cook time:** 5 hours

- 1-pound beef sausages
- ½ cup maple syrup
- 3 tablespoons butter
- 1 teaspoon ground cumin
- ¼ cup of water

1. Toss butter in the skillet and melt it.
2. Then pour the melted butter in the Crock Pot.
3. Add water, cumin, and maple syrup. Stir the liquid until smooth.
4. Add beef sausages and close the lid.
5. Cook the meal on High for 5 hours.

per serving: 630 calories, 15.8 g protein, 29.7g carbohydrates, 50g fat, 0.1g fiber, 103mg cholesterol, 979mg sodium, 307mg potassium.

Garlic Beef Sausages
Yield: 2 servings | **Prep time:** 10 minutes | **Cook time:** 3 hours

- 8 oz beef sausages

- 1 teaspoon garlic powder
- 1 garlic clove, crushed
- 1 teaspoon dried thyme
- 2 tablespoons avocado oil
- ½ cup of water

1. Chop the sausages roughly and sprinkle with garlic powder and dried thyme.
2. Then heat the avocado oil in the skillet.
3. Add the chopped sausages and roast for 1 minute per side.
4. Transfer the sausages in the Crock Pot. Add all remaining ingredients and close the lid.
5. Cook the sausages on High for 3 hours.

per serving: 476 calories, 16.2g protein, 5.7g carbohydrates, 43g fat, 1g fiber, 81mg cholesterol, 916mg sodium, 285mg potassium.

Sausages in Marinara Sauce
Yield: 4 servings | **Prep time:** 15 minutes | **Cook time:** 4.5 hours

- 1-pound beef sausages
- 1 teaspoon olive oil
- ½ cup marinara sauce
- ¼ cup of water

1. Pour olive oil in the skillet. Heat it well.
2. Add beef sausages and roast them for 3 minutes per side on high heat.
3. Then transfer the sausages in the Crock Pot.
4. Add marinara sauce and water.
5. Close the lid and cook the meal on High for 4.5 hours.

per serving: 486 calories, 16.2g protein, 7.4g carbohydrates, 43.1g fat, 0.8g fiber, 81mg cholesterol, 1041mg sodium, 313mg potassium.

Ground Beef Zucchini Squares
Yield: 4 servings | **Prep time:** 25 minutes | **Cook time:** 4.5 hours

- 2 large zucchinis, trimmed
- 2 tablespoons ricotta cheese
- 9 oz ground beef
- 1 teaspoon ground black pepper
- ½ cup of water
- 1 teaspoon butter

1. Slice the zucchini into strips.
2. Then put butter in the Crock Pot and melt it.
3. Add ground beef and ground black pepper.
4. Roast the meat mixture for 5 minutes.
5. After this, add ricotta cheese and carefully mix.
6. Make the cross from 2 zucchini strips.
7. Put the small amount of the ground beef mixture in the center of the zucchini cross and wrap it into squares.
8. Repeat the same steps with all remaining zucchini and meat mixture.
9. Put the zucchini squares in the Crock Pot.
10. Add water and close the lid.
11. Cook the meal on High for 4.5 hours.

per serving: 165 calories, 22.3g protein, 6.2g carbohydrates, 5.9g fat, 1.9g fiber, 62mg cholesterol, 76mg sodium, 697mg potassium.

Beef Stuffing

Yield: 6 servings | **Prep time:** 10 minutes | **Cook time:** 5 hours

- ½ teaspoon cumin seeds
- 12 oz ground beef
- 1 teaspoon garam masala
- 1 teaspoon ginger paste
- 2 oz scallions, chopped
- 1 cup of water
- 1 tablespoon butter
- 1 teaspoon salt

1.   Put all ingredients in the Crock Pot and carefully mix the mixture.
2.   Close the lid and cook the beef stuffing on High for 5 hours.

per serving: 152 calories, 21g protein, 1.2g carbohydrates, 6.6g fat, 0.4g fiber, 67mg cholesterol, 531mg sodium, 315mg potassium.

Asian Style Beef and Broccoli

Yield: 4 servings | **Prep time:** 15 minutes | **Cook time:** 5 hours

- 2 tablespoons soy sauce
- 1 tablespoon liquid honey
- 1 tablespoon sesame seeds
- 1 cup of water
- 1 cup broccoli florets
- 1 garlic clove, diced
- 10 oz beef sirloin, chopped

1.   Mix the beef sirloin with garlic and soy sauce.
2.   Transfer the meat in the Crock Pot and water.
3.   Close the lid and cook it on high for 3 hours.
4.   Then add all remaining ingredients and gently mix.
5.   Cook the meal on High for 2 hours more.

per serving: 174 calories, 23.1g protein, 7.2g carbohydrates, 5.6g fat, 1g fiber, 63mg cholesterol, 507mg sodium, 392mg potassium.

Beef in Wine Sauce

Yield: 4 servings | **Prep time:** 15 minutes | **Cook time:** 6 hours

- 1 tablespoon flour
- 1 tablespoon butter
- 1 cup red wine
- 1 teaspoon brown sugar
- ½ cup of water
- 1 onion, peeled, chopped
- 12 oz beef tenderloin, chopped

1.   Sprinkle the beef with flour.
2.   Then toss the butter in the skillet. Melt it.
3.   Add the beef and roast it on high heat for 3 minutes per side.
4.   Then transfer the meat in the Crock Pot.
5.   Add onion, water, brown sugar, and red wine.
6.   Close the lid and cook the meal on Low for 6 hours.

per serving: 271 calories, 25.2g protein, 6.4g carbohydrates, 10.7g fat, 0.6g fiber, 86mg cholesterol, 76mg sodium, 406mg potassium.

Spaghetti Meatballs

Yield: 4 servings | **Prep time:** 15 minutes | **Cook time:** 4 hours

- 1-pound ground beef
- 1 teaspoon minced garlic
- 1 teaspoon dried dill
- 1 teaspoon ricotta cheese
- ½ cup marinara sauce
- 1 tablespoon avocado oil

1.   Heat the avocado oil in the skillet well.
2.   Then mix the ground beef with minced garlic, dried dill, and ricotta cheese.
3.   Make the small meatballs and put them in the hot oil.
4.   Roast the meatballs on high heat for 3 minutes per side.
5.   Transfer the meatballs in the Crock Pot and add marinara sauce.
6.   Close the lid and cook the meatballs on High for 4 hours.

per serving: 246 calories, 35.2g protein, 4.9g carbohydrates, 8.5g fat, 1g fiber, 102mg cholesterol, 205mg sodium, 579mg potassium.

Beef Bolognese

Yield: 4 servings | **Prep time:** 15 minutes | **Cook time:** 5 hours

- ½ cup onion, diced
- 1 teaspoon dried basil
- 1 teaspoon dried cilantro
- ½ cup tomato juice
- 1 tablespoon sesame oil
- 1-pound ground beef
- 2 oz parmesan, grated

1.   In the mixing bowl mix ground beef with cilantro, basil, and onion.
2.   Pour the sesame oil in the Crock Pot.
3.   Add tomato juice and ground beef mixture.
4.   Cook it on high for 3 hours.
5.   Then add parmesan and carefully mix.
6.   Cook the meal on low for 2 hours more.

per serving: 297 calories, 39.4g protein, 3.2g carbohydrates, 13.5g fat, 0.4g fiber, 111mg cholesterol, 289mg sodium, 548mg potassium.

Jalapeno Mississippi Roast

Yield: 4 servings | **Prep time:** 15 minutes | **Cook time:** 8 hours

- 3 pepperoncini
- 1-pound beef chuck roast
- 2 tablespoons flour
- 1 teaspoon ground black pepper
- ½ teaspoon salt
- 2 tablespoons avocado oil
- 2 cups of water

1.   Put all ingredients in the Crock Pot.
2.   Close the lid and cook the meal on Low for 8 hours.
3.   Then open the lid and shred the beef.

per serving: 440 calories, 30.4g protein, 4.3g carbohydrates, 32.6g fat, 1g fiber, 117mg cholesterol, 369mg sodium, 322mg potassium.

Cocktail Beef Meatballs

Yield: 4 servings | **Prep time:** 15 minutes | **Cook time:** 3.5 hours

- 1 oz walnuts, grinded
- 3 tablespoons breadcrumbs
- 1 teaspoon ground black pepper
- 12 oz ground beef
- 1 tablespoon coconut oil
- ½ cup of water

1. Heat the coconut oil well in the skillet.
2. Then mix walnuts with breadcrumbs, ground black pepper, and ground beef.
3. Make the small meatballs and put them in the hot skillet.
4. Roast the meatballs for 2 minutes per side.
5. Transfer the meatballs in the Crock Pot.
6. Add water and close the lid.
7. Cook the meatballs on High for 3.5 hours.

per serving: 252 calories, 28.3g protein, 4.7g carbohydrates, 13.2g fat, 0.9g fiber, 76mg cholesterol, 94mg sodium, 397mg potassium.

Spring Beef Bowl

Yield: 4 servings | **Prep time:** 15 minutes | **Cook time:** 5 hours

- 3 oz scallions, chopped
- 1 carrot, cut into strips
- 10 oz beef loin, cut into strips
- 1 tablespoon sesame oil
- 1 teaspoon chili powder
- 1 cup of water

1. Pour water in the Crock Pot.
2. Add carrot, beef loin, and chili powder.
3. Close the lid and cook the beef on high for 5 hours.
4. Then transfer the mixture in the bowls.
5. Add sesame oil and scallions. Carefully mix the meal before serving.

per serving: 174 calories, 19.6g protein, 3.4g carbohydrates, 9.5g fat, 1.1g fiber, 50mg cholesterol, 61mg sodium, 361mg potassium.

Beef and Barley Saute

Yield: 6 servings | **Prep time:** 15 minutes | **Cook time:** 8 hours

- ½ cup barley
- 1-pound beef brisket, chopped
- 2 tomatoes, chopped
- 1 onion, sliced
- 1 bell pepper, chopped
- 4 cups of water
- 1 teaspoon ground turmeric

1. Pour water in the Crock Pot.
2. Add barley, beef brisket, tomatoes, onion, and bell pepper.
3. Then add ground turmeric and close the lid.
4. Cook the saute on Low for 8 hours.

per serving: 217 calories, 25.6g protein, 16.3g carbohydrates, 5.3g fat, 3.9g fiber, 68mg cholesterol, 60mg sodium, 546mg potassium.

Beef with Green Peas Sauce

Yield: 4 servings | **Prep time:** 15 minutes | **Cook time:** 5 hours

- 1-pound beef loin, chopped
- 1 cup green peas, frozen
- 1 bay leaf
- 1 tablespoon butter
- 1 teaspoon flour
- 1 teaspoon chili powder
- ½ cup tomato juice
- 2 cup of water

1. Put all ingredients in the Crock Pot and close the lid.
2. Cook the beef on High for 5 hours.
3. Then transfer it in the serving bowls and top with the remaining sauce from the Crock Pot.

per serving: 234 calories, 23.3g protein, 8.9g carbohydrates, 11.3g fat, 2.3g fiber, 68mg cholesterol, 614mg sodium, 175mg potassium.

Korean Style Shredded Beef

Yield: 6 servings | **Prep time:** 20 minutes | **Cook time:** 5 hours

- 1-pound beef sirloin
- 4 cups of water
- 1 tablespoon sriracha
- ¼ cup of soy sauce
- 1 teaspoon brown sugar
- 2 garlic cloves, diced
- 1 teaspoon sesame seeds

1. Pour water in the Crock Pot.
2. Add beef sirloin and garlic. Close the lid and cook it on High for 4 hours.
3. Then shred the beef and add all remaining ingredients.
4. Cook the beef on High for 1 hour more.

per serving: 155 calories, 23.8g protein, 5g carbohydrates, 5g fat, 0.2g fiber, 68mg cholesterol, 672mg sodium, 336mg potassium.

Beef Mac&Cheese

Yield: 4 servings | **Prep time:** 20 minutes | **Cook time:** 4.5 hours

- ½ cup macaroni, cooked
- 10 oz ground beef
- ½ cup marinara sauce
- 1 cup Mozzarella, shredded
- ½ cup of water

1. Mix the ground beef with marinara sauce and water and transfer in the Crock Pot.
2. Cook it on High for 4 hours.
3. After this, add macaroni and Mozzarella. Carefully mix the meal and cook it for 30 minutes more on high.

per serving: 218 calories, 25.4g protein, 12.4g carbohydrates, 1.2g fat, 68g fiber, 63mg cholesterol, 219mg sodium, 408mg potassium.

Garlic-Parmesan Beef

Yield: 2 servings | **Prep time:** 10 minutes | **Cook time:** 4 hours

- 1 oz Parmesan, grated
- 1 carrot, grated
- 8 oz ground beef
- ½ cup of water

- 1 teaspoon olive oil
- 1 teaspoon chili powder
1.   Mix the ground beef with carrot and transfer it in the Crock Pot.
2.   Add olive oil, chili powder, and water.
3.   Close the lid and cook the beef on high for 4 hours.
4.   After this, add parmesan and carefully mix the meal.

per serving: 293 calories, 39.4g protein, 4.2g carbohydrates, 12.7g fat, 1.2g fiber, 111mg cholesterol, 242mg sodium, 580mg potassium.

Buffalo Sauce Beef
Yield: 4 servings | **Prep time:** 10 minutes | **Cook time:** 5 hours

- 1-pound ground beef
- 3 oz buffalo sauce
- ½ cup tomato juice
- 1 tablespoon butter
- 1 onion, diced
- ½ cup of water

1.   Pour water in the Crock Pot.
2.   Add onion, butter, tomato juice, and ground beef.
3.   Close the lid and cook it on high for 4.5 hours.
4.   Then add buffalo sauce and cook the beef for 1 hour more.

per serving: 261 calories, 35g protein, 5.3g carbohydrates, 10g fat, 1.4g fiber, 109mg cholesterol, 859mg sodium, 568mg potassium.

Pickled Pulled Beef
Yield: 4 servings | **Prep time:** 10 minutes | **Cook time:** 5 hours

- 1 cup cucumber pickles, chopped
- 10 oz beef sirloin
- 1 teaspoon ground black pepper
- 1 teaspoon salt
- 2 cups of water
- 2 tablespoons mayonnaise

1.   Pour water in the Crock Pot.
2.   Add beef sirloin, ground black pepper, and salt.
3.   Close the lid and cook the beef on high for 5 hours.
4.   Then drain water and chop the beef.
5.   Put the beef in the big bowl.
6.   Add chopped cucumber pickles and mayonnaise.
7.   Mix the beef well.

per serving: 162 calories, 21.6g protein, 2.1g carbohydrates, 6.9g fat, 0.1g fiber, 65mg cholesterol, 719mg sodium, 294mg potassium.

Hawaiian Pulled Beef
Yield: 4 servings | **Prep time:** 20 minutes | **Cook time:** 9 hours

- 3 oz pineapple, chopped
- ½ cup pineapple juice
- 1-pound beef sirloin
- 1 teaspoon ground black pepper
- ½ teaspoon ground coriander
- 1 tablespoon butter

1.   Pour pineapple juice in the Crock Pot.
2.   Add pineapple, ground black pepper, ground coriander, and butter.
3.   Slice the beef sirloin and put it in the Crock Pot.
4.   Cook the meat on low for 9 hours.
5.   Serve the beef with pineapple gravy from the Crock Pot.

per serving: 265 calories, 34.7g protein, 7.2g carbohydrates, 10g fat, 0.5g fiber, 109mg cholesterol, 96mg sodium, 528mg potassium.

Cilantro Beef Meatballs
Yield: 6 servings | **Prep time:** 20 minutes | **Cook time:** 4 hours

- 2 tablespoons dried cilantro
- 12 oz ground beef
- 2 tablespoons semolina
- 1 teaspoon garlic powder
- 1 teaspoon chili powder
- 1 tablespoon olive oil
- ½ cup of coconut milk

1.   Put the ground beef in the Crock Pot.
2.   Add semolina, garlic powder, chili powder, and dried cilantro.
3.   Make the small balls and put them in the Crock Pot in one layer.
4.   Add olive oil and coconut milk.
5.   Close the lid and cook the meatballs on High for 4 hours.

per serving: 187 calories, 18.2g protein, 4.2g carbohydrates, 10.7g fat, 0.8g fiber, 51mg cholesterol, 45mg sodium, 303mg potassium.

Fajita Beef
Yield: 4 servings | **Prep time:** 10 minutes | **Cook time:** 4.5 hours

- 1 sweet pepper, cut into strips
- 1 red onion, sliced
- 1-pound beef sirloin, cut into strips
- 1 teaspoon fajita seasonings
- ½ cup of water
- 1 tablespoon butter

1.   Put the beef strips in the Crock Pot.
2.   Add fajita seasonings, butter, and water.
3.   Close the lid and cook the beef on high for 3.5 hours.
4.   Add onion and sweet pepper.
5.   Carefully mix the beef mixture and cook for 1 hour on High.

per serving: 259 calories, 35g protein, 5.4g carbohydrates, 10.1g fat, 1g fiber, 109mg cholesterol, 142mg sodium, 554mg potassium.

Chili Beef Strips
Yield: 4 servings | **Prep time:** 10 minutes | **Cook time:** 6 hours

- 1-pound beef loin, cut into strips
- 1 chili pepper, chopped
- 2 tablespoons coconut oil
- 1 teaspoon salt
- 1 teaspoon chili powder

1.   Sprinkle the beef strips with salt and chili powder.

2. Then put the chili pepper in the Crock Pot.
3. Add coconut oil and beef strips.
4. Close the lid and cook the meal on Low for 6 hours.
per serving: 267 calories, 30.4g protein, 0.5g carbohydrates, 16.4g fat, 0.3g fiber, 81mg cholesterol, 650mg sodium, 401mg potassium.

Honey Beef Sausages
Yield: 4 servings | **Prep time:** 10 minutes | **Cook time:** 4.5 hours
- 1-pound beef sausages
- 2 tablespoons of liquid honey
- 1 teaspoon dried dill
- ½ teaspoon salt
- ¼ cup heavy cream
1. In the mixing bowl mix liquid honey with dried dill and salt.
2. Then add cream and whisk until smooth.
3. Pour the liquid in the Crock Pot.
4. Add beef sausages and close the lid.
5. Cook the meal on High for 4.5 hours.
per serving: 507 calories, 15.9g protein, 12.1g carbohydrates, 43.9g fat, 0.1g fiber, 91mg cholesterol, 1207mg sodium, 234mg potassium.

Barbacoa Beef
Yield: 4 servings | **Prep time:** 20 minutes | **Cook time:** 5 hours
- 1-pound beef chuck roast
- 1 teaspoon ground black pepper
- ½ teaspoon salt
- 1 teaspoon ground cumin
- ¼ lime, ½ teaspoon ground clove
- 2 cups of water
1. Put the beef in the Crock Pot.
2. Add ground black pepper, salt, ground cumin, ground clove, and water.
3. Close the lid and cook the meat on High for 5 hours.
4. Then shred the beef.
5. Squeeze the line over the meat and carefully mix.
per serving: 417 calories, 29.9g protein, 1.2g carbohydrates, 31.8g fat, 0.4g fiber, 117mg cholesterol, 369mg sodium, 283mg potassium.

Tender Beef Goulash
Yield: 4 servings | **Prep time:** 10 minutes | **Cook time:** 8 hours
- 1 teaspoon flour
- 2 cups of water
- ¼ cup cream
- 1-pound beef brisket, chopped
- 1 carrot, chopped
- 1 teaspoon ground black pepper
- 1 tablespoon sunflower oil
1. Mix the cream with flour until smooth and pour in the Crock Pot.
2. Add water, chopped beef, carrot, ground black pepper, and sunflower oil.
3. Close the lid and cook the goulash for 8 hours on Low.

per serving: 261 calories, 34.8g protein, 2.8g carbohydrates, 11.4g fat, 0.5g fiber, 104mg cholesterol, 94mg sodium, 520mg potassium.

Tarragon Beef
Yield: 2 servings | **Prep time:** 20 minutes | **Cook time:** 7 hours
- 8 oz beef sirloin
- 1 tablespoon dried tarragon
- ½ teaspoon salt
- 2 tablespoons sunflower oil
- 1 cup of water
1. In the mixing bowl, mix sunflower oil with salt and dried tarragon.
2. After this, brush the beef sirloin with oil mixture and leave for 10-15 minutes to marinate.
3. Then place the meat in the Crock Pot, add water, and close the lid.
4. Cook the beef on Low for 7 hours.
per serving: 337 calories, 34.6g protein, 0.5g carbohydrates, 21.1g fat, 0.1g fiber, 101mg cholesterol, 660mg sodium, 485mg potassium.

Peppercorn Beef Steak
Yield: 4 servings | **Prep time:** 15 minutes | **Cook time:** 8 hours
- 4 beef steaks
- 1 teaspoon salt
- 1 teaspoon peppercorns
- 1 tablespoon butter
- 1 cup of water
- 1 teaspoon dried rosemary
1. Rub the beef steaks with salt and dried rosemary.
2. Then rub the meat with butter and transfer in the Crock Pot.
3. Add water and peppercorns.
4. Close the lid and cook the beef steaks on Low for 8 hours.
per serving: 186 calories, 25.9g protein, 0.5g carbohydrates, 8.3g fat, 0.3g fiber, 84mg cholesterol, 660mg sodium, 354mg potassium.

Delightful Pepperoncini Beef
Yield: 4 servings | **Prep time:** 10 minutes | **Cook time:** 5 hours
- 2 oz pepperoncini
- 1-pound beef chuck roast
- 2 cups of water
- 1 teaspoon minced garlic
1. Chop the beef roughly and mix with minced garlic.
2. Then transfer the beef in the Crock Pot.
3. Add water and pepperoncini.
4. Close the lid and cook the meal on High for 5 hours.
per serving: 418 calories, 29.9g protein, 1.7g carbohydrates, 31.6g fat, 0g fiber, 117mg cholesterol, 216mg sodium, 263mg potassium.

White Beef Chili
Yield: 4 servings | **Prep time:** 10 minutes | **Cook time:** 5 hours

- 1 cup white beans, soaked
- 4 cups of water
- ½ cup plain yogurt
- 1 teaspoon chili powder
- 1 teaspoon ground black pepper
- 1 teaspoon salt
- 12 oz ground beef
- 1 onion, diced
1. Pour water in the Crock Pot.
2. Add white beans, chili powder, ground black pepper, salt, and ground beef.
3. Then add diced onion and close the lid.
4. Cook the meal on High for 4 hours.
5. Then add plain yogurt, carefully mix the meal, and cook it on High for 1 hour more.

per serving: 362 calories, 39.8g protein, 35.9g carbohydrates, 6.3g fat, 8.6g fiber, 78mg cholesterol, 678mg sodium, 1381mg potassium.

Corned Beef
Yield: 4 servings | **Prep time:** 10 minutes | **Cook time:** 8.5 hours
- 1 cup carrot, chopped
- ½ cup celery stalk, chopped
- 1-pound beef brisket
- 1 yellow onion, chopped
- 1 teaspoon mustard seeds
- 1 tablespoon salt
- 4 cups of water
- 1 teaspoon cloves
1. Put all ingredients in the Crock Pot and gently mix.
2. Close the lid and cook the corned beef for 8.5 hours on Low.

per serving: 241 calories, 35.3g protein, 6.3g carbohydrates, 7.5g fat, 1.8g fiber, 101mg cholesterol, 1857mg sodium, 632mg potassium.

Beef Meatloaf
Yield: 6 servings | **Prep time:** 15 minutes | **Cook time:** 6 hours
- 1-pound ground beef
- 1 cup celery stalk, diced
- 3 tablespoons semolina
- 1 teaspoon garlic, diced
- 1 teaspoon cayenne pepper
- 1 tablespoon coconut oil, softened
- 1 teaspoon salt
- ½ cup Monterey Jack cheese, shredded
1. In the mixing bowl mix ground beef with a celery stalk, semolina, garlic, cayenne pepper, and salt.
2. Then grease the Crock Pot bottom with coconut oil.
3. Put the ground beef mixture and flatten it.
4. Top the beef with Monterey jack cheese and close the lid.
5. Cook the meatloaf on Low for 6 hours.

per serving: 218 calories, 26.1g protein, 4.7g carbohydrates, 10g fat, 0.6g fiber, 76mg cholesterol, 502mg sodium, 374mg potassium.

London Broil
Yield: 6 servings | **Prep time:** 15 minutes | **Cook time:** 8 hours
- 2-pounds London broil
- 3 garlic cloves, crushed
- 1 onion, sliced
- 3 cups of water
- ¼ cup of soy sauce
- 1 teaspoon ground black pepper
1. Preheat the grill skillet well.
2. Then put London broil in the hot skillet and roast it on high heat for 3 minutes per side.
3. After this, transfer the meat in the Crock Pot.
4. Add all remaining ingredients from the list above. Close the lid and cook the meal on Low for 8 hours.

per serving: 74 calories, 9.3g protein, 3.9g carbohydrates, 2.4g fat, 0.6g fiber, 0mg cholesterol, 701mg sodium, 61mg potassium.

Stuffed Meatloaf
Yield: 4 servings | **Prep time:** 15 minutes | **Cook time:** 10 hours
- 1 teaspoon ricotta cheese
- 2 oz cheddar cheese, shredded
- 1 teaspoon fresh dill, chopped
- 10 oz ground beef
- 1 tablespoon semolina
- 1 teaspoon onion powder
- 1 tablespoon olive oil
- ½ cup of water
1. In the mixing bowl mix dill with ground beef, semolina, and onion powder.
2. After this, brush the Crock Pot loaf mold with olive oil and put ½ part of the ground beef mixture inside.
3. Flatten it.
4. After this, in the bowl mix ricotta cheese and cheddar cheese.
5. Put the cheese mixture over the ground beef (which is in the mold).
6. Then top the cheese with remaining ground beef and flatten it.
7. Pour water in the Crock Pot.
8. Then insert the loaf mold in the Crock Pot and close the lid.
9. Cook the meatloaf on Low for 10 hours.

per serving: 233 calories, 25.6g protein, 2.8g carbohydrates, 12.8g fat, 0.2g fiber, 79mg cholesterol, 138mg sodium, 320mg potassium.

Beef in Onion Dip
Yield: 4 servings | **Prep time:** 25 minutes | **Cook time:** 6 hours
- 1-pound beef sirloin
- 1 cup onion, sliced
- 1 cup of water
- 3 tablespoons butter
- 1 teaspoon salt
- 1 teaspoon white pepper
- ½ teaspoon ground clove
1. Toss the butter in the pan and melt it.

2. Add beef sirloin and roast it for 4 minutes per side on high heat.
3. After this, transfer the beef sirloin and liquid butter in the Crock Pot.
4. Add onion, water, salt, white pepper, and ground clove.
5. Close the lid and cook the meal on High for 4 hours.
6. Then shred the beef and cook the dip for 2 hours on high more.
 per serving: 301 calories, 34.9g protein, 3.2g carbohydrates, 15.8g fat, 0.9g fiber, 124mg cholesterol, 721mg sodium, 512mg potassium.

Beef Barbecue Cubes
Yield: 2 servings | **Prep time:** 30 minutes | **Cook time:** 5 hours
- 9 oz beef sirloin, chopped
- ½ cup BBQ sauce
- 1 teaspoon dried rosemary
- ¼ cup of water
- 1 tablespoon avocado oil
1. In the big bowl mix avocado oil, water, dried rosemary, and BBQ sauce.
2. Add chopped beef sirloin and carefully mix the mixture.
3. Leave it for 20 minutes to marinate.
4. After this, transfer meat and all remaining liquid in the Crock Pot.
5. Cook it on High for 5 hours.
 per serving: 342 calories, 38.8g protein, 23.4g carbohydrates, 9.1g fat, 1g fiber, 114mg cholesterol, 785mg sodium, 672mg potassium.

Cranberry Beef Saute
Yield: 4 servings | **Prep time:** 15 minutes | **Cook time:** 8 hours
- 1/3 cup cranberries
- 1 cup of water
- ¼ cup red wine
- 12 oz beef sirloin, chopped
- 2 cups tomatoes, chopped
- 1 teaspoon brown sugar
- ½ teaspoon dried thyme
1. Sprinkle the beef sirloin with brown sugar, dried thyme, and transfer in the Crock Pot.
2. Add red wine, water, and tomatoes.
3. After this, put the cranberries in the top of the mixture and close the lid.
4. Cook the saute on Low for 8 hours.
 per serving: 195 calories, 26.6g protein, 5.6g carbohydrates, 5.5g fat, 1.5g fiber, 76mg cholesterol, 63mg sodium, 589mg potassium.

Reuben Beef
Yield: 8 servings | **Prep time:** 15 minutes | **Cook time:** 6 hours
- 3-pounds corned beef brisket
- 1 teaspoon mustard seeds
- 1 tablespoon of liquid smoked
- 1 teaspoon brown sugar
- 1 teaspoon ground paprika
- 1 teaspoon onion powder

- 1 teaspoon garlic powder
1. In the shallow bowl mix garlic powder, onion powder, ground paprika, brown sugar, and mustard seeds.
2. After this, carefully brush the corned beef brisket with liquid smoked and rub with the mustard seeds mixture.
3. Wrap the meat in the foil and place it in the Crock Pot.
4. Cook it on High for 6 hours.
 per serving: 295 calories, 23g protein, 1.1g carbohydrates, 21.4g fat, 0.2g fiber, 106mg cholesterol, 1508mg sodium, 263mg potassium.

Greek-Style Beef Meatballs
Yield: 4 servings | **Prep time:** 25 minutes | **Cook time:** 5 hours
- ½ teaspoon dried mint
- 1 teaspoon minced garlic
- ¼ cup breadcrumbs
- 10 oz ground beef
- 1 tablespoons dried parsley
- 1 egg, beaten
- 2 tablespoons sesame oil
- 1/3 cup plain yogurt
1. Pour sesame oil in the skillet and heat well.
2. Meanwhile, mix dried mint with minced garlic, breadcrumbs, ground beef, and dried parsley.
3. Add egg and carefully stir the mixture until smooth.
4. After this, make the meatballs and put them in the hot sesame oil.
5. Roast the meatballs for 2 minutes per side on high heat.
6. After this, transfer them in the Crock Pot, add plain yogurt, and close the lid.
7. Cook the meatballs on low for 5 hours.
 per serving: 250 calories, 25g protein, 6.7g carbohydrates, 12.9g fat, 0.4g fiber, 105mg cholesterol, 126mg sodium, 370mg potassium.

Beef Tamale Pie
Yield: 4 servings | **Prep time:** 30 minutes | **Cook time:** 4 hours
- 1/2 cup cornflour - masa
- 3 tablespoons butter, softened
- 1/3 cup Cheddar cheese, shredded
- 1 cup of water
- 1 teaspoon ground cumin
- 1 teaspoon salt
- 1-pound ground beef
- 1 cup tomatoes, chopped
- ½ cup hot water
1. Pour water in the pan and bring to boil.
2. Add cornflour and butter. Carefully mix and boil for 3 minutes.
3. Then close the pan with a lid and remove from the heat.
4. After this, Mix ground beef with salt and ground cumin.
5. Put the mixture in the Crock Pot
6. Add chopped tomatoes, and Cheddar cheese.

7. Top the mixture with cooked corn flour – masa and add hot water.
8. Close the lid and cook the pie on High for 4 hours.

per serving: 388 calories, 38.3g protein, 13.4g carbohydrates, 19.6g fat, 1.7g fiber, 134mg cholesterol, 781mg sodium, 631mg potassium.

Beef French Dip

Yield: 4 servings | **Prep time:** 15 minutes | **Cook time:** 8 hours

- 1-pound beef chuck roast
- 1 cup onion, sliced
- ½ cup French onion soup
- 1 teaspoon garlic powder
- ½ cup of water
- 1 tablespoon coconut oil
- 2 oz provolone cheese, shredded

1. Dice the meat and put it in the Crock Pot.
2. Add all remaining ingredients and carefully mix.
3. Close the lid and cook the dip on Low for 8 hours.

per serving: 520 calories, 32.4g protein, 6g carbohydrates, 39g fat, 0.9g fiber, 127mg cholesterol, 386mg sodium, 371mg potassium.

Sausage Dip

Yield: 4 servings | **Prep time:** 15 minutes | **Cook time:** 4.5 hours

- 8 oz beef sausages, chopped
- 1 bell pepper, chopped
- 1 tomato, chopped
- ½ cup tomato sauce
- ¼ cup of water
- 1 tablespoon avocado oil
- 1 teaspoon ground cumin

1. Heat the avocado oil in the skillet.
2. Add beef sausages and roast them for 5 minutes in medium heat. Stir them from time to time.
3. Then transfer the beef sausages in the Crock Pot.
4. Add all remaining ingredients and carefully mix.
5. Close the lid and cook the dip on High for 4.5 hours.
6. Carefully mix the sausage dip before serving.

per serving: 251 calories, 8.8g protein, 6.5g carbohydrates, 21.3g fat, 1.3g fiber, 40mg cholesterol, 620mg sodium, 322mg potassium.

Bavarian Style Sausages

Yield: 4 servings | **Prep time:** 15 minutes | **Cook time:** 4 hours

- 12 oz beef sausages
- ½ cup beer
- ¼ cup tomato sauce
- 1 tablespoon garlic, crushed
- 1 tablespoon olive oil
- 1 teaspoon cumin seeds

1. In the mixing bowl, mix olive oil with cumin seeds, crushed garlic, and tomato sauce.

2. Then sprinkle the beef sausages with olive oil mixture and put in the Crock Pot.
3. Add tomato sauce and beer.
4. Close the lid and cook the meal on high for 4 hours.

per serving: 361 calories, 12.3g protein, 5.2g carbohydrates, 31.2g fat, 0.4g fiber, 60mg cholesterol, 786mg sodium, 238mg potassium.

Beer Sausages

Yield: 4 servings | **Prep time:** 15 minutes | **Cook time:** 7 hours

- 1-pound beef sausages
- 3 tablespoons butter
- 1 teaspoon ground black pepper
- 1 teaspoon salt
- 1 cup beer

1. Toss the butter in the skillet and melt it.
2. Add beef sausages and roast them on high heat for 2 minutes per side.
3. Transfer the beef sausages in the Crock Pot.
4. Add ground black pepper, salt, and beer.
5. Close the lid and cook the meal on Low for 7 hours.

per serving: 552 calories, 16.1g protein, 5.5g carbohydrates, 49.8g fat, 0.1g fiber, 103mg cholesterol, 1558mg sodium, 240mg potassium.

Paprika Beef

Yield: 4 servings | **Prep time:** 10 minutes | **Cook time:** 5 hours

- 1-pound beef sirloin
- 1 tablespoon ground paprika
- ½ cup of water
- 1 tablespoon sunflower oil

1. Rub the beef sirloin with ground paprika and sprinkle with sunflower oil.
2. Put the meat in the Crock Pot.
3. Add water and close the lid.
4. Cook the beef on High for 5 hours.

per serving: 247 calories, 34.7g protein, 1g carbohydrates, 10.8g fat, 0.7g fiber, 101mg cholesterol, 76mg sodium, 498mg potassium.

Kebab Cubes

Yield: 4 servings | **Prep time:** 15 minutes | **Cook time:** 5 hours

- 1 teaspoon curry powder
- 1 teaspoon dried mint
- 1 teaspoon cayenne pepper
- ½ cup plain yogurt
- 1-pound beef tenderloin, cubed

1. In the mixing bowl, mix beef cubes with plain yogurt, cayenne pepper, dried mint, and curry powder.
2. Then put the mixture in the Crock Pot. Add water if there is not enough liquid and close the lid.
3. Cook the meal on High for 5 hours.

per serving: 259 calories, 34.7g protein, 2.7g carbohydrates, 10.9g fat, 0.3g fiber, 106mg cholesterol, 89mg sodium, 495mg potassium.

Sausages in Sweet Currant Sauce

Yield: 4 servings | **Prep time:** 15 minutes | **Cook time:** 4.5 hours

- 1 tablespoon butter
- 1 cup fresh currant
- 1 tablespoon brown sugar
- 1 cup of water
- 1-pound beef sausages
- 1 tablespoon sunflower oil

1. Mix currants with brown sugar and blend with the help of the immersion blender until smooth.
2. Pour the liquid in the Crock Pot.
3. Add all remaining ingredients and close the lid.
4. Cook the sausages on High for 4.5 hours.

per serving: 530 calories, 16.1g protein, 9.1g carbohydrates, 47.6g fat, 1.2g fiber, 88mg cholesterol, 936mg sodium, 296mg potassium.

Super-Fast Golubkis

Yield: 4 servings | **Prep time:** 20 minutes | **Cook time:** 8 hours

- 7 oz ground beef
- 1 teaspoon garam masala
- 2 cups of water
- ½ cup basmati rice
- 2 cups white cabbage, shredded
- 1 cup tomatoes, chopped
- 1 teaspoon tomato paste

1. In the mixing bowl, mix ground beef, garam masala, basmati rice, tomato paste, and tomatoes.
2. Then put ½ part of ground beef mixture in the Crock Pot.
3. Top it with shredded white cabbage.
4. Then add remaining ground beef mixture and top with remaining shredded cabbage.
5. Add water and close the lid.
6. Cook the meal on Low for 8 hours.

per serving: 195 calories, 17.6g protein, 22.5g carbohydrates, 3.4g fat, 1.8g fiber, 44mg cholesterol, 48mg sodium, 407mg potassium.

Kale Tamales

Yield: 4 servings | **Prep time:** 20 minutes | **Cook time:** 5 hours

- 3 oz corn husks
- 1 cup kale, chopped
- 1 cup mushrooms, chopped
- 1 onion, diced
- ½ cup ricotta cheese
- 1 teaspoon cayenne pepper
- 1 cup of water
- 1 tablespoon sunflower oil

1. Pour sunflower oil in the pan. Preheat it.
2. Add onion and mushrooms and cook for 5 minutes or until the vegetables are tender.
3. Then transfer the mixture in the mixing bowl.
4. Add kale, cayenne pepper, and ricotta cheese. Carefully mix the mixture.
5. Then fill the corn husks with kale mixture and roll in the shape of tamales.
6. Put them in the Crock Pot.
7. Add water and close the lid.

8. Cook the tamales on Low for 5 hours.

per serving: 98 calories, 4.9g protein, 6.7g carbohydrates, 6.1g fat, 1.1g fiber, 10mg cholesterol, 50mg sodium, 226mg potassium.

BBQ Beer Beef Tenderloin

Yield: 4 servings | **Prep time:** 10 minutes | **Cook time:** 10 hours

- ¼ cup beer
- 1-pound beef tenderloin
- ½ cup BBQ sauce
- 1 teaspoon fennel seeds
- 1 teaspoon olive oil

1. Mix BBQ sauce with beer, fennel seeds, and olive oil.
2. Pour the liquid in the Crock Pot.
3. Add beef tenderloin and close the lid.
4. Cook the meal on Low for 10 hours.

per serving: 299 calories, 33g protein, 12.1g carbohydrates, 11.7g fat, 0.4g fiber, 104mg cholesterol, 418mg sodium, 482mg potassium.

Cajun Beef

Yield: 4 servings | **Prep time:** 10 minutes | **Cook time:** 5 hours

- 1-pound beef ribs
- 1 tablespoon Cajun seasonings
- 3 tablespoons lemon juice
- 1 tablespoon coconut oil, melted
- ½ cup of water

1. Rub the beef ribs with Cajun seasonings and sprinkle with lemon juice.
2. Then pour the coconut oil in the Crock Pot.
3. Add beef ribs and water.
4. Close the lid and cook the beef on high for 5 hours.

per serving: 243 calories, 34.5g protein, 0.2g carbohydrates, 10.6g fat, 0.1g fiber, 101mg cholesterol, 115mg sodium, 471mg potassium.

Old Fashioned Shredded Beef

Yield: 4 servings | **Prep time:** 15 minutes | **Cook time:** 6 hours

- ½ cup of canned soup
- 1 cup of water
- 1-pound beef tenderloin
- 1 teaspoon peppercorns

1. Pour water in the Crock Pot.
2. Add peppercorns and beef tenderloin.
3. Close the lid and cook the meat on High for 5 hours.
4. After this, drain water and shred the meat with the help of the forks.
5. Add canned soup and stir well.
6. Cook the beef on High for 1 hour.

per serving: 247 calories, 33.4g protein, 1.8g carbohydrates, 10.9g fat, 0.1g fiber, 106mg cholesterol, 291mg sodium, 427mg potassium.

Chipotle Beef Strips

Yield: 4 servings | **Prep time:** 15 minutes | **Cook time:** 7 hours

- 1 tablespoon sunflower oil

- 1 teaspoon minced garlic
- 1 tablespoon chipotle paste
- 2 tablespoons fish sauce
- ¼ cup marinara sauce
- 1 teaspoon ground black pepper
- 1/3 cup water
- 1-pound beef brisket, cut into strips

1. Mix beef brisket with ground black pepper, marinara sauce, fish sauce, chipotle paste, and minced garlic.
2. Add the sunflower oil and transfer the meat mixture in the Crock Pot.
3. Add water and close the lid.
4. Cook the beef strips on Low for 7 hours.

per serving: 273 calories, 35.5g protein, 4.6g carbohydrates, 11.6g fat, 0.6g fiber, 103mg cholesterol, 880mg sodium, 542mg potassium.

Beef Burger
Yield: 4 servings | **Prep time:** 20 minutes | **Cook time:** 6 hours

- 1 teaspoon ground black pepper
- 12 oz ground beef
- ¼ cup Cheddar cheese, shredded
- 1 teaspoon salt
- 1 tablespoon sunflower oil
- ¼ cup cream

1. Mix ground beef with salt, and ground black pepper.
2. Then add shredded cheese and carefully mix the meat mixture.
3. Pour sunflower oil in the Crock Pot.
4. Then make the burgers and place them in the Crock Pot.
5. Add cream and close the lid.
6. Cook the meal on Low for 6 hours.

per serving: 228 calories, 27.7g protein, 0.9g carbohydrates, 12g fat, 0.1g fiber, 86mg cholesterol, 686mg sodium, 362mg potassium.

Mussaman Curry
Yield: 4 servings | **Prep time:** 15 minutes | **Cook time:** 5 hours

- 16 oz beef sirloin, cubed
- 1 tablespoon curry powder
- 2 tablespoons coconut aminos
- 2 tablespoons soy sauce
- 1 tablespoon sesame oil
- 2 tablespoons peanut butter
- ¼ cup peanuts, chopped
- 1 cup coconut cream

1. Mix curry powder with coconut aminos, soy sauce, sesame oil, and coconut cream.
2. After this, mix the curry mixture with beef and transfer in the Crock Pot.
3. Add all remaining ingredients and mix well.
4. Close the lid and cook the curry on High for 5 hours.

per serving: 494 calories, 40.8g protein, 9.4g carbohydrates, 33.5g fat, 3.2g fiber, 101mg cholesterol, 582mg sodium, 773mg potassium.

Spanish Beef Roast

Yield: 5 servings | **Prep time:** 10 minutes | **Cook time:** 4.5 hours

- 2-pounds beef rump roast
- 1 teaspoon smoked paprika
- 1 tablespoon lemon juice
- 1 capsicum, chopped
- 1 cup potatoes, chopped
- ½ cup onion, chopped
- ¼ cup fresh parsley
- 3 cups of water

1. Mix beef with smoked paprika, lemon juice, and parsley and transfer in the Crock Pot.
2. Add all remaining ingredients and close the lid.
3. Cook the meat on High for 4.5 hours.

per serving: 288 calories, 41.1g protein, 6.8g carbohydrates, 9.8g fat, 1.6g fiber, 120mg cholesterol, 115mg sodium, 194mg potassium.

3-Ingredients Beef Roast
Yield: 6 servings | **Prep time:** 10 minutes | **Cook time:** 5 hours

- 2-pounds beef chuck roast, chopped
- 1 teaspoon ground cumin
- 1 cup of water

1. Put all ingredients from the list above in the Crock Pot.
2. Close the lid and cook the meal on High for 5 hours.

per serving: 550 calories, 39.6g protein, 0.2g carbohydrates, 42.1g fat, 0g fiber, 156mg cholesterol, 99mg sodium, 351mg potassium.

Soy Sauce Marinated Meatballs
Yield: 4 servings | **Prep time:** 15 minutes | **Cook time:** 5 hours

- ¼ cup of soy sauce
- 12 oz ground beef
- 1 onion, minced
- 1 teaspoon cayenne pepper
- ½ teaspoon dried mint
- 1 tablespoon coconut oil
- ¼ cup of water

1. In the mixing bowl mix ground beef with minced onion, cayenne pepper, and dried mint.
2. Make the small balls.
3. Melt the coconut oil in the skillet.
4. Add meatballs and roast them for 3 minutes per side.
5. After this, transfer the meatballs in the Crock Pot.
6. Add water and soy sauce.
7. Close the lid and cook the meatballs on low for 5 hours.

per serving: 208 calories, 27.2g protein, 4.1g carbohydrates, 8.8g fat, 0.9g fiber, 76mg cholesterol, 956mg sodium, 428mg potassium.

Bulgogi
Yield: 6 servings | **Prep time:** 15 minutes | **Cook time:** 8 hours

- 1-pound beef chuck roast
- 5 tablespoons soy sauce
- 2 tablespoons rice vinegar

- 2 tablespoons cornflour
- 2 tablespoons sesame oil
- 1 teaspoon ground black pepper
- 1 teaspoon chili powder
- 2 cups beef stock
- 1 onion, sliced
- 1 teaspoon sriracha
1.   Chop the beef and put it in the Crock Pot.
2.   Then add soy sauce, rice vinegar, cornflour, sesame oil, ground black pepper, chili powder, onion, and sriracha.
3.   Mix the mixture well and add beef stock.
4.   Close the lid and cook the meal on low for 8 hours.
 per serving: 350 calories, 22g protein, 5.3g carbohydrates, 25.9g fat, 0.9g fiber, 78mg cholesterol, 1072mg sodium, 292mg potassium.

Sautéed Beef Liver
Yield: 4 servings | **Prep time:** 15 minutes | **Cook time:** 5 hours
- 12 oz beef liver, cut into strips
- 1 cup of water
- ½ cup cream
- 1 teaspoon salt
- 1 teaspoon ground black pepper
- 1 onion, sliced
- 1 tablespoon flour
- 1 tablespoon butter
1.   Sprinkle the beef liver with ground black pepper and salt.
2.   Then sprinkle it with flour.
3.   After this, put the sliced onion in the Crock Pot in one layer.
4.   Add the layer of the liver.
5.   Then add water, butter, and cream.
6.   Close the lid and cook the meal on high for 5 hours.
 per serving: 213 calories, 23.4g protein, 9.7g carbohydrates, 8.6g fat, 0.8g fiber, 337mg cholesterol, 680mg sodium, 360mg potassium.

Beef Heart Saute
Yield: 4 servings | **Prep time:** 15 minutes | **Cook time:** 6 hours
- 1-pound beef heart, chopped
- 1 teaspoon fresh ginger, minced
- 2 tablespoons apple cider vinegar
- 1 sweet pepper, chopped
- 1 red onion, chopped
- 2 cups tomatoes
- 2 tablespoons sunflower oil
- 1 cup of water
1.   Heat the sunflower oil until hot in the skillet.
2.   Add chopped beef heart and roast it for 10 minutes on medium heat.
3.   Then transfer it in the Crock Pot.
4.   Add all remaining ingredients and close the lid.
5.   Cook the saute on low for 6 hours.
 per serving: 289 calories, 33.7g protein, 8.9g carbohydrates, 12.7g fat, 2.1g fiber, 240mg cholesterol, 75mg sodium, 570mg potassium.

Wine-Braised Beef Heart
Yield: 4 servings | **Prep time:** 15 minutes | **Cook time:** 5 hours
- 10 oz beef heart
- 1/3 cup red wine
- ½ cup beef broth
- ½ cup potatoes, chopped
- 3 oz fennel bulb, chopped
- 1 teaspoon salt
- 1 teaspoon peppercorns
- 1 teaspoon brown sugar
- Cooking spray
1.   Spray the skillet with cooking spray.
2.   Then chop the beef heart roughly and put it in the skillet.
3.   Roast the beef heart on high heat for 6 minutes (for 3 minutes per side).
4.   Transfer the beef heart in the Crock Pot.
5.   Add all remaining ingredients and close the lid.
6.   Cook the meal on High for 5 hours.
 per serving: 162 calories, 21.4g protein, 6.3g carbohydrates, 3.6g fat, 1.3g fiber, 150mg cholesterol, 732mg sodium, 373mg potassium.

Beef Heart in Creamy Gravy
Yield: 4 servings | **Prep time:** 10 minutes | **Cook time:** 6 hours
- 12 oz beef heart, cut into slices
- 1 cup cream
- 1 teaspoon cornflour
- 1 teaspoon salt
- 3 garlic cloves, diced
- 1 tablespoon butter
1.   Sprinkle the beef heart with salt and cornflour.
2.   Then put butter in the Crock Pot.
3.   Add a beef heart, garlic, and cream.
4.   Close the lid and cook the meal on Low for 6 hours.
 per serving: 210 calories, 24.9g protein, 3.2g carbohydrates, 10.3g fat, 0.1g fiber, 199mg cholesterol, 672mg sodium, 220mg potassium.

Beef and Tater Tots Casserole
Yield: 4 servings | **Prep time:** 15 minutes | **Cook time:** 4.5 hours
- 8 oz ground beef
- 4 oz tater tots
- 1 cup of coconut milk
- 1 cup cheddar cheese, shredded
- 1 tablespoon sesame oil
- 1 teaspoon cayenne pepper
1.   Brush the Crock Pot bottom with sesame oil.
2.   After this, mix the ground beef with cayenne pepper.
3.   Put the ground beef mixture in the Crock Pot in one layer.
4.   Top it with tater tots.
5.   Add coconut milk and cheddar cheese. Cook the casserole on High for 4.5 hours.
 per serving: 443 calories, 26.2g protein, 11.8g carbohydrates, 33.1g fat, 2.2g fiber, 80mg cholesterol, 358mg sodium, 511mg potassium.

Beef Stifado

Yield: 4 servings | **Prep time:** 15 minutes | **Cook time:** 7 hours

- 1-pound beef stew meat
- 1 onion, chopped
- 1 tablespoon sunflower oil
- 1 cup tomatoes, canned, diced
- 1 teaspoon ground nutmeg
- 1 cup red wine
- ½ cup ketchup
- 1 teaspoon dried rosemary

1. Mix red wine with ketchup and dried rosemary and pour it in the Crock Pot.
2. Then add tomatoes and ground nutmeg.
3. Add onion.
4. Heat the sunflower oil in the skillet well.
5. Add beef stew meat and roast it on high heat for 3 minutes per side.
6. Then add the meat in the Crock Pot, close the lid, and cook on Low for 7 hours.

per serving: 343 calories, 35.7g protein, 13.9g carbohydrates, 11g fat, 1.5g fiber, 101mg cholesterol, 415mg sodium, 781mg potassium.

Marinated Beef Neck Bones

Yield: 6 servings | **Prep time:** 15 minutes | **Cook time:** 5 hours

- 2-pounds beef neck bones, chopped
- ½ cup apple cider vinegar
- 1 lemon, chopped
- ½ cup of water
- 1 teaspoon cayenne pepper
- 1 teaspoon salt
- 2 tablespoons olive oil
- 1 bay leaf

1. Heat the olive oil in the skillet until hot.
2. Add beef neck bones and roast them for 3 minutes per side.
3. Transfer the meat in the Crock Pot.
4. Add all remaining ingredients and carefully mix.
5. Close the lid and cook the meal on high for 5 hours.

per serving: 511 calories, 35.7g protein, 1.4g carbohydrates, 39.2g fat, 0.4g fiber, 98mg cholesterol, 491mg sodium, 462mg potassium.

Beef San Marco Steak

Yield: 4 servings | **Prep time:** 10 minutes | **Cook time:** 5 hours

- 4 beef steaks
- 2 tablespoons avocado oil
- 1 teaspoon minced garlic
- 1 teaspoon dried oregano
- 1 tablespoon balsamic vinegar
- ½ cup onion soup, canned
- ¼ cup red wine

1. Rub the beef steaks with minced ginger, dried oregano, and sprinkle with balsamic vinegar.
2. Transfer the beef steaks in the Crock Pot.
3. Add all remaining ingredients from the list above and close the lid.

4. Cook the meal on High for 5 hours.

per serving: 197 calories, 26.9g protein, 3.3g carbohydrates, 6.7g fat, 0.7g fiber, 76mg cholesterol, 322mg sodium, 409mg potassium.

Ginger Beef Balls

Yield: 4 servings | **Prep time:** 15 minutes | **Cook time:** 4 hours

- 1 teaspoon ground ginger
- 1 teaspoon garlic powder
- 1 teaspoon chili flakes
- ¼ cup butter
- ¼ cup of water
- 12 oz ground beef
- 1 egg, beaten

1. In the mixing bowl mix ground beef, egg, chili flakes, garlic powder, and ground ginger.
2. Make the small balls.
3. After this, melt the butter in the skillet.
4. Add meatballs and roast them for 3 minutes per side.
5. Transfer the meatballs in the Crock Pot. Add water and close the lid.
6. Cook the meatballs on High for 4 hours.

per serving: 279 calories, 27.5g protein, 0.9g carbohydrates, 17.9g fat, 0.1g fiber, 147mg cholesterol, 154mg sodium, 376mg potassium.

Pork&Lamb

Lamb in Curry Sauce

Yield: 4 servings | **Prep time:** 15 minutes | **Cook time:** 5 hours

- 1 teaspoon curry paste
- 1-pound lamb fillet, sliced
- 1 tablespoon pomegranate juice
- ½ cup of water
- ½ cup of coconut milk
- 1 onion, sliced
- 1 teaspoon lemongrass
- 1 tablespoon coconut oil

1. Melt the coconut oil in the skillet.
2. Add lamb fillet and roast it for 2 minutes per side on low heat.
3. After this, transfer the lamb in the Crock Pot.
4. In the bowl mix curry paste, pomegranate juice, coconut milk, water, and lemongrass.
5. Pour the liquid over the lamb.
6. Add sliced onion and cook the meal on High for 5 hours.

per serving: 329 calories, 32.9g protein, 4.7g carbohydrates, 19.6g fat, 1.3g fiber, 102mg cholesterol, 93mg sodium, 503mg potassium.

Rosemary Lamb Shoulder

Yield: 3 servings | **Prep time:** 30 minutes | **Cook time:** 9 hours

- 9 oz lamb shoulder
- 1 tablespoon fresh rosemary
- ½ cup apple cider vinegar
- 1 tablespoon olive oil
- 1 cup of water
- 1 teaspoon ground black pepper
- 2 garlic cloves, peeled

1. Rub the lamb shoulder with olive oil and fresh rosemary.
2. Then put the lamb shoulder in the apple cider vinegar and leave for 30 minutes to marinate.
3. After this, transfer the lamb shoulder in the Crock Pot.
4. Add water, ground black pepper, and garlic cloves.
5. Close the lid and cook the meat on low for 9 hours.

per serving: 215 calories, 24.1g protein, 2.2g carbohydrates, 11.1g fat, 0.7g fiber, 77mg cholesterol, 70mg sodium, 342mg potassium.

Lamb Saute

Yield: 5 servings | **Prep time:** 15 minutes | **Cook time:** 4.5 hours

- 1 cup tomatoes, chopped
- 1 cup bell pepper, chopped
- 1 chili pepper, chopped
- 1 tablespoon avocado oil
- 12 oz lamb fillet, chopped
- ½ cup cremini mushrooms, sliced
- 1 cup of water

1. Heat the avocado oil in the skillet well.

2. Add chopped lamb and roast it for 5 minutes. Stir the meat from time to time.
3. After this, transfer the meat in the Crock Pot and add all remaining ingredients.
4. Close the lid and cook the saute on High for 4.5 hours.

per serving: 147 calories, 19.9g protein, 3.7g carbohydrates, 5.5g fat, 0.9g fiber, 61mg cholesterol, 56mg sodium, 402mg potassium.

Aromatic Lamb

Yield: 4 servings | **Prep time:** 10 minutes | **Cook time:** hours

- 1 tablespoon minced garlic
- 1 teaspoon ground black pepper
- ½ teaspoon salt
- 1 teaspoon sesame oil
- 1-pound lamb sirloin, chopped
- ½ cup of water

1. Mix the lamb with minced garlic, ground black pepper, and salt.
2. Then sprinkle the meat with sesame oil and transfer in the Crock Pot.
3. Add water and cook the meat on low for 8 hours.

per serving: 246 calories, 32.3g protein, 1g carbohydrates, 11.6g fat, 0.2g fiber, 104mg cholesterol, 373mg sodium, 393mg potassium.

Sweet Lamb Tagine

Yield: 6 servings | **Prep time:** 10 minutes | **Cook time:** 10 hours

- 12 oz lamb fillet, chopped
- 1 cup apricots, pitted, chopped
- 1 cup red wine
- 1 jalapeno pepper, sliced
- 1 teaspoon ground nutmeg
- 1 cup of water
- 1 teaspoon ground ginger

1. Mix lamb with ground nutmeg and ground ginger.
2. Transfer the lamb meat in the Crock Pot.
3. Add water, jalapeno pepper, red wine, and apricots.
4. Close the lid and cook the tagine for 10 hours on Low.

per serving: 154 calories, 16.4g protein, 4.4g carbohydrates, 4.5g fat, 0.7g fiber, 51mg cholesterol, 47mg sodium, 307mg potassium.

Lamb Meatballs

Yield: 4 servings | **Prep time:** 10 minutes | **Cook time:** 4 hours

- 2 tablespoons minced onion
- 9 oz lamb fillet, minced
- 1 teaspoon Italian seasonings
- 1 teaspoon flour
- 1 tablespoon olive oil
- ½ teaspoon salt
- ½ cup of water

1. In the bowl mix minced lamb, minced onion, Italian seasonings, flour, and salt.

2. Make the small meatballs.
3. After this, preheat the olive oil in the skillet.
4. Add meatballs and roast them on high heat for 30 seconds per side.
5. Then transfer the meatballs in the Crock Pot.
6. Add water and cook the meal on high for 4 hours.
 per serving: 157 calories, 18g protein, 1.1g carbohydrates, 8.6g fat, 0.1g fiber, 58mg cholesterol, 341mg sodium, 223mg potassium.

Hot Lamb Strips
Yield: 6 servings | **Prep time:** 7 minutes | **Cook time:** 5 hours
- 14 oz lamb fillet, cut into strips 1 teaspoon cayenne pepper
- 2 tablespoons butter, melted
- 1 tablespoon hot sauce
- ½ cup of water
1. Mix lamb strips with hot sauce and cayenne pepper.
2. Transfer them in the Crock Pot.
3. After this, add water and butter.
4. Close the lid and cook the lamb on High for 5 hours.
 per serving: 158 calories, 18.7g protein, 0.2g carbohydrates, 8.8g fat, 0.1g fiber, 70mg cholesterol, 142mg sodium, 232mg potassium.

Braised Lamb Shank
Yield: 4 servings | **Prep time:** 10 minutes | **Cook time:** 10 hours
- 4 lamb shanks
- 1 cup of water
- ½ cup tomato juice
- 1 tablespoon cornflour
- 1 teaspoon salt
- 1 teaspoon cayenne pepper
- 1 onion, chopped
- ½ carrot, chopped
1. Mix tomato juice with cornflour and pour the liquid in the Crock Pot.
2. Add lamb shanks, water, salt, cayenne pepper, onion, and carrot.
3. Close the lid and cook the meat on low for 10 hours.
 per serving: 427 calories, 33.8g protein, 25.3g carbohydrates, 19.2g fat, 5.2g fiber, 114mg cholesterol, 1894mg sodium, 150mg potassium.

Sweet Lamb Ribs
Yield: 3 servings | **Prep time:** 10 minutes | **Cook time:** 9 hours
- 8 oz lamb ribs, chopped
- 1 teaspoon tomato paste
- 2 teaspoons liquid honey
- ½ cup butter
- ¼ cup of water
1. Rub the lamb ribs with tomato paste and liquid honey.
2. Then place them in the Crock Pot.
3. Add butter and water.

4. Close the lid and cook the meat on low for 9 hours.
 per serving: 414 calories, 15.8g protein, 4.2g carbohydrates, 37.4g fat, 0.1g fiber, 132mg cholesterol, 274mg sodium, 30mg potassium.

Lamb Chops
Yield: 4 servings | **Prep time:** 10 minutes | **Cook time:** 5 hours
- 1 teaspoon ground black pepper
- ½ teaspoon salt
- 1 teaspoon sesame oil
- 4 lamb chops
- 1/3 cup water
1. Sprinkle the lamb chops with sesame oil, salt, and ground black pepper.
2. Place the lamb chops in the Crock Pot and add water.
3. Close the lid and cook the meal on High for 5 hours.
 per serving: 169 calories, 23.9g protein, 0.3g carbohydrates, 7.4g fat, 0.1g fiber, 77mg cholesterol, 356mg sodium, 292mg potassium.

BBQ Bratwurst
Yield: 5 servings | **Prep time:** 10 minutes | **Cook time:** 4 hours
- 1-pound bratwurst
- 4 tablespoons BBQ sauce
- 1 teaspoon olive oil
- ¼ cup of water
- 1 teaspoon chili powder
1. Roast the bratwurst in the olive oil for 1 minute per side.
2. Then transfer the bratwurst in the Crock Pot.
3. Add water and BBQ sauce.
4. Close the lid and cook the meal on High for 4 hours.
 per serving: 330 calories, 12.5g protein, 7.4g carbohydrates, 27.5g fat, 0.3g fiber, 67mg cholesterol, 913mg sodium, 352mg potassium.

Cilantro Pork Chops
Yield: 4 servings | **Prep time:** 10 minutes | **Cook time:** 8 hours
- 4 pork chops
- 1 teaspoon dried cilantro
- 1 teaspoon olive oil
- 1 teaspoon lemon juice
- ½ teaspoon salt
- ¼ cup of coconut milk
1. In the shallow bowl mix dried cilantro, olive oil, salt, and lemon juice.
2. Brush the pork chops with cilantro mixture from both sides and transfer in the Crock Pot.
3. Add coconut milk and cook on Low for 8 hours.
 per serving: 301 calories, 18.3g protein, 0.9g carbohydrates, 24.6g fat, 0.3g fiber, 69mg cholesterol, 349mg sodium, 317mg potassium.

Tender Goulash
Yield: 4 servings | **Prep time:** 10 minutes | **Cook time:** 9 hours

- 1 onion, chopped
- 1 teaspoon cornflour
- 1 teaspoon ground turmeric
- 1 teaspoon ground paprika
- 1-pound pork chunk, chopped
- 1 teaspoon tomato paste
- 1 teaspoon salt
- 1 cup of water

1. Mix water with cornflour until smooth and pour in the Crock Pot.
2. Add onion, ground turmeric, paprika, pork chunk, tomato paste, and salt.
3. Gently stir the goulash mixture and cook it on Low for 9 hours.

per serving: 256 calories, 30.3g protein, 4g carbohydrates, 12.1g fat, 1g fiber, 89mg cholesterol, 924mg sodium, 83mg potassium.

Swedish Style Meatballs
Yield: 4 servings | **Prep time:** 10 minutes | **Cook time:** 5.5 hours

- ½ cup of water
- ½ cup cream
- 1 tablespoon flour
- 9 oz minced pork
- 1 teaspoon ground black pepper
- 1 teaspoon salt
- 1 tablespoon breadcrumbs
- 1 tablespoon fresh parsley, chopped

1. Make the meatballs: mix minced pork with ground black pepper, salt, and breadcrumbs.
2. Make the small meatballs and place them in the Crock Pot in one layer.
3. After this, mix water with cream and flour.
4. Pour the liquid over the meatballs and cook them on High for 5.5 hours.

per serving: 126 calories, 17.5g protein, 4.1g carbohydrates, 4.1g fat, 0.3g fiber, 52mg cholesterol, 642mg sodium, 297mg potassium.

Garlic Pork Ribs
Yield: 3 servings | **Prep time:** 10 minutes | **Cook time:** 5.5 hours

- 8 oz pork ribs, chopped
- 1 teaspoon garlic powder
- 1 teaspoon avocado oil
- ½ teaspoon salt
- ½ cup of water

1. Preheat the skillet until hot.
2. Then sprinkle the pork ribs with garlic powder and avocado oil and put in the hot skillet.
3. Roast the ribs for 3 minutes per side or until they are light brown.
4. Then transfer the pork ribs in the Crock Pot and sprinkle with salt.
5. Add water and cook the ribs on high for 5.5 hours.

per serving: 212 calories, 20.2g protein, 0.8g carbohydrates, 13.6g fat, 0.2g fiber, 78mg cholesterol, 433mg sodium, 233mg potassium.

Sweet and Sour Pulled Pork

Yield: 4 servings | **Prep time:** 10 minutes | **Cook time:** 6 hours

- 1-pound pork sirloin
- 2 cups of water
- 2 tablespoons ketchup
- 2 tablespoons lemon juice
- 1 teaspoon cayenne pepper
- 1 teaspoon liquid honey

1. Pour water in the Crock Pot.
2. Add pork sirloin and close the lid.
3. Cook the meat on high for 6 hours.
4. Then drain water and shred the meat.
5. Add ketchup, lemon juice, cayenne pepper, and liquid honey.
6. Stir the mixture carefully and transfer in the serving plates.

per serving: 207 calories, 23.3g protein, 3.7g carbohydrates, 10.2g fat, 0.2g fiber, 80mg cholesterol, 154mg sodium, 49mg potassium.

Sandwich Pork Chops
Yield: 2 servings | **Prep time:** 10 minutes | **Cook time:** 4.5 hours

- 2 pork chops
- 1 teaspoon mayonnaise
- 1 teaspoon ground black pepper
- ¼ teaspoon garlic powder
- ½ cup of water

1. Pour water in the Crock Pot.
2. Add garlic powder and ground black pepper.
3. Then add pork chops and cook them on High for 4.5 hours.
4. Remove the cooked pork chops from the water and brush with mayonnaise.

per serving: 269 calories, 18.2g protein, 1.5g carbohydrates, 20.7g fat, 0.3g fiber, 69mg cholesterol, 76mg sodium, 293mg potassium.

BBQ Meatballs
Yield: 4 servings | **Prep time:** 10 minutes | **Cook time:** 7 hours

- 3 tablespoons BBQ sauce
- 10 oz minced pork
- 1 garlic clove, diced
- 1 teaspoon chili powder
- 3 tablespoons water
- 1 teaspoon salt
- 1 teaspoon dried cilantro
- 4 tablespoons coconut oil

1. In the bowl mix minced pork, garlic, chili powder, water, salt, and dried cilantro.
2. Make the medium size meatballs and arrange them in the Crock Pot in one layer.
3. Add coconut oil and close the lid.
4. Cook the meatballs on low for 7 hours.
5. When the meatballs are cooked, brush them gently with BBW sauce.

per serving: 239 calories, 18.7g protein, 4.9g carbohydrates, 16.2g fat, 0.3g fiber, 52mg cholesterol, 760mg sodium, 339mg potassium.

Cranberry Minced Meat

Yield: 5 servings | **Prep time:** 10 minutes | **Cook time:** 6 hours

- ¼ cup cranberry sauce
- 1-pound pork mince
- 1 tablespoon butter
- ¼ cup of water
- 1 teaspoon chili powder
- 1 teaspoon dried parsley
1. Melt butter and pour in the Crock Pot.
2. Add pork mince, chili powder, and dried parsley.
3. Then add water and cranberry sauce. Stir the mixture well.
4. Close the lid and cook the meal on Low for 6 hours.

per serving: 274 calories, 0.1g protein, 57.1g carbohydrates, 6g fat, 1.3g fiber, 6mg cholesterol, 22mg sodium, 22mg potassium.

Pork Casserole
Yield: 4 servings | **Prep time:** 10 minutes | **Cook time:** 8 hours

- 1 cup cauliflower, chopped
- 1 teaspoon ground black pepper
- 1 teaspoon cayenne pepper
- 7 oz pork mince
- 1 cup Cheddar cheese, shredded
- ½ cup cream
- 1 teaspoon sesame oil
1. Brush the Crock Pot bowl with sesame oil from inside.
2. Then mix minced pork with ground black pepper and cayenne pepper.
3. Place the meat in the Crock Pot and flatten gently.
4. After this, top it with cauliflower and Cheddar cheese.
5. Add cream and close the lid.
6. Cook the casserole on Low for 8 hours.

per serving: 288 calories, 7.9g protein, 34g carbohydrates, 14.3g fat, 1.4g fiber, 35mg cholesterol, 193mg sodium, 130mg potassium

Pesto Pork Chops
Yield: 4 servings | **Prep time:** 10 minutes | **Cook time:** 8 hours

- 4 pork chops
- 4 teaspoons pesto sauce
- 4 tablespoons butter
1. Brush pork chops with pesto sauce.
2. Put butter in the Crock Pot.
3. Add pork chops and close the lid.
4. Cook the meat on low for 8 hours.
5. Then transfer the cooked pork chops in the plates and sprinkle with butter-pesto gravy from the Crock Pot.

per serving: 380 calories, 18.6g protein, 0.3g carbohydrates, 33.6g fat, 0.1g fiber, 101mg cholesterol, 89mg sodium, 279mg potassium

Meat and Mushrooms Saute
Yield: 4 servings | **Prep time:** 10 minutes | **Cook time:** 5 hours

- 8 oz pork sirloin, sliced
- 1 cup white mushrooms, chopped
- 1 onion, sliced
- 1 cup cream
- 1 teaspoon ground black pepper
- 1 teaspoon salt
1. Put all ingredients in the Crock Pot and carefully mix with the help of the spatula.
2. Then close the lid and cook the saute on High for 5 hours.

per serving: 156 calories, 13g protein, 5.4g carbohydrates, 9g fat, 0.9g fiber, 47mg cholesterol, 634mg sodium, 125mg potassium

Fall Pork
Yield: 4 servings | **Prep time:** 8 minutes | **Cook time:** 10 hours

- 9 oz pork tenderloin, chopped
- ½ cup carrot, chopped
- ½ cup pumpkin, chopped
- 2 cups of water
- 1 cup tomatoes, chopped
- 1 teaspoon Italian seasonings
- 1 teaspoon salt
1. Put all ingredients in the Crock Pot.
2. Close the lid and cook the meal on Low for 10 hours.
3. Carefully mix the cooked meal before serving.

per serving: 119 calories, 17.5g protein, 5.7g carbohydrates, 2.8g fat, 1.8g fiber, 47mg cholesterol, 635mg sodium, 484mg potassium

Indian Style Cardamom Pork
Yield: 4 servings | **Prep time:** 10 minutes | **Cook time:** 6 hours

- 1-pound pork steak, tenderized
- 1 teaspoon ground cardamom
- ½ cup of coconut milk
- 1 teaspoon chili powder
- 1 teaspoon ground turmeric
- 1 teaspoon cashew butter
- ¼ cup of water
1. Cut the pork steak into 4 servings and rub with ground cardamom, chili powder. And ground turmeric.
2. Place the meat in the Crock Pot.
3. Add cashew butter, water, and coconut milk.
4. Close the lid and cook the pork on high for 6 hours.

per serving: 295 calories, 21g protein, 7.2g carbohydrates, 21.1g fat, 1.9g fiber, 69mg cholesterol, 569mg sodium, 118mg potassium

Pork Rolls
Yield: 2 servings | **Prep time:** 10 minutes | **Cook time:** 4.5 hours

- 2 pork chops
- 2 oz Mozzarella, sliced
- 1 teaspoon cayenne pepper
- ¼ teaspoon salt
- 1 tablespoon mayonnaise
- ½ cup of water

1. Beat the pork chops gently and sprinkle with cayenne pepper and salt.
2. Then brush one side of pork chops with mayonnaise and top with mozzarella.
3. Roll the pork chops and secure the prepared rolls with toothpicks.
4. Place the pork rolls in the Crock Pot.
5. Add water and cook them on High for 4.5 hours.
per serving: 308 calories, 15.1g protein, 19.8g carbohydrates, 18.7g fat, 1.9g fiber, 30mg cholesterol, 1103mg sodium, 19mg potassium

Pork Ribs in Soy Sauce
Yield: 5 servings | **Prep time:** 10 minutes | **Cook time:** 5 hours
- 1-pound pork ribs
- ½ cup of soy sauce
- ½ cup of water
- 1 onion, sliced
- 1 garlic clove, sliced
- 1 teaspoon sesame seeds
- ½ teaspoon sugar
- ½ teaspoon chili powder
1. Put all ingredients in the Crock Pot and carefully stir them with the help of the spatula.
2. After this, close the lid and cook the pork ribs on high for 5 hours.
3. When the pork ribs are cooked, transfer them in the bowls and top with soy sauce liquid.
per serving: 277 calories, 26.1g protein, 4.9g carbohydrates, 16.4g fat, 0.8g fiber, 93mg cholesterol, 1494mg sodium, 359mg potassium

Pineapple Pork
Yield: 4 servings | **Prep time:** 10 minutes | **Cook time:** 4.5 hours
- ½ cup pineapple, canned, chopped
- 10 oz pork sirloin, sliced
- ½ cup of water
- 1 teaspoon smoked paprika
- ½ teaspoon chili flakes
- 1 teaspoon butter
1. Melt the butter in the skillet and add sliced pork sirloin.
2. Sprinkle it with smoked paprika and chili flakes and roast for 5 minutes on high heat.
3. Then transfer the meat in the Crock Pot, add water and pineapple.
4. Close the lid and cook the meal on High for 4.5 hours.
per serving: 147 calories, 14.8g protein, 3g carbohydrates, 8g fat, 0.5g fiber, 47mg cholesterol, 46mg sodium, 36mg potassium

Apple Pork
Yield: 4 servings | **Prep time:** 10 minutes | **Cook time:** 8 hours
- 1-pound pork tenderloin, chopped
- 1 teaspoon ground cinnamon
- 1 tablespoon maple syrup
- 1 cup apples, chopped
- 1 cup of water

1. Mix apples with ground cinnamon and put in the Crock Pot.
2. Add water, maple syrup, and pork tenderloin.
3. Close the lid and cook the meal on Low for 8 hours.
per serving: 206 calories, 29.9g protein, 11.5g carbohydrates, 4.1g fat, 1.7g fiber, 83mg cholesterol, 67mg sodium, 550mg potassium

Taco Pork
Yield: 5 servings | **Prep time:** 10 minutes | **Cook time:** 5 hours
- 1-pound pork shoulder, chopped
- 1 tablespoon taco seasonings
- 1 tablespoon lemon juice
- 1 cup of water
1. Mix pork shoulder with taco seasonings and place in the Crock Pot.
2. Add water and cook it on High for 5 hours.
3. After this, transfer the cooked meat in the bowl and shred gently with the help of the fork.
4. Add lemon juice and shake gently.
per serving: 274 calories, 21.1g protein, 1.7g carbohydrates, 19.4g fat, 0g fiber, 82mg cholesterol, 232mg sodium, 303mg potassium

Salsa Meat
Yield: 4 servings | **Prep time:** 10 minutes | **Cook time:** 4 hours
- 1-pound pork sirloin, sliced
- 1 cup tomatillo salsa
- 2 garlic cloves, diced
- 1 teaspoon apple cider vinegar
- ½ cup of water
1. Put all ingredients in the Crock Pot and carefully mix.
2. Then close the lid and cook the salsa meat on high for 4 hours.
per serving: 214 calories, 23.8g protein, 2.3g carbohydrates, 11.2g fat, 0.4g fiber, 71mg cholesterol, 169mg sodium, 75mg potassium

Tomato Pork Sausages
Yield: 5 servings | **Prep time:** 10 minutes | **Cook time:** 7 hours
- 1-pound pork sausages, chopped
- 2 cups tomatoes, chopped
- ½ cup of water
- 1 tablespoon butter
- 1 teaspoon salt
- 1 teaspoon chili powder
1. Mix pork sausages with chili powder and salt and transfer in the Crock Pot.
2. Add butter, water, and tomatoes.
3. Close the lid and cook the meal on Low for 7 hours.
per serving: 342 calories, 18.3g protein, 3.1g carbohydrates, 28.3g fat, 1g fiber, 82mg cholesterol, 1170mg sodium, 448mg potassium

Thyme Pork Belly
Yield: 6 servings | **Prep time:** 10 minutes | **Cook time:** 10 hours

- 10 oz pork belly
- 1 teaspoon salt
- 1 teaspoon ground thyme
- 1 teaspoon ground black pepper
- 1 teaspoon garlic powder
- ½ cup of water

1. In the shallow bowl mix salt, ground thyme, ground black pepper, and garlic powder.
2. Then rub the pork belly with the spice mixture and place it in the Crock Pot.
3. Add water and close the lid.
4. Cook the pork belly on Low for 10 hours.
5. Then slice the cooked pork belly into servings.

per serving: 221 calories, 22g protein, 0.7g carbohydrates, 12.7g fat, 0.2g fiber, 55mg cholesterol, 1152mg sodium, 11mg potassium

Horseradish Pork Chops
Yield: 4 servings | **Prep time:** 10 minutes | **Cook time:** 5 hours

- 4 pork chops
- 5 tablespoons horseradish
- ½ cup of water
- 1 onion, sliced
- 1 tablespoon avocado oil

1. Mix avocado oil with horseradish and rub the pork chops/
2. Put the pork chops and all remaining horseradish mixture in the Crock Pot.
3. Add onion and water.
4. Cook the pork chops on high for 5 hours.

per serving: 281 calories, 18.5g protein, 4.9g carbohydrates, 20.5g fat, 1.4g fiber, 69mg cholesterol, 117mg sodium, 373mg potassium

Oregano Pork Strips
Yield: 4 servings | **Prep time:** 5 minutes | **Cook time:** 7 hours

- 12 oz pork tenderloin, cut into strips
- 1 tablespoon dried oregano
- 1 cup of water
- 1 teaspoon salt

1. Place pork strips in the Crock Pot.
2. Add all remaining ingredients and close the lid.
3. Cook the pork strips on Low for 7 hours.
4. Serve the cooked meal with hot gravy from the Crock Pot.

per serving: 125 calories, 22.4g protein, 0.7g carbohydrates, 3.1g fat, 0.5g fiber, 62mg cholesterol, 632mg sodium, 378mg potassium

Cumin Pork
Yield: 6 servings | **Prep time:** 10 minutes | **Cook time:** 5 hours

- 1-pound pork shoulder, chopped
- 1 teaspoon cumin seeds
- 1 teaspoon garlic powder
- 1 teaspoon ground nutmeg
- 1 carrot, diced
- 2 cup of water
- 1 teaspoon salt

1. Roast the cumin seeds in the skillet for 2-3 minutes or until the seeds start to smell.
2. Then place them in the Crock Pot.
3. Add all remaining ingredients and close the lid.
4. Cook the pork on high for 5 hours.

per serving: 230 calories, 17.8g protein, 1.7g carbohydrates, 16.4g fat, 0.4g fiber, 68mg cholesterol, 449mg sodium, 295mg potassium

Pork Meatloaf
Yield: 4 servings | **Prep time:** 10 minutes | **Cook time:** 4 hours

- 8 oz pork mince
- ¼ cup onion, diced
- 1 teaspoon ground black pepper
- 1 teaspoon chili powder
- 1 egg, beaten
- 1 teaspoon olive oil
- ½ teaspoon salt
- 1 teaspoon tomato paste
- Cooking spray

1. Spray the bottom of the Crock Pot with cooking spray.
2. After this, mix the pork mince, onion, ground black pepper, chili powder, egg, olive oil, and salt.
3. Transfer the mixture in the Crock Pot and flatten it.
4. Then brush the surface of the meatloaf with tomato paste and cook it on High for 4 hours.

per serving: 188 calories, 1.7g protein, 36.9g carbohydrates, 4.7g fat, 1.1g fiber, 41mg cholesterol, 314mg sodium, 58mg potassium

Jamaican Pork Mix
Yield: 4 servings | **Prep time:** 10 minutes | **Cook time:** 4 hours

- 1 cup corn kernels, frozen
- 1 cup of water
- 1 teaspoon Jamaican spices
- 10 oz pork sirloin, chopped
- 1 tomato, chopped
- 1 teaspoon salt
- 1 teaspoon avocado oil

1. Roast the chopped pork sirloin in the avocado oil for 1 minute per side.
2. Then mix the meat with Jamaican spices and transfer in the Crock Pot.
3. Add all remaining ingredients and close the lid.
4. Cook the meal on High for 4 hours.

per serving: 174 calories, 23.5g protein, 7.9g carbohydrates, 5.4g fat, 1.3g fiber, 65mg cholesterol, 629mg sodium, 412mg potassium

Sweet Pork Strips
Yield: 2 servings | **Prep time:** 20 minutes | **Cook time:** 5 hours

- 6 oz pork loin, cut into strips
- 1 tablespoon maple syrup
- 1 teaspoon ground paprika
- ½ teaspoon salt
- 1 teaspoon butter
- 1 cup of water

1. Pour water in the Crock Pot.
2. Add salt and pork strips.
3. Cook the meat on High for 4 hours.
4. Then drain water and transfer the meat in the skillet.
5. Add butter, ground paprika, and roast the meat for 2 minutes per side.
6. Then sprinkle the meat with maple syrup and carefully mix.

per serving: 252 calories, 23.4g protein, 7.3g carbohydrates, 13.9g fat, 0.4g fiber, 73mg cholesterol, 652mg sodium, 407mg potassium

Pork and Zucchini Bowl
Yield: 4 servings | **Prep time:** 10 minutes | **Cook time:** 5 hours

- 12 oz pork stew meat, cubed
- 1 cup zucchini, chopped
- 1 teaspoon white pepper
- 1 teaspoon dried dill
- 1 teaspoon salt
- ½ cup sour cream
- 1 cup of water
- 1 chili pepper, chopped

1. Put meat in the Crock Pot.
2. Add white pepper, dried dill, salt, sour cream, water, and chili pepper.
3. Close the lid and cook the meal on High for 4 hours.
4. Then add zucchini and cook the meal on High for 1 hour more.

per serving: 249 calories, 26.3g protein, 2.8g carbohydrates, 14.3g fat, 0.5g fiber, 86mg cholesterol, 652mg sodium, 452mg potassium

Pork and Lentils Mash
Yield: 4 servings | **Prep time:** 10 minutes | **Cook time:** 4 hours

- 8 oz pork mince
- ½ cup red lentils
- 2.5 cups water
- 1 teaspoon chili powder
- 1 teaspoon salt
- 1 onion, diced
- 1 teaspoon olive oil

1. Pour olive oil in the skillet.
2. Add onion and roast the mixture for 4-5 minutes or until the onion is light brown.
3. Transfer it in the Crock Pot.
4. Add red lentils, pork mince, and all remaining ingredients.
5. Carefully mix the mixture and cook it on High for 4 hours.
6. Then stir the meal well and transfer it in the serving bowls.

per serving: 263 calories, 6.6g protein, 52.5g carbohydrates, 3.8g fat, 8.7g fiber, 0mg cholesterol, 595mg sodium, 283mg potassium

Cocoa Pork Chops
Yield: 4 servings | **Prep time:** 10 minutes | **Cook time:** 2.5 hours

- 4 pork chops
- 1 tablespoon cocoa powder
- ½ cup cream
- 1 tablespoon butter
- 1 teaspoon ground black pepper
- ½ teaspoon salt
- ¼ cup of water

1. Beat the pork chops gently with the help of the kitchen hammer.
2. Then sprinkle the meat with ground black pepper and salt. Transfer it in the Crock Pot.
3. After this, mix water with cocoa powder and cream and pour it in the Crock Pot.
4. Add butter and close the lid.
5. Cook the pork chops on high for 2.5 hours.

per serving: 305 calories, 18.6g protein, 2g carbohydrates, 24.6g fat, 0.5g fiber, 82mg cholesterol, 378mg sodium, 328mg potassium

Pepsi Pork Tenderloin
Yield: 4 servings | **Prep time:** 35 minutes | **Cook time:** 6 hours

- 1-pound pork tenderloin
- 1 cup Pepsi
- 1 teaspoon cumin seeds
- 1 teaspoon olive oil
- 2 tablespoons soy sauce

6. Chop the pork tenderloin roughly and put it in the mixing bowl.
7. Add cumin seeds, soy sauce, Pepsi, and olive oil. Leave the meat for 30 minutes to marinate.
8. After this, transfer the meat and all Pepsi liquid in the Crock Pot and close the lid.
9. Cook the meat on low for 6 hours.

per serving: 179 calories, 30.3g protein, 0.8g carbohydrates, 5.3g fat, 0.1g fiber, 83mg cholesterol, 523mg sodium, 514mg potassium

Wine Pork Shoulder
Yield: 4 servings | **Prep time:** 10 minutes | **Cook time:** 10 hours

- 1-pound pork shoulder, roughly chopped
- 1 cup red wine
- 1 cup celery stalk, chopped
- ½ cup red onion, chopped
- 1 teaspoon dried thyme
- 1 teaspoon salt
- 1 teaspoon ground paprika

1. Sprinkle the pork shoulder with dried thyme, salt, and ground paprika.
2. Transfer it in the Crock Pot.
3. Add all remaining ingredients and close the lid.
4. Cook the meal on low for 10 hours.

per serving: 392 calories, 26.9g protein, 4.2g carbohydrates, 24.4g fat, 1g fiber, 102mg cholesterol, 683mg sodium, 533mg potassium

Apple Juice Pulled Pork
Yield: 4 servings | **Prep time:** 15 minutes | **Cook time:** 9 hours

- ½ cup apple juice
- 12 oz pork shoulder
- 1 cup of water

- 1 teaspoon ground black pepper
- ½ teaspoon salt
- 1 teaspoon butter
1. Put all ingredients in the Crock Pot and close the lid.
2. Cook the meat on low for 9 hours.
3. Then open the lid and shred the meat with the help of the forks.

per serving: 272 calories, 19.9g protein, 3.8g carbohydrates, 19.2g fat, 0.2g fiber, 79mg cholesterol, 359mg sodium, 319mg potassium

Braised Ham
Yield: 4 servings | **Prep time:** 10 minutes | **Cook time:** 10 hours
- 12 oz smoked shoulder ham
- 1 tablespoon mustard
- 2 cups of water
- ¼ cup maple syrup
- ¼ cup beer
1. Rub the smoked shoulder ham with mustard and transfer in the Crock Pot.
2. Add water and beer.
3. Close the lid and cook the ham on low for 10 hours.
4. When the time is finished, sprinkle the meat with maple syrup and slice.

per serving: 221 calories, 15.7g protein, 15.7g carbohydrates, 9.9g fat, 0.4g fiber, 50mg cholesterol, 747mg sodium, 64mg potassium

Carrot and Pork Cubes
Yield: 2 servings | **Prep time:** 10 minutes | **Cook time:** 4 hours
- 8 oz pork tenderloin, cubed
- 1 cup carrot, cubed
- 1 tablespoon tomato paste
- 1 tablespoon avocado oil
- 1 teaspoon salt
- 1 teaspoon white pepper
1. Pour the avocado oil in the skillet and preheat it well.
2. Then put the pork tenderloins in the hot oil and roast on high heat for 3 minutes per side.
3. Transfer the roasted meat in the Crock Pot and add all remaining ingredients.
4. Close the lid and cook the pork on high for 4 hours.

per serving: 203 calories, 30.7g protein, 8g carbohydrates, 4.9g fat, 2.3g fiber, 83mg cholesterol, 1274mg sodium, 770mg potassium

Pork Roast with Apples
Yield: 4 servings | **Prep time:** 10 minutes | **Cook time:** 8 hours
- 1-pound pork shoulder, boneless
- 1 teaspoon brown sugar
- 1 teaspoon allspices
- 1 teaspoon thyme
- 1 cup apples, chopped
- 1 yellow onion, sliced
- 2 cups of water

1. Sprinkle the pork shoulder with allspices, thyme, and brown sugar. Transfer it in the Crock Pot.
2. Add all remaining ingredients and close the lid.
3. Cook the pork roast on Low for 8 hours.

per serving: 376 calories, 26.9g protein, 11.5g carbohydrates, 24.5g fat, 2.1g fiber, 102mg cholesterol, 83mg sodium, 482mg potassium

Fennel Seeds Pork Chops
Yield: 4 servings | **Prep time:** 10 minutes | **Cook time:** 6 hours
- 4 pork chops
- 1 tablespoon fennel seeds
- 3 tablespoons avocado oil
- 1 teaspoon garlic, diced
- ½ cup of water
1. Mix fennel seeds with avocado oil and garlic. Mash the mixture.
2. Then rub the pork chops with fennel seeds mixture and transfer in the Crock Pot.
3. Add water and close the lid.
4. Cook the meat on low for 6 hours.

per serving: 276 calories, 18.4g protein, 1.6g carbohydrates, 21.4g fat, 1.1g fiber, 69mg cholesterol, 59mg sodium, 336mg potassium

Pork Ragu with Basil
Yield: 4 servings | **Prep time:** 10 minutes | **Cook time:** 4 hours
- 8 oz pork loin, chopped
- 1 cup russet potatoes
- ½ cup carrot, chopped
- 3 oz fennel bulb, chopped
- 1 tablespoon dried basil
- 1 teaspoon salt
- 3 cups of water
- ½ cup plain yogurt
- 1 teaspoon tomato paste
1. In the mixing bowl mix tomato paste with plain yogurt, salt, dried basil, and pork loin.
2. Transfer the mixture in the Crock Pot and close the lid.
3. Cook the meat on high for 2 hours.
4. Then add water and all remaining ingredients. Carefully mix the mixture.
5. Close the lid and cook the ragu on low for 5 hours.

per serving: 198 calories, 18.3g protein, 11.2g carbohydrates, 8.4g fat, 2g fiber, 47mg cholesterol, 667mg sodium, 613mg potassium

Spaghetti Meatballs
Yield: 4 servings | **Prep time:** 20 minutes | **Cook time:** 3 hours
- 2 cups ground pork
- 1 teaspoon ground black pepper
- ½ teaspoon salt
- 1 teaspoon dried cilantro
- ½ cup tomato juice
- 1 teaspoon butter
- ¼ cup of water
1. In the mixing bowl mix ground pork with ground black pepper.

2. Then add salt and dried cilantro.
3. Make the small balls from the mixture and press them gently.
4. Put butter in the Crock Pot.
5. Add water and meatballs.
6. Close the lid and cook the meatballs on high for 3 hours.

per serving: 141 calories, 11.2g protein, 1.6g carbohydrates, 9.8g fat, 0.3g fiber, 42mg cholesterol, 411mg sodium, 231mg potassium

Pork Ribs Braised in Wine
Yield: 4 servings | **Prep time:** 10 minutes | **Cook time:** 6 hours

- 1-pound pork ribs, roughly chopped
- ½ cup wine
- 2 garlic cloves, crushed
- 1 teaspoon brown sugar
- 1 teaspoon clove
- ½ teaspoon chili flakes

1. Rub the pork ribs with chili flakes and put in the Crock Pot.
2. Add garlic, brown sugar, and clove.
3. Then add the wine and close the lid.
4. Cook the meal on Low for 6 hours.

per serving: 341 calories, 30.2g protein, 2.4g carbohydrates, 20.2g fat, 0.2g fiber, 117mg cholesterol, 69mg sodium, 369mg potassium

Pork and Oysters Mushrooms Saute
Yield: 4 servings | **Prep time:** 10 minutes | **Cook time:** 8 hours

- 1-pound pork tenderloin, chopped
- 6 oz oysters mushrooms, chopped
- 1 cup onion, sliced
- 2 cups of water
- 1 cup cream
- 1 teaspoon ground black pepper
- 1 teaspoon salt

1. Mix pork tenderloin with ground black pepper and salt and put in the Crock Pot.
2. Top the meat with oysters mushrooms and sliced onion.
3. Then add water and cream.
4. Close the lid and cook the meal on low for 8 hours.

per serving: 223 calories, 31.9g protein, 6.3g carbohydrates, 7.5g fat, 1.2g fiber, 94mg cholesterol, 673mg sodium, 685mg potassium

Hawaiian Meatballs in Pineapple Sauce
Yield: 4 servings | **Prep time:** 15 minutes | **Cook time:** 5 hours

- 12 oz ground pork
- ½ cup pineapple juice
- 1 teaspoon dried cilantro
- 1 teaspoon chili flakes
- ½ teaspoon salt
- 1 tablespoon flour
- 2 tablespoons butter

1. In the mixing bowl mix ground pork, dried cilantro, chili flakes, and salt.
2. Make the small meatballs.
3. Then put the butter in the skillet and melt it.
4. Add the meatballs and roast them for 2 minutes per side.
5. Transfer the roasted meatballs in the Crock Pot.
6. Mix pineapple juice with flour and pour the liquid in the Crock Pot.
7. Cook the meatballs on low for 5 hours.

per serving: 196 calories, 22.6g protein, 5.5g carbohydrates, 8.8g fat, 0.1g fiber, 77mg cholesterol, 381mg sodium, 404mg potassium

Hamburger Style Stuffing
Yield: 4 servings | **Prep time:** 10 minutes | **Cook time:** 3 hours

- 1-pound ground pork
- ½ cup Cheddar cheese, shredded
- ½ cup fresh cilantro, chopped
- ¼ cup onion, minced
- 1 cup of water
- ¼ cup tomato juice
- 1 bell pepper, diced
- 1 teaspoon salt

1. Mix ground pork with cilantro, onion, and diced pepper.
2. Then transfer the mixture in the Crock Pot.
3. Add all remaining ingredients and mix.
4. Close the lid and cook the stuffing on High for 3 hours.

per serving: 235 calories, 33.7g protein, 3.8g carbohydrates, 8.8g fat, 0.7g fiber, 98mg cholesterol, 778mg sodium, 604mg potassium

Winter Pork with Green Peas
Yield: 4 servings | **Prep time:** 10 minutes | **Cook time:** 7 hours

- 1-pound pork shoulder, boneless, chopped
- 1 cup green peas
- 3 cups of water
- 1 cup carrot, chopped
- 1 teaspoon chili powder
- 1 teaspoon dried thyme

1. Sprinkle the pork shoulder with chili powder and dried thyme. Transfer the meat in the Crock Pot.
2. Add carrot, water, and green peas.
3. Close the lid and cook the meal on low for 7 hours.

per serving: 374 calories, 28.7g protein, 8.5g carbohydrates, 24.5g fat, 2.8g fiber, 102mg cholesterol, 110mg sodium, 566mg potassium

Dijon Mustard Pork
Yield: 2 servings | **Prep time:** 15 minutes | **Cook time:** 8 hours

- 8 oz pork tenderloin
- 2 tablespoons Dijon mustard
- 1 tablespoon avocado oil
- ½ teaspoon ground paprika
- ½ cup of water

1. Mix Dijon mustard with avocado oil and ground paprika.

2. Then rub the pork tenderloin with mustard mixture and put in the Crock Pot.
3. Add water and close the lid.
4. Cook the meal on Low for 8 hours.
 per serving: 183 calories, 30.5g protein, 1.5g carbohydrates, 5.6g fat, 1g fiber, 83mg cholesterol, 244mg sodium, 534mg potassium

BBQ Ribs
Yield: 4 servings | **Prep time:** 15 minutes | **Cook time:** 4 hours
- 1-pound pork ribs, roughly chopped
- 1 teaspoon minced garlic
- ½ cup BBQ sauce
- 1 tablespoon olive oil
- ¼ cup plain yogurt
1. Mix BBQ sauce with plain yogurt and minced garlic and pour it in the Crock Pot.
2. Then pour olive oil in the skillet and heat well.
3. Add pork ribs and roast them for 3 minutes per side on high heat.
4. Transfer the pork ribs in the Crock Pot and carefully mix.
5. Close the lid and cook them on High for 4 hours.
 per serving: 398 calories, 31g protein, 12.6g carbohydrates, 23.9g fat, 0.2g fiber, 118mg cholesterol, 426mg sodium, 430mg potassium

Meatballs in Vodka Sauce
Yield: 4 servings | **Prep time:** 15 minutes | **Cook time:** 6 hours
- 1-pound ground pork
- 1 onion, diced
- 1 teaspoon ground black pepper
- 1 tablespoon semolina
- 1 cup vodka sauce
- 2 tablespoons sesame oil
1. In the mixing bowl mix ground pork with onion, ground black pepper, and semolina.
2. Make the small meatballs.
3. Brush the Crock Pot bottom with sesame oil and put the meatballs inside in one layer.
4. Add vodka sauce and close the lid.
5. Cook the meatballs on low for 6 hours.
 per serving: 299 calories, 32.9g protein, 10.3g carbohydrates, 13.4g fat, 0.8g fiber, 85mg cholesterol, 286mg sodium, 529mg potassium

Bacon-Wrapped Pork Tenderloin
Yield: 4 servings | **Prep time:** 20 minutes | **Cook time:** 4 hours
- 3 oz bacon, sliced
- 1-pound pork tenderloin
- 1 tablespoon maple syrup
- 1 teaspoon white pepper
- 1 tablespoon avocado oil
- 1 teaspoon salt
- ½ cup of water
- 1 tablespoon mayonnaise
1. Cut the pork tenderloin into 4 servings.
2. Then sprinkle the meat with white pepper, salt, and mayonnaise.

3. Wrap the pork cuts in the bacon and sprinkle with maple syrup and avocado oil.
4. Put the meat in the Crock Pot.
5. Add water and close the lid.
6. Cook the meal on High for 4 hours.
 per serving: 311 calories, 37.7g protein, 5.1g carbohydrates, 14.6g fat, 0.3g fiber, 107mg cholesterol, 1165mg sodium, 626mg potassium

Sesame Short Ribs
Yield: 4 servings | **Prep time:** 35 minutes | **Cook time:** 8 hours
- 4 tablespoons mirin
- 1 tablespoon sesame oil
- 1 teaspoon sesame seeds
- ¼ cup of soy sauce
- 1-pound pork ribs
- ½ teaspoon brown sugar
- ¼ cup of water
1. In the mixing bowl mix sesame oil with mirin, sesame seeds, brown sugar, and soy sauce.
2. Add the pork ribs in the soy sauce mixture and leave for 30 minutes to marinate.
3. After this, transfer the ingredients in the Crock Pot.
4. Add water and close the lid.
5. Cook the short ribs on Low for 8 hours.
 per serving: 379 calories, 31.2g protein, 8.8g carbohydrates, 23.9g fat, 0.2g fiber, 117mg cholesterol, 1095mg sodium, 365mg potassium

Sour Cream Roast
Yield: 4 servings | **Prep time:** 10 minutes | **Cook time:** 4.5 hours
- 1-pound pork shoulder, boneless, chopped
- 1 tablespoon lemon zest, grated
- 4 tablespoons lemon juice
- 1 cup sour cream
- ¼ cup of water
1. Sprinkle the pork shoulder with lemon zest and lemon juice.
2. Transfer the meat in the Crock Pot.
3. Add sour cream and water.
4. Close the lid and cook it on high for 4.5 hours.
 per serving: 459 calories, 28.4g protein, 3.1g carbohydrates, 36.4g fat, 0.2g fiber, 127mg cholesterol, 111mg sodium, 480mg potassium

Cajun Pork Loin
Yield: 3 servings | **Prep time:** 10 minutes | **Cook time:** 7 hours
- 12 oz pork loin
- 1 tablespoon Cajun seasonings
- 2 tablespoons sunflower oil
- ½ cup of water
- 3 garlic cloves, sliced
1. Rub the pork loin with Cajun seasonings and sprinkle with sunflower oil.
2. Transfer the meat in the Crock Pot.
3. Add water and garlic cloves.
4. Close the lid and cook the meat on low for 7 hours.

per serving: 361 calories, 31.2g protein, 1g carbohydrates, 25.1g fat, 0.1g fiber, 91mg cholesterol, 122mg sodium, 492mg potassium

Cayenne Pepper Strips

Yield: 4 servings | **Prep time:** 10 minutes | **Cook time:** 4 hours

- 1-pound pork sirloin, cut into strips
- 1 teaspoon cayenne pepper
- 2 tablespoons ketchup
- 1 tablespoon avocado oil
- 1 cup of water

1. Mix ketchup with cayenne pepper and avocado oil.
2. Then carefully brush the pork strips with ketchup mixture and put in the Crock Pot.
3. Add water and close the lid.
4. Cook the meat on high for 4 hours.

per serving: 204 calories, 23.3g protein, 2.3g carbohydrates, 10.6g fat, 0.3g fiber, 80mg cholesterol, 151mg sodium, 49mg potassium

Hot Sloppy Joes

Yield: 4 servings | **Prep time:** 15 minutes | **Cook time:** 6 hours

- 2 cups ground pork
- 2 tablespoons hot sauce
- ½ cup bell pepper, chopped
- 1 cup white onion, diced
- 1 tablespoon tomato paste
- ½ cup tomato juice
- 1 teaspoon ground cumin
- ¼ cup of water

1. Put the ground pork in the Crock Pot.
2. Add hot sauce, bell pepper, white onion, tomato paste, tomato juice, and ground cumin.
3. Carefully mix the meat mixture and add water.
4. Close the lid and cook the meal on Low for 6 hours.
5. Stir the meal well before serving.

per serving: 376 calories, 31.2g protein, 6.2g carbohydrates, 24.6g fat, 1.2g fiber, 110mg cholesterol, 364mg sodium, 625mg potassium

Layered Casserole

Yield: 4 servings | **Prep time:** 15 minutes | **Cook time:** 7 hours

- ½ cup Mozzarella, shredded
- 1 cup ground pork
- 1 teaspoon ground black pepper
- 1 teaspoon salt
- 1 teaspoon coconut oil, softened
- 1 teaspoon garlic powder
- 1 cup green peas, frozen
- 1 cup of water

1. Grease the Crock Pot bottom with softened coconut oil.
2. Then mix ground pork with ground black pepper, salt, and garlic powder.
3. Put the ground pork in the Crock Pot in one layer.
4. Add the layer of green peas and Mozzarella.
5. Then add water and close the lid.

6. Cook the casserole on Low for 7 hours.

per serving: 119 calories, 9g protein, 6.2g carbohydrates, 6.5g fat, 2.1g fiber, 28mg cholesterol, 626mg sodium, 181mg potassium

Poached Pork Roast

Yield: 4 servings | **Prep time:** 10 minutes | **Cook time:** 7 hours

- 2 cups onion, diced
- 1-pound pork loin
- 1 tablespoon sunflower oil
- 1 teaspoon salt
- 1 teaspoon ground black pepper
- 2 cups of water
- 1 tablespoon flour

1. Sprinkle the pork loin with flour.
2. Then heat the sunflower oil in the skillet well.
3. Add pork loin and roast it for 3 minutes per side on high heat.
4. Transfer the meat in the Crock Pot.
5. Add all remaining ingredients and close the lid.
6. Cook the pork roast on low for 7 hours.

per serving: 337 calories, 31.9g protein, 7.2g carbohydrates, 19.4g fat, 1.4g fiber, 91mg cholesterol, 658mg sodium, 574mg potassium

Seasoned Poached Pork Belly

Yield: 4 servings | **Prep time:** 15 minutes | **Cook time:** 4 hours

- 10 oz pork belly
- 1 teaspoon minced garlic
- 1 teaspoon ginger paste
- ¼ cup apple cider vinegar
- 1 cup of water

1. Rub the pork belly with minced garlic and garlic paste.
2. Then sprinkle it with apple cider vinegar and transfer in the Crock Pot.
3. Add water and close the lid.
4. Cook the pork belly on High for 4 hours.
5. Then slice the cooked pork belly and sprinkle with hot gravy from the Crock Pot.

per serving: 333 calories, 32.8g protein, 0.7g carbohydrates, 19.1g fat, 0.1g fiber, 82mg cholesterol, 1148mg sodium, 20mg potassium

Maple Syrup Sliced Belly

Yield: 4 servings | **Prep time:** 10 minutes | **Cook time:** 8 hours

- 8 oz pork belly, sliced
- ¼ cup maple syrup
- 3 tablespoons butter, melted
- 1 teaspoon ground coriander
- ½ teaspoon garlic powder
- ¼ teaspoon salt
- 1 tablespoon sesame oil

6. Mix butter with maple syrup, ground coriander, garlic powder, and salt.
7. After this, add sesame oil and whisk the mixture until smooth.
8. Mix the sliced pork belly with maple syrup mixture and put it in the Crock Pot.

9. Add all remaining maple syrup liquid and close the lid.
10. Cook the meal on Low for 8 hours. Add water in pork belly if needed.
per serving: 421 calories, 26.3g protein, 13.5g carbohydrates, 27.4g fat, 0g fiber, 88mg cholesterol, 1126mg sodium, 47mg potassium

Garlic Pork Chops
Yield: 6 servings | **Prep time:** 15 minutes | **Cook time:** 4 hours
- 6 pork chops
- 2 tablespoons minced garlic
- 2 tablespoons olive oil
- 1 cup of water
- 1 teaspoon cayenne pepper
- ½ teaspoon smoked paprika

1. In the shallow bowl mix smoked paprika, cayenne pepper, olive oil, and minced garlic.
2. Rub the pork chops with garlic mixture carefully and leave for 10-15 minutes to marinate.
3. Then transfer the pork chops in the Crock Pot.
4. Add water and all remaining garlic mixture.
5. Cook the pork chops on high for 4 hours.
per serving: 302 calories, 18.2g protein, 1.2g carbohydrates, 24.6g fat, 0.6g fiber, 69mg cholesterol, 58mg sodium, 297mg potassium

Ground Pork Pie
Yield: 4 servings | **Prep time:** 20 minutes | **Cook time:** 4.5 hours
- 1 teaspoon tomato paste
- 1 cup ground pork
- 1 teaspoon salt
- 1 teaspoon ground black pepper
- 1 tablespoon avocado oil
- 4 oz puff pastry

1. Mix ground pork with salt and ground black pepper.
2. Then add tomato paste and stir the ingredients well.
3. Brush the Crock Pot bottom with avocado oil.
4. Then put the puff pastry inside and flatten it in the shape of the pie crust.
5. Put the ground pork mixture over the puff pastry, flatten it in one layer and close the lid.
6. Cook the pie on High for 4.5 hours.
per serving: 396 calories, 22.3g protein, 13.g carbohydrates, 27.5g fat, 0.8g fiber, 74mg cholesterol, 711mg sodium, 332mg potassium

Pork Balls with Eggs
Yield: 4 servings | **Prep time:** 20 minutes | **Cook time:** 4 hours
- 4 quail eggs, hard-boiled, peeled
- 8 oz ground pork
- 1 tablespoon semolina
- 2 teaspoon dried dill
- 1 teaspoon salt
- ½ teaspoon cayenne pepper
- 1 tablespoon avocado oil
- ½ cup of water

1. In the mixing bowl mix ground pork with semolina, dried dill, salt, and cayenne pepper.
2. Then make 4 balls from the ground pork mixture and fill them with quail eggs.
3. Pour the avocado oil in the skillet and preheat it well.
4. Add the prepared pork balls and roast them on high heat for 2 minutes per side.
5. Then put the pork balls in the Crock Pot.
6. Add water and close the lid.
7. Cook the meal on High for 4 hours.
per serving: 113 calories, 17.4g protein, 4.5g carbohydrates, 2.5g fat, 2.4g fiber, 41mg cholesterol, 622mg sodium, 276mg potassium

Bacon Potatoes with Cheese Inside
Yield: 4 servings | **Prep time:** 15 minutes | **Cook time:** 3.5 hours
- 2 russet potatoes, halved
- 4 bacon slices, roasted
- 4 Cheddar cheese slices
- 4 teaspoons butter, softened
- 4 tablespoons plain yogurt
- ½ cup of water

1. Pour water in the Crock Pot.
2. Then arrange the potato halves in the Crock Pot in one layer.
3. Mix butter with plain yogurt.
4. Top the potato halves with bacon and cheese and close the lid.
5. Cook the potatoes on High for 3.5 hours.
6. Then transfer them in the plates and top with butter-yogurt mixture.
per serving: 334 calories, 16.7g protein, 18.4g carbohydrates, 21.3g fat, 2.6g fiber, 61mg cholesterol, 658mg sodium, 606mg potassium

Stuffed Mushrooms with Ground Pork
Yield: 4 servings | **Prep time:** 20 minutes | **Cook time:** 4 hours
- 2 cups cremini mushrooms caps
- 1 cup ground pork
- 1 onion, minced
- ¼ cup butter
- 1 teaspoon salt
- ¼ cup of water

1. Mix ground pork with minced onion and salt.
2. Then fill the cremini mushroom caps with ground pork mixture and put in the Crock Pot.
3. Add butter and water.
4. Cook the mushroom caps on High for 4 hours.
per serving: 355 calories, 21.5g protein, 4.1g carbohydrates, 27.8g fat, 0.6g fiber, 104mg cholesterol, 722mg sodium, 327mg potassium

Ketchup Pork Ribs
Yield: 4 servings | **Prep time:** 10 minutes | **Cook time:** 4 hours
- 1-pound pork ribs, roughly chopped
- 4 tablespoons ketchup
- 1 tablespoon fresh dill

- 1 tablespoon avocado oil
- ½ cup beef broth
1. Mix pork ribs with ketchup and avocado oil.
2. Put them in the Crock Pot.
3. Add beef broth and dill.
4. Close the pork ribs on High for 4 hours.

per serving: 336 calories, 31.1g protein, 4.5g carbohydrates, 20.8g fat, 0.3g fiber, 117mg cholesterol, 330mg sodium, 447mg potassium

Mayo Pork Salad
Yield: 4 servings | **Prep time:** 15 minutes | **Cook time:** 4 hours

- 7 oz pork loin
- 1 teaspoon salt
- 1 cup of water
- 1 cup arugula, chopped
- 2 eggs, hard-boiled, peeled, chopped
- 3 tablespoons mayonnaise
1. Pour water in the Crock Pot.
2. Add pork loin and close the lid.
3. Cook the meat on high for 4 hours.
4. After this, drain water and cut the pork loin into strips.
5. Put the pork strips in the big salad bowl.
6. Add arugula and chopped eggs.
7. Add mayonnaise and carefully mix the salad.

per serving: 196 calories, 16.6g protein, 3g carbohydrates, 12.8g fat, 0.1g fiber, 124mg cholesterol, 724mg sodium, 259mg potassium

Radish and Pork Ragu
Yield: 4 servings | **Prep time:** 10 minutes | **Cook time:** 7 hours

- 2 cups radish, halved
- 1 cup of water
- 1 tablespoon dried dill
- ½ teaspoon dried basil
- 1 teaspoon salt
- 2 tablespoons sesame oil
- 1 teaspoon sesame seeds
- 8 oz pork tenderloin, sliced
1. Put all ingredients in the Crock Pot.
2. Carefully mix them and close the lid.
3. Cook the pork ragu on Low for 7 hours.

per serving: 157 calories, 15.5g protein, 2.6g carbohydrates, 9.3g fat, 1.1g fiber, 41mg cholesterol, 640mg sodium, 404mg potassium

Pork in Onion Gravy
Yield: 4 servings | **Prep time:** 10 minutes | **Cook time:** 9 hours

- 2 cups onion, sliced
- 2 tablespoons butter
- 1 teaspoon smoked paprika
- ½ teaspoon dried parsley
- 1 cup cream
- 12 oz pork loin, sliced
1. Grease the Crock Pot bottom with butter.
2. Put the onion inside in one layer.
3. After this, add sliced pork loin and sprinkle it with smoked paprika and dried parsley.

4. Add cream and close the lid.
5. Cook the meal on Low for 9 hours.

per serving: 320 calories, 24.5g protein, 7.6g carbohydrates, 21.1g fat, 1.4g fiber, 95mg cholesterol, 116mg sodium, 481mg potassium

Meatballs with Melted Core
Yield: 4 servings | **Prep time:** 20 minutes | **Cook time:** 4 hours

- 4 oz Cheddar cheese, shredded
- 1 tablespoon cream cheese
- 1 cup ground pork
- 1 tablespoon cornflour
- ½ teaspoon smoked paprika
- ½ teaspoon onion powder
- 1 tablespoon olive oil
- ½ cup chicken stock
1. Mix ground pork with cornflour, smoked paprika, and onion powder.
2. Then make the ground pork meatballs.
3. After this, make the small balls from the shredded cheese.
4. Fill the pork meatballs with cheese balls and put in the Crock Pot.
5. Sprinkle them with olive oil.
6. Add chicken stock and cream cheese.
7. Close the lid and cook the meatballs on High for 4 hours.

per serving: 395 calories, 27.6g protein, 2.3g carbohydrates, 30.2g fat, 0.3g fiber, 106mg cholesterol, 336mg sodium, 331mg potassium

Cucumber and Pork Cubes Bowl
Yield: 4 servings | **Prep time:** 20 minutes | **Cook time:** 4 hours

- 3 cucumbers, chopped
- 1 jalapeno pepper, diced
- 1 red onion, diced
- 3 tablespoons soy sauce
- 1 tablespoon olive oil
- 8 oz pork tenderloin
- 1 cup of water
1. Pour water in the Crock Pot.
2. Add pork tenderloin and cook it on High for 4 hours.
3. Meanwhile, mix the red onion with jalapeno pepper and cucumbers in the salad bowl.
4. In the shallow bowl mix soy sauce and olive oil.
5. When the pork is cooked, chop it roughly and add in the cucumber salad.
6. Sprinkle the salad with oil-soy sauce mixture and shake well.

per serving: 163 calories, 17.4g protein, 11.9g carbohydrates, 5.8g fat, 1.9g fiber, 41mg cholesterol, 716mg sodium, 645mg potassium

Bacon Casserole
Yield: 4 servings | **Prep time:** 10 minutes | **Cook time:** 8 hours

- 4 oz bacon, chopped
- 2 cups potatoes, chopped
- 1 cup cheddar cheese, shredded
- 1 teaspoon ground black pepper

- 1 cup of water
- 1 tablespoon butter, softened
1.   Grease the Crock Pot bottom with butter.
2.   Then add chopped potatoes.
3.   Top the potatoes with bacon and sprinkle with ground black pepper.
4.   Add water and cheddar cheese.
5.   Close the lid and cook the casserole on Low for 8 hours.

per serving: 346 calories, 18.9g protein, 12.9g carbohydrates, 24.2g fat, 1.9g fiber, 68mg cholesterol, 857mg sodium, 501mg potassium

Pork Liver Kebabs
Yield: 6 servings | **Prep time:** 15 minutes | **Cook time:** 3.5 hours

- 15 oz pork liver, roughly chopped
- 1 teaspoon onion powder
- 1 teaspoon garlic powder
- 2 bell peppers, roughly chopped
- 1 tablespoon cornflour
- ½ teaspoon salt
- 1 cup of water
- 1 tablespoon coconut oil
1.   Sprinkle the pork liver with onion powder, garlic powder, cornflour, and salt.
2.   Then string the liver int skewers (wooden sticks) and sprinkle with coconut oil.
3.   Arrange the skewers in the Crock Pot.
4.   Add water and close the lid.
5.   Cook them on High for 3.5 hours.

per serving: 157 calories, 19g protein, 7.3g carbohydrates, 5.5g fat, 0.7g fiber, 252mg cholesterol, 231mg sodium, 194mg potassium

Pork and Cheese Patties
Yield: 6 servings | **Prep time:** 15 minutes | **Cook time:** 4.5 hours

- 2 oz chives, chopped
- 10 oz ground pork
- 3 oz parmesan, grated
- 1 teaspoon chili flakes
- 1 egg yolk
- 1 tablespoon coconut oil
- 1/3 cup water
1.   In the mixing bowl mix chives, ground pork, parmesan, chili flakes, and egg yolk.
2.   Make the small patties and put them in the Crock Pot.
3.   Add water and coconut oil.
4.   Close the lid and cook the patties on high for 4.5 hours.

per serving: 145 calories, 17.7g protein, 1g carbohydrates, 7.8g fat, 0.2g fiber, 80mg cholesterol, 161mg sodium, 231mg potassium

Ground Pork with Macaroni
Yield: 4 servings | **Prep time:** 15 minutes | **Cook time:** 2.5 hours

- 5 oz macaroni, cooked
- ½ cup ground pork
- 1 onion, diced
- ½ cup tomato juice
- 1 teaspoon ground black pepper
- 4 oz provolone cheese, shredded
- 1 tablespoon avocado oil
1.   Pour avocado oil in the skillet and heat it.
2.   Add ground pork and ground black pepper.
3.   Roast the meat for 5 minutes on medium heat.
4.   Then transfer it in the Crock Pot.
5.   Add provolone cheese, tomato juice, and diced onion. Mix the mixture.
6.   Add cooked macaroni and mix the meal well.
7.   Close the lid and cook the meal on High for 2.5 hours.

per serving: 369 calories, 22.6g protein, 31.5g carbohydrates, 16.7g fat, 2.1g fiber, 56mg cholesterol, 362mg sodium, 387mg potassium

Egg Salad with Ground Pork
Yield: 2 servings | **Prep time:** 15 minutes | **Cook time:** 4 hours

- 2 eggs, hard-boiled, peeled, chopped
- ¼ cup ground pork
- 1 teaspoon ground turmeric
- 1 teaspoon salt
- ¼ cup plain yogurt
- 1 tablespoon coconut oil
- 2 tomatoes, chopped
1.   Put the coconut oil in the Crock Pot.
2.   Add ground pork, ground turmeric, salt, and yogurt.
3.   Close the lid and cook the meat on High for 4 hours.
4.   After this, transfer the ground pork and all remaining liquid from the Crock Pot in the salad bowl.
5.   Add all remaining ingredients from the list above and mix the salad.

per serving: 198 calories, 11g protein, 8g carbohydrates, 13.9g fat, 1.7g fiber, 175mg cholesterol, 1262mg sodium, 450mg potassium

Yogurt Casserole
Yield: 6 servings | **Prep time:** 10 minutes | **Cook time:** 8 hours

- 1 cup ground pork
- 1 garlic clove, diced
- 5 oz potato, cooked, mashed
- 1 cup plain yogurt
- 1 teaspoon avocado oil
- ½ teaspoon ground black pepper
- ½ cup Mozzarella, shredded
1.   Put all ingredients in the Crock Pot and gently mix.
2.   Close the lid and cook the casserole on Low for 8 hours.

per serving: 134 calories, 10.2g protein, 7.4g carbohydrates, 6.5g fat, 0.6g fiber, 28mg cholesterol, 63mg sodium, 296mg potassium

Baked Pork with Capers Gravy
Yield: 4 servings | **Prep time:** 10 minutes | **Cook time:** 5 hours

- 2 teaspoons capers
- 1 cup of water
- 1-pound pork tenderloin

- 1 chili pepper
- 1 tablespoon tomato paste
- ½ teaspoon dried dill
- 1 teaspoon cornflour
- ½ teaspoon salt

1. Sprinkle the pork tenderloin with salt and dried dill.
2. Put the pork tenderloin in the Crock Pot.
3. After this, in the mixing bowl mix capers, water, chili pepper, tomato paste, and cornflour. Pour the liquid over the meat and close the lid.
4. Cook the pork on high for 5 hours.

per serving: 169 calories, 30g protein, 1.5g carbohydrates, 4.1g fat, 0.3g fiber, 83mg cholesterol, 404mg sodium, 528mg potassium

Shredded Pork
Yield: 4 servings | **Prep time:** 10 minutes | **Cook time:** 5 hours

- 10 oz pork loin
- ½ cup cream
- 1 cup of water
- 1 teaspoon coriander seeds
- 1 teaspoon salt

1. Put all ingredients in the Crock Pot.
2. Cook it on High for 5 hours.
3. Then open the lid and shredded pork with the help of 2 forks.

per serving: 191 calories, 19.6g protein, 0.9g carbohydrates, 11.5g fat, 0g fiber, 62mg cholesterol, 367mg sodium, 312mg potassium

Shredded Meat Dip with Pickles
Yield: 4 servings | **Prep time:** 15 minutes | **Cook time:** 4 hours

- 1 tablespoon ketchup
- 2 oz dill pickles, shredded
- 1 cup of water
- 9 oz pork tenderloin
- 1 teaspoon ground cinnamon
- 1 teaspoon brown sugar

1. Pour water in the Crock Pot.
2. Add pork tenderloin and ground cinnamon.
3. Cook the meat on High for 4 hours.
4. Then remove the meat from the Crock Pot and put it in the big bowl.
5. Shred the meat with the help of the fork.
6. Add ketchup, brown sugar, and dill pickles.
7. Carefully mix the meal.

per serving: 101 calories, 16.8g protein, 2.5g carbohydrates, 2.3g fat, 0.5g fiber, 47mg cholesterol, 251mg sodium, 290mg potassium

Pork Chops Stuffed with Olives
Yield: 4 servings | **Prep time:** 20 minutes | **Cook time:** 4 hours

- 4 pork chops
- 4 kalamata olives, sliced
- 4 teaspoons sesame oil
- 1 teaspoon minced garlic
- 1 teaspoon dried parsley
- ½ cup chicken stock

1. Make the horizontal cut in every pork chop.
2. Then mix minced garlic with sliced olives and dried parsley.
3. Fill every pork chop with olive mixture and secure them with toothpicks.
4. Put the stuffed pork chops in the Crock Pot.
5. Add all remaining ingredients from the list above and close the lid.
6. Cook the pork chops on high for 4 hours.

per serving: 303 calories, 18.2g protein, 0.6g carbohydrates, 25g fat, 0.2g fiber, 69mg cholesterol, 190mg sodium, 282mg potassium

Scalloped Potato Casserole
Yield: 4 servings | **Prep time:** 20 minutes | **Cook time:** 8 hours

- 2 pork chops, sliced
- 3 potatoes, sliced
- 1 egg, beaten
- 1 tablespoon butter, softened
- 2 tablespoons breadcrumbs
- 1 oz Parmesan, grated
- ½ cup of coconut milk

1. Grease the Crock Pot bottom with butter.
2. Then put the pork chops inside.
3. Add sliced potatoes over the meat.
4. Then sprinkle the potatoes with egg and breadcrumbs.
5. Add parmesan and coconut milk.
6. Close the lid and cook the casserole on Low for 8 hours.

per serving: 385 calories, 16.5g protein, 29.5g carbohydrates, 22.9g fat, 4.6g fiber, 88mg cholesterol, 169mg sodium, 889mg potassium

Country Style Pie
Yield: 8 servings | **Prep time:** 15 minutes | **Cook time:** 4 hours

- 1 cup cherry tomatoes, halved
- 1 teaspoon dried basil
- 1 zucchini, grated
- ½ cup ground pork
- ½ cup tomato sauce
- 1 tablespoon sunflower oil
- 6 oz puff pastry

1. Brush the Crock Pot bottom with sunflower oil.
2. Then put the puff pastry inside and flatten it in the shape of the pie crust.
3. In the mixing bowl mix dried basil with ground pork, tomato sauce, and zucchini.
4. Put the meat mixture over the puff pastry.
5. Then top the meat with halved cherry tomatoes.
6. Close the lid and cook the pie on High for 4 hours.

per serving: 202 calories, 7.3g protein, 12.1g carbohydrates, 14g fat, 1.1g fiber, 18mg cholesterol, 151mg sodium, 252mg potassium

Meat Buns
Yield: 4 servings | **Prep time:** 15 minutes | **Cook time:** 3.5 hours

- 4 oz pork loin, boiled
- 1 teaspoon cream cheese

- ½ teaspoon cayenne pepper
- 4 oz puff pastry
- 1 egg yolk, beaten
- 3 tablespoons coconut oil, melted

1. Grind the pork loin and mix it with cayenne pepper and cream cheese.
2. Then roll up the puff pastry and cut it into squares.
3. Put the grinded pork loin in the center of every puff pastry square and roll them in the buns.
4. Then brush the Crock Pot with coconut oil from inside.
5. Add the buns. Brush the buns with beaten egg.
6. Close the lid and cook them on High for 3.5 hours.

per serving: 330 calories, 10.6g protein, 13.1g carbohydrates, 26.4g fat, 0.6g fiber, 76mg cholesterol, 93mg sodium, 147mg potassium

Blanked Hot Dogs
Yield: 4 servings | **Prep time:** 20 minutes | **Cook time:** 4 hours

- 4 mini (cocktail) pork sausages
- 1 teaspoon cumin seeds
- 1 tablespoon olive oil
- 1 egg, beaten
- 4 oz puff pastry

1. Roll up the puff pastry and cut into strips.
2. Put the pork sausages on every strip.
3. Roll the puff pastry and brush with egg.
4. Then top the blanked hot dogs with cumin seeds.
5. Brush the Crock Pot with olive oil from inside.
6. Add the blanked hot dogs and close the lid.
7. Cook them on high for 4 hours.

per serving: 225 calories, 4.4g protein, 14.1g carbohydrates, 16.9g fat, 0.6g fiber, 41mg cholesterol, 120mg sodium, 42mg potassium

Braised Pork Knuckle
Yield: 7 servings | **Prep time:** 10 minutes | **Cook time:** 10 hours

- 3-pound pork knuckles
- 1 tablespoon liquid honey
- 1 cup red wine
- 2 cups of water
- 1 teaspoon dried mint
- 1 teaspoon salt
- 1 cinnamon stick

1. Put all ingredients in the Crock Pot.
2. Close the lid and cook the pork knuckle on Low for 10 hours.

per serving: 412 calories, 60.6g protein, 3.4g carbohydrates, 13g fat, 0g fiber, 179mg cholesterol, 446mg sodium, 770mg potassium

Garlic Pork Knuckle
Yield: 4 servings | **Prep time:** 15 minutes | **Cook time:** 8 hours

- 1 tablespoon minced garlic
- 1 teaspoon garlic powder
- 3 cups of water
- 1 tablespoon olive oil
- 1 tablespoon mirin
- 1-pound pork knuckle

1. Rub the pork knuckle with minced garlic and sprinkle with garlic powder.
2. Then sprinkle the meat with mirin and olive oil. Put the meat in the Crock Pot.
3. Add water and close the lid.
4. Cook the pork knuckle on Low for 8 hours.

per serving: 323 calories, 31g protein, 3g carbohydrates, 20.1g fat, 0.1g fiber, 93mg cholesterol, 105mg sodium, 481mg potassium

Tender Butter Knuckle
Yield: 4 servings | **Prep time:** 15 minutes | **Cook time:** 8 hours

- 1-pound pork knuckle
- 1/3 cup butter
- 1 teaspoon dried rosemary
- 1 teaspoon dried thyme
- ½ cup of coconut milk

1. Mix the butter with dried rosemary and thyme.
2. Carefully rub the pork knuckle and put it in the Crock Pot.
3. Add coconut milk and close the lid.
4. Cook the meal on Low for 8 hours.

per serving: 448 calories, 33.2g protein, 2g carbohydrates, 34.1g fat, 0.9g fiber, 137mg cholesterol, 195mg sodium, 543mg potassium

Schweinshaxe
Yield: 4 servings | **Prep time:** 10 minutes | **Cook time:** 10 hours

- 1 tablespoon juniper berries
- ½ cup beer
- 1-pound pork knuckle
- ½ teaspoon sugar
- 1 lemon, halved
- 2 cups of water
- 1 tablespoon sunflower oil

1. Put all ingredients in the Crock Pot and close the lid.
2. Cook the meal on Low for 10 hours.

per serving: 311 calories, 29.1g protein, 2.9g carbohydrates, 18.9g fat, 0.4g fiber, 102mg cholesterol, 90mg sodium, 422mg potassium

BBQ Pork Knuckles
Yield: 4 servings | **Prep time:** 10 minutes | **Cook time:** 9 hours

- 14 oz pork knuckle
- ½ cup BBQ sauce
- ¼ cup tomato sauce
- ½ cup chicken stock
- 1 tablespoon ground cumin
- ¼ cup of water

1. Put all ingredients in the Crock Pot and close the lid.
2. Cook the meal on Low for 9 hours.

per serving: 286 calories, 25.7g protein, 12.9g carbohydrates, 14g fat, 0.6g fiber, 89mg cholesterol, 603mg sodium, 488mg potassium

Ham Terrine

Yield: 4 servings | **Prep time:** 20 minutes | **Cook time:** 8 hours

- 2 smoked ham hock, cooked
- 1 onion, chopped
- 1 carrot, grated
- 1 tablespoon fresh parsley, chopped
- 1 tablespoon mustard
- 3 oz prosciutto, sliced
- 1 teaspoon sunflower oil
- 1 cup of water

1. Chop the ham hock into small pieces and mix with onion, carrot, parsley, and mustard.
2. Then brush the loaf mold with sunflower oil from inside.
3. Make the pie crust from prosciutto in the loaf mold.
4. Add ham hock mixture over the prosciutto and wrap it.
5. Pour water in the Crock Pot.
6. Then insert the loaf mild with terrine inside and close the lid.
7. Cook the meal on Low for 8 hours.

per serving: 179 calories, 17.9g protein, 5.4g carbohydrates, 9.3g fat, 1.4g fiber, 52mg cholesterol, 296mg sodium, 334mg potassium

Pork Cobbler
Yield: 4 servings | **Prep time:** 15 minutes | **Cook time:** 4.5 hours

- ½ cup flour
- 3 tablespoons coconut oil
- 6 oz ground pork
- 1 carrot, grated
- ½ cup tomato juice
- 1 teaspoon salt
- 1 teaspoon chili flakes
- ¼ cup Cheddar cheese, shredded

1. In the mixing bowl mix ground pork, carrot, tomato juice, salt, and chili flakes.
2. Then mix flour with coconut oil.
3. Separate the flour mixture into 3 parts. Crumble every flour part. Make the layer of flour crumbs in the Crock Pot.
4. Top it with ground pork mixture. Then top the ground pork mixture with the second part of the crumble flour mixture. Repeat the same steps till you use all ingredients.
5. Top the cobbler with Cheddar cheese.
6. Add tomato juice and close the lid. Cook the cobbler on High for 4.5 hours.

per serving: 246 calories, 14.9g protein, 14.8g carbohydrates, 14.2g fat, 0.9g fiber, 38mg cholesterol, 742mg sodium, 322mg potassium

Succulent Pork Ribs
Yield: 4 servings | **Prep time:** 10 minutes | **Cook time:** 8 hours

- 12 oz pork ribs, roughly chopped
- ¼ cup of orange juice
- 1 cup of water
- 1 teaspoon ground nutmeg
- 1 teaspoon salt

1. Pour water and orange juice in the Crock Pot.

2. Then sprinkle the pork ribs with ground nutmeg and salt.
3. Put the pork ribs in the Crock Pot and close the lid.
4. Cook the meat on low for 8 hours.

per serving: 242 calories, 22.7g protein, 1.9g carbohydrates, 15.3g fat, 0.1g fiber, 88mg cholesterol, 633mg sodium, 279mg potassium

Lime Pork
Yield: 2 servings | **Prep time:** 15 minutes | **Cook time:** 8 hours

- 8 oz pork loin
- 1 lime
- 1 teaspoon lime zest
- ½ cup of water
- 1 teaspoon ground tarragon
- 1 teaspoon olive oil

1. Cut the lime into halves and put in the Crock Pot.
2. Chop the pork loin roughly and put in the Crock Pot.
3. Add lime zest, water, oil, and ground tarragon.
4. Close the lid and cook the pork on low for 8 hours.

per serving: 305 calories, 31.2g protein, 3.7g carbohydrates, 18.2g fat, 1.1g fiber, 91mg cholesterol, 73mg sodium, 516mg potassium

Pork Chops under Peach Blanket
Yield: 4 servings | **Prep time:** 10 minutes | **Cook time:** 4.5 hours

- 4 pork chops
- 2 tablespoons butter, softened
- 1 teaspoon salt
- 1 onion, sliced
- 1 cup of water
- 1 cup peaches, pitted, halved

1. Sprinkle the pork chops with salt.
2. Grease the Crock Pot bottom with butter.
3. Put the pork chops inside in one layer.
4. Then top them with sliced onion and peaches.
5. Add water and close the lid.
6. Cook the meal on High for 4.5 hours.

per serving: 333 calories, 18.7g protein, 6.1g carbohydrates, 25.8g fat, 1.2g fiber, 84mg cholesterol, 681mg sodium, 389mg potassium

Pork Honey Bites
Yield: 4 servings | **Prep time:** 20 minutes | **Cook time:** 4 hours

- 1 tablespoon liquid honey
- 2 tablespoons lemon juice
- 1 teaspoon sesame seeds
- ½ teaspoon ground cumin
- 4 pork chops, cut into cubes
- ½ cup of water
- 1 teaspoon peppercorns
- 1 teaspoon coconut oil

1. Pour water in the Crock Pot.
2. Add peppercorns, ground cumin, and pork chops.

3. Close the lid and cook the meat on High for 4 hours.
4. After this, toss the coconut oil in the skillet. Melt it.
5. Add cooked pork chops bites and sprinkle them with lemon juice, liquid honey, and sesame seeds.
6. Roast the meat on high heat for 2 minutes per side.

per serving: 290 calories, 18.3g protein, 5.1g carbohydrates, 21.5g fat, 0.3g fiber, 69mg cholesterol, 59mg sodium, 303mg potassium

Rosemary and Bacon Pork Chops

Yield: 4 servings | **Prep time:** 20 minutes | **Cook time:** 4 hours

- 4 pork chops
- 4 bacon slices
- 1 teaspoon dried rosemary
- 1 tablespoon olive oil
- ½ cup of water

1. Rub the pork chops with rosemary and olive oil.
2. Then wrap the pork chops in the bacon and put in the hot skillet.
3. Roast the pork chops for 1 minute per side.
4. Then transfer them in the Crock Pot. Add water.
5. Close the lid and cook the meat on High for 4 hours.

per serving: 390 calories, 25g protein, 0.5g carbohydrates, 31.4g fat, 0.1g fiber, 90mg cholesterol, 496mg sodium, 386mg potassium

Lettuce and Pork Wraps

Yield: 2 servings | **Prep time:** 20 minutes | **Cook time:** 3.5 hours

- 2 lettuce leaves
- 4 oz ground pork
- 1 teaspoon ketchup
- 1 tablespoon butter
- 3 tablespoons water
- 1 teaspoon white pepper

1. Mix ground pork with water, butter, and white pepper.
2. Put the meat mixture in the Crock Pot.
3. Close the lid and cook it on High for 3.5 hours.
4. After this, mix ground pork with ketchup.
5. Fill the lettuce leaves with ground pork.

per serving: 138 calories, 15.1g protein, 1.5g carbohydrates, 7.8g fat, 0.3g fiber, 57mg cholesterol, 10mg sodium, 270mg potassium

Pork Tomatoes

Yield: 2 servings | **Prep time:** 15 minutes | **Cook time:** 4.5 hours

- 2 tomatoes
- ¼ cup ground pork
- ¼ cup of rice, cooked
- 2 oz Parmesan
- 1 tablespoon cream cheese
- ½ teaspoon chili powder
- ½ cup of water

1. Cut the caps from tomatoes and remove the flesh to get the tomato cups.

2. After this, mix ground pork with rice, cream cheese, and chili pepper.
3. Fill the tomato cups with ground pork mixture.
4. Grate the parmesan.
5. Top the tomato cups with parmesan and put in the Crock Pot.
6. Add water and cook on High for 4.5 hours.

per serving: 246 calories, 14.8g protein, 24.8g carbohydrates, 10.3g fat, 2g fiber, 35mg cholesterol, 304mg sodium, 337mg potassium

Habanero Pork Chops

Yield: 4 servings | **Prep time:** 10 minutes | **Cook time:** 7 hours

- 1 habanero pepper, chopped
- 1 teaspoon tabasco
- 2 tablespoons maple syrup
- 1 teaspoon lemon zest
- 4 pork chops
- 1 tablespoon butter
- ½ cup of water

1. Put all ingredients in the Crock Pot and close the lid.
2. Cook the meat on low for 7 hours.

per serving: 313 calories, 18.3g protein, 7.8g carbohydrates, 22.8g fat, 0.2g fiber, 76mg cholesterol, 87mg sodium, 336mg potassium

Pork Marbella

Yield: 4 servings | **Prep time:** 10 minutes | **Cook time:** 8 hours

- 2 oz prunes, chopped
- 12 oz pork loin
- ¼ cup red wine
- 1 teaspoon capers
- ½ teaspoon sugar
- 1 teaspoon dried oregano
- 1 garlic clove, peeled
- 1 tablespoon sunflower oil
- ¼ cup of water

1. Slice the pork loin and put it in the Crock Pot.
2. Add all remaining ingredients and gently mix.
3. Cook the meal on Low for 8 hours.
4. Then carefully mix the meat and cool it to the room temperature.

per serving: 287 calories, 23.7g protein, 10.5g carbohydrates, 15.4g fat, 1.2g fiber, 68mg cholesterol, 76mg sodium, 488mg potassium

Ginger Ground Pork

Yield: 3 servings | **Prep time:** 10 minutes | **Cook time:** 6 hours

- 1.5 cup ground pork
- 1 oz minced ginger
- 2 tablespoons coconut oil
- 1 tablespoon tomato paste
- ½ teaspoon chili powder

1. Mix ground pork with minced ginger, tomato paste, and chili powder.
2. Put the ground pork in the Crock Pot.
3. Add coconut oil and close the lid.
4. Cook the meal on Low for 6 hours.

per serving: 193 calories, 7.8g protein, 7.9g carbohydrates, 15.1g fat, 1.6g fiber, 25mg cholesterol, 39mg sodium, 189mg potassium

Sweet Pork Shoulder

Yield: 2 servings | **Prep time:** 10 minutes | **Cook time:** 8 hours

- 8 oz pork shoulder
- 3 tablespoons agave syrup
- 1 tablespoon sunflower oil
- ½ cup of water

1. Brush the pork shoulder with sunflower oil and agave syrup.
2. Put it in the Crock Pot. Add water.
3. Cook the meat on low for 8 hours.

per serving: 489 calories, 26.4g protein, 25.2g carbohydrates, 31.3g fat, 0g fiber, 102mg cholesterol, 100mg sodium, 393mg potassium

Tender Glazed Pork Ribs

Yield: 4 servings | **Prep time:** 15 minutes | **Cook time:** 7 hours

- 1-pound baby back pork ribs
- 1 orange, sliced
- 1 teaspoon liquid honey
- 1 tablespoon tamarind ½ cup apple juice
- 1 anise pod
- 1 tablespoon tomato sauce

1. Put the baby back ribs in the Crock Pot.
2. Add tamarind, apple juice, tomato sauce, and anise pod.
3. Then add sliced orange and close the lid.
4. Cook the pork ribs on low for 6 hours.
5. Then sprinkle the meat with liquid honey and cook on high for 1 hour.

per serving: 368 calories, 18.6g protein, 11.7g carbohydrates, 27.2g fat, 1.3g fiber, 90mg cholesterol, 107mg sodium, 140mg potassium

Soft Pork Skewers

Yield: 4 servings | **Prep time:** 10 minutes | **Cook time:** 4.5 hours

- 15 oz pork loin, cubed
- 1 tablespoon olive oil
- ¼ cup apple cider vinegar
- 1 teaspoon hot sauce
- ¼ cup of water
- ½ lemon

1. String the pork loin cubes in the wooden skewers and sprinkle with olive oil and hot sauce.
2. Put the skewers in the Crock Pot.
3. Add apple cider vinegar, water, and lemon.
4. Close the lid and cook the skewers on High for 4.5 hours.

per serving: 293 calories, 29.1g protein, 0.8g carbohydrates, 18.3g fat, 0.2g fiber, 85mg cholesterol, 99mg sodium, 473mg potassium

Apricot Pork Saute

Yield: 4 servings | **Prep time:** 10 minutes | **Cook time:** 4 hours

- 12 oz pork loin, cubed
- 2 cups apricots, pitted, chopped

- 1 cup of water
- 1 tablespoon coconut oil
- 1 teaspoon peppercorns
- 1 teaspoon ground turmeric
- 1 teaspoon salt
- ½ teaspoon smoked paprika

1. Put all ingredients in the Crock Pot.
2. Carefully mix the saute and close the lid.
3. Cook the meal on High for 4 hours.

per serving: 276 calories, 24.4g protein, 9.3g carbohydrates, 15.8g fat, 1.9g fiber, 68mg cholesterol, 637mg sodium, 588mg potassium

Cider Pork Roast

Yield: 4 servings | **Prep time:** 10 minutes | **Cook time:** 8 hours

- 1-pound pork roast
- 1 cup cider
- 1 apple, chopped
- 1 teaspoon peppercorns
- ½ cup of water
- 1 teaspoon chili flakes

1. Put all ingredients in the Crock Pot.
2. Close the lid and cook the meat on low for 8 hours.

per serving: 294 calories, 32.6g protein, 15.3g carbohydrates, 10.9g fat, 1.6g fiber, 98mg cholesterol, 67mg sodium, 597mg potassium

Fish&Seafood

Onion Cod Fillets

Yield: 4 servings | **Prep time:** 10 minutes | **Cook time:** 3 hours

- 1 onion, minced
- 4 cod fillets
- 1 teaspoon salt
- 1 teaspoon dried cilantro
- ½ cup of water
- 1 teaspoon butter, melted

1. Sprinkle the cod fillets with salt, dried cilantro, and butter.
2. Then place them in the Crock Pot and top with minced onion.
3. Add water and close the lid.
4. Cook the fish on high for 3 hours.

per serving: 109 calories, 20.3g protein, 2.6g carbohydrates, 2g fat, 0.6g fiber, 58mg cholesterol, 660mg sodium, 41mg potassium

Tender Tilapia in Cream Sauce

Yield: 4 servings | **Prep time:** 10 minutes | **Cook time:** 5 hours

- 4 tilapia fillets
- ½ cup heavy cream
- 1 teaspoon garlic powder
- 1 teaspoon ground black pepper
- ½ teaspoon salt
- 1 teaspoon cornflour

1. Mix cornflour with cream until smooth.
2. Then pour the liquid in the Crock Pot.
3. After this, sprinkle the tilapia fillets with garlic powder, ground black pepper, and salt.
4. Place the fish fillets in the Crock Pot and close the lid.
5. Cook the fish on Low for 5 hours.

per serving: 151 calories, 21.6g protein, 1.7g carbohydrates, 6.6g fat, 0.3g fiber, 76mg cholesterol, 337mg sodium, 28mg potassium

Lemon Scallops

Yield: 4 servings | **Prep time:** 10 minutes | **Cook time:** 1 hour

- 1-pound scallops
- 1 teaspoon salt
- 1 teaspoon ground white pepper
- ½ teaspoon olive oil
- 3 tablespoons lemon juice
- 1 teaspoon lemon zest, grated
- 1 tablespoon dried oregano
- ½ cup of water

1. Sprinkle the scallops with salt, ground white pepper, lemon juice, and lemon zest and leave for 10-15 minutes to marinate.
2. After this, sprinkle the scallops with olive oil and dried oregano.
3. Put the scallops in the Crock Pot and add water.
4. Cook the seafood on High for 1 hour.

per serving: 113 calories, 19.3g protein, 4.1g carbohydrates, 1.7g fat, 0.7g fiber, 37mg cholesterol, 768mg sodium, 407mg potassium

Haddock Chowder

Yield: 5 servings | **Prep time:** 10 minutes | **Cook time:** 6 hours

- 1-pound haddock, chopped
- 2 bacon slices, chopped, cooked
- ½ cup potatoes, chopped
- 1 teaspoon ground coriander
- ½ cup heavy cream
- 4 cups of water
- 1 teaspoon salt

1. Put all ingredients in the Crock Pot and close the lid.
2. Cook the chowder on Low for 6 hours.

per serving: 203 calories, 27.1g protein, 2.8g carbohydrates, 8.6g fat, 0.4g fiber, 97mg cholesterol, 737mg sodium, 506mg potassium

Shrimp Scampi

Yield: 4 servings | **Prep time:** 5 minutes | **Cook time:** 4 hours

- 1-pound shrimps, peeled
- 2 tablespoons lemon juice
- 2 tablespoons coconut oil
- 1 cup of water
- 1 teaspoon dried parsley
- ½ teaspoon white pepper

1. Put all ingredients in the Crock Pot and gently mix.
2. Close the lid and cook the scampi on Low for 4 hours.

per serving: 196 calories, 25.9g protein, 2.1g carbohydrates, 8.8g fat, 0.1g fiber, 239mg cholesterol, 280mg sodium, 207mg potassium

Nutmeg Trout

Yield: 4 servings | **Prep time:** 10 minutes | **Cook time:** 3 hours

- 1 tablespoon ground nutmeg
- 1 tablespoon butter, softened
- 1 teaspoon dried cilantro
- 1 teaspoon dried oregano
- 1 teaspoon fish sauce
- 4 trout fillets
- ½ cup of water

1. In the shallow bowl mix butter with cilantro, dried oregano, and fish sauce. Add ground nutmeg and whisk the mixture.
2. Then grease the fish fillets with nutmeg mixture and put in the Crock Pot.
3. Add remaining butter mixture and water.
4. Cook the fish on high for 3 hours.

per serving: 154 calories, 16.8g protein, 1.2g carbohydrates, 8.8g fat, 0.5g fiber, 54mg cholesterol, 178mg sodium, 305mg potassium

Clams in Coconut Sauce

Yield: 2 servings | **Prep time:** 10 minutes | **Cook time:** 2 hours

- 1 cup coconut cream
- 1 teaspoon minced garlic
- 1 teaspoon chili flakes
- 1 teaspoon salt

- 1 teaspoon ground coriander
- 8 oz clams

1. Pour coconut cream in the Crock Pot.
2. Add minced garlic, chili flakes, salt, and ground coriander.
3. Cook the mixture on high for 1 hour.
4. Then add clams and stir the meal well. Cook it for 1 hour on high more.

per serving: 333 calories, 3.5g protein, 19.6g carbohydrates, 28.9g fat, 3.1g fiber, 0mg cholesterol, 1592mg sodium, 425mg potassium.

Sweet Milkfish Saute
Yield: 4 servings | **Prep time:** 10 minutes | **Cook time:** 3 hours

- 2 mangos, pitted, peeled, chopped
- 12 oz milkfish fillet, chopped
- ½ cup tomatoes, chopped
- ½ cup of water
- 1 teaspoon ground cardamom

1. Mix mangos with tomatoes and ground cardamom.
2. Transfer the ingredients in the Crock Pot.
3. Then add milkfish fillet and water.
4. Cook the saute on High for 3 hours.
5. Carefully stir the saute before serving.

per serving: 268 calories, 24g protein, 26.4g carbohydrates, 8.1g fat, 3.1g fiber, 57mg cholesterol, 82mg sodium, 660mg potassium.

Thyme Mussels
Yield: 4 servings | **Prep time:** 10 minutes | **Cook time:** 2.5 hours

- 1-pound mussels
- 1 teaspoon dried thyme
- 1 teaspoon ground black pepper
- ½ teaspoon salt
- 1 cup of water
- ½ cup sour cream

1. In the mixing bowl mix mussels, dried thyme, ground black pepper, and salt.
2. Then pour water in the Crock Pot.
3. Add sour cream and cook the liquid on High for 1.5 hours.
4. After this, add mussels and cook them for 1 hour on High or until the mussels are opened.

per serving: 161 calories, 14.5g protein, 5.9g carbohydrates, 8.6g fat, 0.2g fiber, 44mg cholesterol, 632mg sodium, 414mg potassium.

Cinnamon Catfish
Yield: 2 servings | **Prep time:** 10 minutes | **Cook time:** 2.5 hours

- 2 catfish fillets
- 1 teaspoon ground cinnamon
- 1 tablespoon lemon juice
- ½ teaspoon sesame oil
- 1/3 cup water

1. Sprinkle the fish fillets with ground cinnamon, lemon juice, and sesame oil.
2. Put the fillets in the Crock Pot in one layer.
3. Add water and close the lid.
4. Cook the meal on High for 2.5 hours.

per serving: 231 calories, 25g protein, 1.1g carbohydrates, 13.3g fat, 0.6g fiber, 75mg cholesterol, 88mg sodium, 528mg potassium.

Hot Salmon
Yield: 4 servings | **Prep time:** 10 minutes | **Cook time:** 3 hours

- 1-pound salmon fillet, sliced
- 2 chili peppers, chopped
- 1 tablespoon olive oil
- 1 onion, diced
- ½ cup cream
- ½ teaspoon salt

1. Mix salmon with salt, onion, and olive oil.
2. Transfer the ingredients in the Crock Pot.
3. Add cream and onion.
4. Cook the salmon on high for 3 hours.

per serving: 211 calories, 22.6g protein, 3.7g carbohydrates, 12.2g fat, 0.7g fiber, 56mg cholesterol, 352mg sodium, 491mg potassium.

Sage Shrimps
Yield: 4 servings | **Prep time:** 10 minutes | **Cook time:** 1 hour

- 1-pound shrimps, peeled
- 1 teaspoon dried sage
- 1 teaspoon minced garlic
- 1 teaspoon white pepper
- 1 cup tomatoes chopped
- ½ cup of water

1. Put all ingredients in the Crock Pot and close the lid.
2. Cook the shrimps on High for 1 hour.

per serving: 146 calories, 26.4g protein, 4.1g carbohydrates, 2.1g fat, 0.8g fiber, 239mg cholesterol, 280mg sodium, 310mg potassium.

Fish Salpicao
Yield: 4 servings | **Prep time:** 5 minutes | **Cook time:** 1 hour

- 1 teaspoon ground black pepper
- 1 teaspoon cayenne pepper
- 1 tablespoon avocado oil
- 1-pound cod fillet
- 1 teaspoon salt
- 1 garlic clove, diced

1. Put all ingredients in the Crock Pot and carefully mix.
2. Then close the lid and cook the meal on High for 1 hour.

per serving: 100 calories, 20.5g protein, 1g carbohydrates, 1.6g fat, 0.4g fiber, 56mg cholesterol, 653mg sodium, 30mg potassium.

Miso Cod
Yield: 4 servings | **Prep time:** 10 minutes | **Cook time:** 4 hours

- 1-pound cod fillet, sliced
- 1 teaspoon miso paste
- ½ teaspoon ground ginger
- 2 cups chicken stock
- ½ teaspoon ground nutmeg

1. In the mixing bowl mix chicken stock, ground nutmeg, ground ginger, and miso paste.
2. Then pour the liquid in the Crock Pot.
3. Add cod fillet and close the lid.
4. Cook the fish on Low for 4 hours.
per serving: 101 calories, 20.8g protein, 1.1g carbohydrates, 1.5g fat, 0.2g fiber, 56mg cholesterol, 506mg sodium, 14mg potassium.

Coconut Catfish
Yield: 3 servings | **Prep time:** 10 minutes | **Cook time:** 2.5 hours
- 3 catfish fillets
- 1 teaspoon coconut shred
- ½ cup of coconut milk
- 1 teaspoon sesame seeds
- 2 tablespoons fish sauce
- 1 cup of water
- 2 tablespoons soy sauce
1. Pour water in the Crock Pot.
2. Add soy sauce, fish sauce, sesame seeds, and coconut milk.
3. Then add coconut shred and catfish fillets.
4. Cook the fish on high for 2.5 hours.
per serving: 329 calories, 27.3g protein, 3.9g carbohydrates, 22.7g fat, 1.2g fiber, 75mg cholesterol, 1621mg sodium, 682mg potassium.

Hot Calamari
Yield: 4 servings | **Prep time:** 10 minutes | **Cook time:** 1 hour
- 12 oz calamari, sliced
- ¼ cup of soy sauce
- 1 teaspoon cayenne pepper
- 1 garlic clove, crushed
- 1 teaspoon mustard
- ½ cup of water
- 1 teaspoon sesame oil
1. In the bowl mix slices calamari, soy sauce, cayenne pepper, garlic, mustard, and sesame oil. Leave the ingredients for 10 minutes to marinate.
2. Then transfer the mixture in the Crock Pot, add water, and close the lid.
3. Cook the meal on high for 1 hour.
per serving: 103 calories, 14.6g protein, 4.6g carbohydrates, 2.6g fat, 0.4g fiber, 198mg cholesterol, 937mg sodium, 262mg potassium.

Curry Squid
Yield: 5 servings | **Prep time:** 10 minutes | **Cook time:** 3 hours
- 15 oz squid, peeled, sliced
- 1 teaspoon curry paste
- ½ cup of coconut milk
- ¼ cup of water
- 1 teaspoon dried dill
- 1 teaspoon ground nutmeg
1. Mix coconut milk with water and curry paste.
2. Then pour the liquid in the Crock Pot.
3. Add dried dill and ground nutmeg.
4. After this, add the sliced squid and close the lid.
5. Cook the meal on low for 3 hours.

per serving: 143 calories, 13.9g protein, 4.6g carbohydrates, 7.6g fat, 0.7g fiber, 198mg cholesterol, 42mg sodium, 281mg potassium.

Rosemary Seabass
Yield: 3 servings | **Prep time:** 10 minutes | **Cook time:** 4 hours
- 3 seabass fillets
- 1 teaspoon dried rosemary
- 1 carrot, grated
- 2 teaspoons sesame oil
- ½ cup of water
1. Rub the seabass fillets with dried rosemary and sesame oil.
2. Then place them in the Crock Pot in one layer.
3. Top the fillets with grated carrot.
4. Add water and close the lid.
5. Cook the fish on low for 4 hours.
per serving: 271 calories, 26.3g protein, 2.3g carbohydrates, 17.2g fat, 1.6g fiber, 0mg cholesterol, 16mg sodium, 69mg potassium.

Butter Salmon
Yield: 2 servings | **Prep time:** 10 minutes | **Cook time:** 1.5 hours
- 8 oz salmon fillet
- 3 tablespoons butter
- 1 teaspoon dried sage
- ¼ cup of water
1. Churn butter with sage and preheat the mixture until liquid.
2. Then cut the salmon fillets into 2 servings and put in the Crock Pot.
3. Add water and melted butter mixture.
4. Close the lid and cook the salmon on High for 1.5 hours.
per serving: 304 calories, 22.2g protein, 0.2g carbohydrates, 24.3g fat, 0.1g fiber, 96mg cholesterol, 174mg sodium, 444mg potassium.

Seabass Balls
Yield: 4 servings | **Prep time:** 20 minutes | **Cook time:** 2 hours
- 1 teaspoon ground coriander
- ½ teaspoon salt
- 2 tablespoons flour
- ½ cup chicken stock
- 1 teaspoon dried dill
- 10 oz seabass fillet
- 1 tablespoon sesame oil
1. Dice the seabass fillet into tiny pieces and mix with salt, ground coriander, flour, and dill.
2. Make the medium size balls.
3. Preheat the skillet well.
4. Add sesame oil and heat it until hot.
5. Add the fish balls and roast them on high heat for 1 minute per side.
6. Then transfer the fish balls in the Crock Pot. Arrange them in one layer.
7. Add water and close the lid.
8. Cook the meal on High for 2 hours.
per serving: 191 calories, 16.6g protein, 3.2g carbohydrates, 12.2g fat, 0.7g fiber, 0mg cholesterol, 387mg sodium, 15mg potassium.

Cod Sticks

Yield: 2 servings | **Prep time:** 15 minutes | **Cook time:** 1.5 hour

- 2 cod fillets
- 1 teaspoon ground black pepper
- 1 egg, beaten
- 1/3 cup breadcrumbs
- 1 tablespoon coconut oil
- ¼ cup of water

1. Cut the cod fillets into medium sticks and sprinkle with ground black pepper.
2. Then dip the fish in the beaten egg and coat in the breadcrumbs.
3. Pour water in the Crock Pot.
4. Add coconut oil and fish sticks.
5. Cook the meal on High for 1.5 hours.

per serving: 254 calories, 25.3g protein, 13.8g carbohydrates, 11g fat, 1.1g fiber, 137mg cholesterol, 234mg sodium, 78mg potassium.

Cumin Snapper

Yield: 4 servings | **Prep time:** 15 minutes | **Cook time:** 4 hours

- 1-pound snapper, peeled, cleaned
- 1 teaspoon ground cumin
- ½ teaspoon salt
- ½ teaspoon garlic powder
- 1 teaspoon dried oregano
- 1 tablespoon sesame oil
- ¼ cup of water

1. Cut the snapper into 4 servings.
2. After this, in the shallow bowl mix ground cumin, salt, garlic powder, and dried oregano.
3. Sprinkle fish with spices and sesame oil.
4. Arrange the snapper in the Crock Pot. Add water.
5. Cook the fish on Low for 4 hours.

per serving: 183 calories, 29.9g protein, 0.7g carbohydrates, 5.6g fat, 0.3g fiber, 54mg cholesterol, 360mg sodium, 20mg potassium.

Fish Pie

Yield: 6 servings | **Prep time:** 15 minutes | **Cook time:** 7 hours

- 7 oz yeast dough
- 1 tablespoon cream cheese
- 8 oz salmon fillet, chopped
- 1 onion, diced
- 1 teaspoon salt
- 1 tablespoon fresh dill
- 1 teaspoon olive oil

1. Brush the Crock Pot bottom with olive oil.
2. Then roll up the dough and place it in the Crock Pot.
3. Flatten it in the shape of the pie crust.
4. After this, in the mixing bowl mix cream cheese, salmon, onion, salt, and dill.
5. Put the fish mixture over the pie crust and cover with foil.
6. Close the lid and cook the pie on Low for 7 hours.

per serving: 158 calories, 9.5g protein, 18.6g carbohydrates, 5g fat, 1.3g fiber, 19mg cholesterol, 524mg sodium, 191mg potassium.

Cardamom Trout

Yield: 4 servings | **Prep time:** 10 minutes | **Cook time:** 2.5 hours

- 1 teaspoon ground cardamom
- 1-pound trout fillet
- 1 teaspoon butter, melted
- 1 tablespoon lemon juice
- ¼ cup of water
- 1.2 teaspoon salt

1. In the shallow bowl mix butter, lemon juice, and salt.
2. Then sprinkle the trout fillet with ground cardamom and butter mixture.
3. Place the fish in the Crock Pot and add water.
4. Cook the meal on High for 2.5 hours.

per serving: 226 calories, 30.3g protein, 0.4g carbohydrates, 10.6g fat, 0.2g fiber, 86mg cholesterol, 782mg sodium, 536mg potassium.

Rosemary Sole

Yield: 2 servings | **Prep time:** 10 minutes | **Cook time:** 2 hours

- 8 oz sole fillet
- 1 tablespoon dried rosemary
- 1 tablespoon avocado oil
- 1 tablespoon apple cider vinegar
- 5 tablespoons water

1. Pour water in the Crock Pot.
2. Then rub the sole fillet with dried rosemary and sprinkle with avocado oil and apple cider vinegar.
3. Put the fish fillet in the Crock Pot and cook it on High for 2 hours.

per serving: 149 calories, 27.6g protein, 1.5g carbohydrates, 2.9g fat, 1g fiber, 77mg cholesterol, 122mg sodium, 434mg potassium.

Cheesy Fish Dip

Yield: 6 servings | **Prep time:** 10 minutes | **Cook time:** 5 hours

- ½ cup cream
- ½ cup Mozzarella, shredded
- 8 oz tuna, canned, shredded
- 2 oz chives, chopped

1. Put all ingredients in the Crock Pot and gently mix.
2. Then close the lid and cook the fish dip in Low for 5 hours.

per serving: 93 calories, 11.2g protein, 1.1g carbohydrates, 4.7g fat, 0.2g fiber, 17mg cholesterol, 40mg sodium, 161mg potassium.

Tuna Casserole

Yield: 4 servings | **Prep time:** 15 minutes | **Cook time:** 7 hours

- 1 cup mushrooms, sliced
- ½ cup corn kernels, frozen
- 8 oz tuna, chopped
- 1 teaspoon Italian seasonings
- 1 cup chicken stock

● ½ cup Cheddar cheese, shredded
● 1 tablespoon sesame oil
1. Heat the sesame oil in the skillet.
2. Add mushrooms and roast them for 5 minutes on medium heat.
3. Then transfer the mushrooms in the Crock Pot and flatten in one layer.
4. After this, mix Italian seasonings with tuna and put over the mushrooms.
5. Then top the fish with corn kernels and cheese.
6. Add chicken stock.
7. Cook the casserole on Low for 7 hours.
 per serving: 219 calories, 19.9g protein, 4.7g carbohydrates, 13.4g fat, 0.7g fiber, 33mg cholesterol, 311mg sodium, 315mg potassium.

Lemon Trout
Yield: 4 servings | **Prep time:** 15 minutes | **Cook time:** 5 hours
• 1-pound trout, peeled, cleaned
• 1 lemon, sliced
• 1 teaspoon dried thyme
• 1 teaspoon ground black pepper
• 1 tablespoon olive oil
• ½ teaspoon salt
• ½ cup of water
1. Rub the fish with dried thyme, ground black pepper, and salt.
2. Then fill the fish with sliced lemon and sprinkle with olive oil.
3. Place the trout in the Crock Pot and add water.
4. Cook the fish on Low for 5 hours.
 per serving: 252 calories, 30.4g protein, 1.9g carbohydrates, 13.2g fat, 0.6g fiber, 84mg cholesterol, 368mg sodium, 554mg potassium.

Braised Salmon
Yield: 4 servings | **Prep time:** 10 minutes | **Cook time:** 1 hour
● 1 cup of water
● 2-pound salmon fillet
● 1 teaspoon salt
● 1 teaspoon ground black pepper
1. Put all ingredients in the Crock Pot and close the lid.
2. Cook the salmon on High for 1 hour.
 per serving: 301 calories, 44.1g protein, 0.3g carbohydrates, 14g fat, 0.1g fiber, 100mg cholesterol, 683mg sodium, 878mg potassium.

Seabass Ragout
Yield: 4 servings | **Prep time:** 15 minutes | **Cook time:** 3.5 hours
• 7 oz shiitake mushrooms
• 1 onion, diced
• 1 tablespoon coconut oil
• 1 teaspoon ground coriander
• ½ teaspoon salt
• 1 cup of water
• 12 oz seabass fillet, chopped
1. Heat the coconut oil in the skillet.
2. Add onion and mushrooms and roast the vegetables for 5 minutes on medium heat.

3. Then transfer the vegetables in the Crock Pot and add water.
4. Add fish fillet, salt, and ground coriander.
5. Cook the meal on High for 3.5 hours.
 per serving: 241 calories, 20.4g protein, 9.4g carbohydrates, 14g fat, 2.3g fiber, 0mg cholesterol, 413mg sodium, 99mg potassium.

Sweet and Sour Shrimps
Yield: 2 servings | **Prep time:** 10 minutes | **Cook time:** 50 minutes
● 8 oz shrimps, peeled
● ½ cup of water
● 2 tablespoons lemon juice
● 1 tablespoon maple syrup
1. Pour water in the Crock Pot.
2. Add shrimps and cook them on High for 50 minutes.
3. Then drain water and ass lemon juice and maple syrup.
4. Carefully stir the shrimps and transfer them in the serving bowls.
 per serving: 165 calories, 26g protein, 8.8g carbohydrates, 2.1g fat, 0.1g fiber, 239mg cholesterol, 282mg sodium, 232mg potassium.

Orange Cod
Yield: 4 servings | **Prep time:** 10 minutes | **Cook time:** 3 hours
• 1-pound cod fillet, chopped
• 2 oranges, chopped
• 1 tablespoon maple syrup
• 1 cup of water
• 1 garlic clove, diced
• 1 teaspoon ground black pepper
1. Mix cod with ground black pepper and transfer in the Crock Pot.
2. Add garlic, water, maple syrup, and oranges.
3. Close the lid and cook the meal on High for 3 hours.
 per serving: 150 calories, 21.2g protein, 14.8g carbohydrates, 1.2g fat, 2.4g fiber, 56mg cholesterol, 73mg sodium, 187mg potassium.

Chili Salmon
Yield: 4 servings | **Prep time:** 5 minutes | **Cook time:** 5 hours
● 1-pound salmon fillet, chopped
● 3 oz chili, chopped, canned
● ½ cup of water
● ½ teaspoon salt
1. Place all ingredients in the Crock Pot and close the lid.
2. Cook the meal on Low for 5 hours.
 per serving: 174 calories, 23.2g protein, 2.5g carbohydrates, 8.2g fat, 0.9g fiber, 54mg cholesterol, 453mg sodium, 513mg potassium.

Trout Cakes
Yield: 2 servings | **Prep time:** 10 minutes | **Cook time:** 2 hours
• 7 oz trout fillet, diced
• 1 tablespoon semolina

- 1 teaspoon dried oregano
- ¼ teaspoon ground black pepper
- 1 teaspoon cornflour
- 1 egg, beaten
- 1/3 cup water
- 1 teaspoon sesame oil

1. In the bowl mix diced trout, semolina, dried oregano, ground black pepper, and cornflour.
2. Then add egg and carefully mix the mixture.
3. Heat the sesame oil well.
4. Then make the fish cakes and put them in the hot oil.
5. Roast them for 1 minute per side and transfer in the Crock Pot.
6. Add water and cook the trout cakes for 2 hours on High.

per serving: 266 calories, 30g protein, 5.6g carbohydrates, 13.1g fat, 0.7g fiber, 155mg cholesterol, 99mg sodium, 519mg potassium.

Salmon Croquettes
Yield: 6 servings | **Prep time:** 15 minutes | **Cook time:** 2 hours

- 1-pound salmon fillet, minced
- 1 tablespoon mayonnaise
- 2 tablespoons panko breadcrumbs
- ½ teaspoon ground black pepper
- 1 egg, beaten
- 1 teaspoon smoked paprika
- ½ cup of water

1. In the bowl mix minced salmon with mayonnaise panko breadcrumbs, ground black pepper, egg, and smoked paprika.
2. Then make the small croquettes and place them in the Crock Pot.
3. Add water and close the lid.
4. Cook the meal on high for 2 hours.

per serving: 127 calories, 15.9g protein, 2.2g carbohydrates, 6.3g fat, 0.4g fiber, 61mg cholesterol, 73mg sodium, 311mg potassium.

Spiced Mackerel
Yield: 4 servings | **Prep time:** 10 minutes | **Cook time:** 4 hours

- 1-pound mackerel, peeled, cleaned
- 1 teaspoon salt
- 1 teaspoon ground black pepper
- ½ teaspoon ground clove
- 1 cup of water
- 1 tablespoon olive oil

1. Sprinkle the fish with salt, ground black pepper, ground clove, and olive oil.
2. Then put the fish in the Crock Pot. Add water.
3. Close the lid and cook the mackerel on high for 4 hours.

per serving: 329 calories, 27.1g protein, 0.5g carbohydrates, 23.8g fat, 0.2g fiber, 85mg cholesterol, 678mg sodium, 465mg potassium.

Mackerel Chops
Yield: 6 servings | **Prep time:** 15 minutes | **Cook time:** 5 hours

- 24 oz mackerel fillet

- 1 teaspoon dried lemongrass
- ½ teaspoon ground nutmeg
- 1 teaspoon smoked paprika
- 1 teaspoon salt
- 1 tablespoon apple cider vinegar
- 1 tablespoon fish sauce
- ½ cup of water

1. Cut the mackerel fillet into 6 servings.
2. Then sprinkle every mackerel fillet with dried lemongrass, ground nutmeg, smoked paprika, salt, apple cider vinegar, and fish sauce.
3. Put the fish fillets in the Crock Pot. Add water.
4. Cook the meal on Low for 5 hours.

per serving: 301 calories, 27.3g protein, 0.5g carbohydrates, 20.3g fat, 0.2g fiber, 85mg cholesterol, 714mg sodium, 476mg potassium.

Mini Fish Balls
Yield: 6 servings | **Prep time:** 20 minutes | **Cook time:** 2.5 hours

- 4 oz corn kernels, cooked
- 1-pound salmon fillet, minced
- 1 tablespoon semolina
- ½ zucchini, grated
- 1 teaspoon ground black pepper
- ½ teaspoon salt
- 1 tablespoon sesame oil
- ½ cup of water

1. Mix corn kernels, salmon, semolina, grated zucchini, ground black pepper, and salt in the bowl.
2. Make the small balls.
3. Then heat the sesame oil well.
4. Put the small balls in the hot oil and roast for 1.5 minutes per side.
5. Then arrange the fish balls one-by-one in the Crock Pot.
6. Add water and close the lid.
7. Cook the meal on High for 2.5 hours.

per serving: 218 calories, 18.5g protein, 21.4g carbohydrates, 8.2g fat, 3.1g fiber, 33mg cholesterol, 245mg sodium, 618mg potassium.

Cod Fingers
Yield: 5 servings | **Prep time:** 15 minutes | **Cook time:** 2.5 hours

- 3 cod fillets
- ½ cup panko bread crumbs
- ½ teaspoon salt
- 3 eggs, beaten
- 4 tablespoons butter

1. Slice the cod fillet into sticks and sprinkle with salt.
2. Then dip the fish sticks in the eggs and coat well with panko bread crumbs.
3. Put butter in the Crock Pot and melt it.
4. Put the fish sticks in the Crock Pot in one layer and close the lid.
5. Cook them on High for 2.5 hours.

per serving: 216 calories, 16.9g protein, 8g carbohydrates, 13g fat, 0.5g fiber, 156mg cholesterol, 456mg sodium, 59mg potassium.

Thai Style Flounder

Yield: 6 servings | **Prep time:** 15 minutes | **Cook time:** 6 hours

- 24 oz flounder, peeled, cleaned
- 1 lemon, sliced
- 1 teaspoon ground ginger
- ½ teaspoon cayenne pepper
- ½ teaspoon chili powder
- 1 teaspoon salt
- 1 teaspoon ground turmeric
- 1 tablespoon sesame oil
- 1 cup of water

1. Chop the flounder roughly and put in the Crock Pot.
2. Add water and all remaining ingredients.
3. Close the lid and cook the fish on low for 6 hours.

per serving: 159 calories, 27.6g protein, 1.6g carbohydrates, 4.2g fat, 0.5g fiber, 77mg cholesterol, 511mg sodium, 425mg potassium.

Snapper Ragout
Yield: 6 servings | **Prep time:** 10 minutes | **Cook time:** 6 hours

- 1-pound snapper, chopped
- 1 cup tomatoes, chopped
- 1 cup onion, chopped
- 1 cup mushrooms, chopped
- 2 cups of water
- ½ cup sour cream
- 1 teaspoon salt
- 1 teaspoon chili powder

1. Put all ingredients in the Crock Pot.
2. Gently stir them with the help of the spoon.
3. Close the lid and cook the meal on low for 6 hours.

per serving: 155 calories, 21.4g protein, 4.4g carbohydrates, 5.5g fat, 1g fiber, 44mg cholesterol, 450mg sodium, 568mg potassium.

Garlic Perch
Yield: 4 servings | **Prep time:** 15 minutes | **Cook time:** 4 hours

- 1-pound perch
- 1 teaspoon minced garlic
- 1 tablespoon butter, softened
- 1 tablespoon fish sauce
- ½ cup of water

1. In the shallow bowl mix minced garlic, butter, and fish sauce.
2. Rub the perch with a garlic butter mixture and arrange it in the Crock Pot.
3. Add remaining garlic butter mixture and water.
4. Cook the fish on high for 4 hours.

per serving: 161 calories, 28.5g protein, 0.4g carbohydrates, 4.2g fat, 0g fiber, 138mg cholesterol, 458mg sodium, 407mg potassium.

Tomato Squid
Yield: 4 servings | **Prep time:** 10 minutes | **Cook time:** 2 hours

- 1-pound squid tubes, cleaned
- 1 cup tomatoes, chopped
- ½ cup bell pepper, chopped
- 1 teaspoon cayenne pepper
- 1 cup of water
- 1 teaspoon avocado oil

1. Chop the squid tube roughly and mix with avocado oil and cayenne pepper.
2. Put the squid in the Crock Pot.
3. Add water, bell pepper, and tomatoes.
4. Close the lid and cook the squid on High for 2 hours.

per serving: 76 calories, 12.6g protein, 3.2g carbohydrates, 1.8g fat, 0.9g fiber, 351mg cholesterol, 546mg sodium, 148mg potassium.

Apricot and Halibut Saute
Yield: 2 servings | **Prep time:** 5 minutes | **Cook time:** 5 hours

- 6 oz halibut fillet, chopped
- ½ cup apricots, pitted, chopped
- ½ cup of water
- 1 tablespoon soy sauce
- 1 teaspoon ground cumin

1. Put all ingredients in the Crock Pot.
2. Close the lid and cook the fish sauté on Low for 5 hours.

per serving: 407 calories, 28.7g protein, 5.3g carbohydrates, 28.7g fat, 0.9g fiber, 94mg cholesterol, 619mg sodium, 684mg potassium.

Sweet Salmon
Yield: 4 servings | **Prep time:** 15 minutes | **Cook time:** 1.5 hours

- 1-pound salmon fillet
- 1 teaspoon Italian seasonings
- 1 tablespoon butter
- 1 tablespoon maple syrup
- ½ teaspoon salt
- 1 cup of water

1. Pour water in the Crock Pot.
2. Add salt, salmon, and Italian seasonings.
3. Cook the fish on high for 1.5 hours.
4. Then melt the butter in the skillet and add maple syrup. Stir the mixture until smooth.
5. Add the cooked salmon and roast it on high heat for 2 minutes per side.

per serving: 192 calories, 22g protein, 3.5g carbohydrates, 10.2g fat, 0g fiber, 58mg cholesterol, 364mg sodium, 448mg potassium.

Marinated Salmon with Sesame Seeds
Yield: 2 servings | **Prep time:** 10 minutes | **Cook time:** 2 hours

- 8 oz salmon fillet
- ½ cup of soy sauce
- 1 garlic clove, diced
- 1 teaspoon coriander seeds
- 1 teaspoon olive oil
- 1 tablespoon sesame seeds
- ¼ cup of water

1. Cut salmon fillet into 2 pieces and put in the Crock Pot.

2.   Add all remaining ingredients in the Crock Pot and close the lid.
3.   Cook the salmon on High for 2 hours.
4.   Serve the cooked fish with hot soy sauce marinade.

per serving: 232 calories, 26.9g protein, 6.4g carbohydrates, 11.6g fat, 1.1g fiber, 50mg cholesterol, 3645mg sodium, 602mg potassium.

Butter Crab
Yield: 4 servings | **Prep time:** 10 minutes | **Cook time:** 4.5 hours

- 1-pound crab meat, roughly chopped
- 1 tablespoon fresh parsley, chopped
- 3 tablespoons butter
- 2 tablespoons water

1.   Melt butter and pour it in the Crock Pot.
2.   Add water, parsley, and crab meat.
3.   Cook the meal on Low for 4.5 hours.

per serving: 178 calories, 14.3g protein, 2.1g carbohydrates, 10.7g fat, 0g fiber, 84mg cholesterol, 771mg sodium, 8mg potassium.

Braised Lobster
Yield: 4 servings | **Prep time:** 10 minutes | **Cook time:** 3 hours

- 2-pound lobster, cleaned
- 1 cup of water
- 1 teaspoon Italian seasonings

1.   Put all ingredients in the Crock Pot.
2.   Close the lid and cook the lobster in High for 3 hours.
3.   Remove the lobster from the Crock Pot and cool it till room temperature

per serving: 206 calories, 43.1g protein, 0.1g carbohydrates, 2.2g fat, 0g fiber, 332mg cholesterol, 1104mg sodium, 524mg potassium.

Crab Bake
Yield: 4 servings | **Prep time:** 10 minutes | **Cook time:** 1.5 hours

- 1 cup Cheddar cheese, shredded
- 1-pound crab meat, cooked, chopped
- 1 teaspoon white pepper
- 1 teaspoon dried cilantro
- 1 cup cream

1.   Put crab meat in the Crock Pot and flatten it in one layer.
2.   Sprinkle it with white pepper and dried cilantro.
3.   After this, pour the cream and sprinkle the crab meat with Cheddar cheese.
4.   Close the lid and cook the meal on High for 1.5 hours.

per serving: 255 calories, 21.8g protein, 4.6g carbohydrates, 14.7g fat, 0.1g fiber, 102mg cholesterol, 904mg sodium, 57mg potassium.

Tacos Stuffing
Yield: 4 servings | **Prep time:** 10 minutes | **Cook time:** 3 hours

- 1-pound trout fillet, sliced
- ¼ cup fresh cilantro, chopped
- 1 teaspoon taco seasoning
- 1 teaspoon olive oil
- 1 tablespoon tomato paste
- ½ cup of water
- 2 tablespoons lemon juice

1.   Pour water in the Crock Pot.
2.   Add tomato paste and stir the liquid until the tomato paste is dissolved.
3.   Add sliced trout and taco seasonings.
4.   Cook the fish on high for 3 hours.
5.   Then drain water and mix the fish with olive oil, fresh cilantro, and lemon juice.
6.   Shake the stuffing well.

per serving: 233 calories, 30.5g protein, 1.5g carbohydrates, 10.9g fat, 0.2g fiber, 84mg cholesterol, 136mg sodium, 581mg potassium.

Shrimp Skewers
Yield: 4 servings | **Prep time:** 10 minutes | **Cook time:** 50 minutes

- 1-pound shrimps, peeled
- ½ cup chicken stock
- 1 teaspoon ground coriander
- 1 teaspoon salt
- 1 teaspoon fennel seeds
- 1 teaspoon tomato paste

1.   Sting the shrimps on the skewers and put in the Crock Pot.
2.   Add all remaining ingredients and close the lid.
3.   Cook the meal on High for 50 minutes.

per serving: 139 calories, 26.1g protein, 2.3g carbohydrates, 2.1g fat, 0.3g fiber, 239mg cholesterol, 955mg sodium, 216mg potassium.

Fish Soufflé
Yield: 4 servings | **Prep time:** 10 minutes | **Cook time:** 4 hours

- 3 oz white sandwich bread, chopped
- 1 cup cream
- ¼ cup Mozzarella, shredded
- 8 oz salmon, chopped
- 1 teaspoon ground black pepper
- ½ cup of water

3.   Pour water and cream in the Crock Pot,
4.   Then add salmon and bread.
5.   Top the mixture with Mozzarella and ground black pepper.
6.   Close the lid and cook the soufflé for 4 hours on Low.

per serving: 181 calories, 13.9g protein, 13.1g carbohydrates, 8.3g fat, 0.4g fiber, 37mg cholesterol, 164mg sodium, 247mg potassium.

Sriracha Cod
Yield: 4 servings | **Prep time:** 10 minutes | **Cook time:** 6 hours

- 4 cod fillets
- 2 tablespoons sriracha
- 1 tablespoon olive oil
- 1 teaspoon tomato paste
- ½ cup of water

1.   Sprinkle the cod fillets with sriracha, olive oil, and tomato paste.
2.   Put the fish in the Crock Pot and add water.

3. Cook it on Low for 6 hours.
per serving: 129 calories, 20.1g protein, 1.8g carbohydrates, 4.5g fat, 0.1g fiber, 55mg cholesterol, 125mg sodium, 14mg potassium.

Curry Clams
Yield: 4 servings | **Prep time:** 5 minutes | **Cook time:** 1.5 hour

- 1-pound clams
- 1 teaspoon curry paste
- ¼ cup of coconut milk
- 1 cup of water

1. Mix coconut milk with curry paste and water and pour it in the Crock Pot.
2. Add clams and close the lid.
3. Cook the meal on High for 1.5 hours or until the clams are opened.

per serving: 97 calories, 1.1g protein, 13.6g carbohydrates, 4.5g fat, 0.8g fiber, 0mg cholesterol, 415mg sodium, 141mg potassium.

Salmon Pudding
Yield: 4 servings | **Prep time:** 10 minutes | **Cook time:** 6 hours

- 1-pound salmon fillet, chopped
- ½ cup milk
- 2 tablespoons breadcrumbs
- 1 teaspoon coconut oil
- 1 teaspoon fish sauce
- 1 teaspoon salt
- 2 eggs, beaten

1. Mix all ingredients in the Crock Pot and close the lid.
2. Cook the pudding on Low for 6 hours.

per serving: 220 calories, 26.3g protein, 4.2g carbohydrates, 11.1g fat, 0.2g fiber, 134mg cholesterol, 817mg sodium, 494mg potassium.

Butter Crab Legs
Yield: 4 servings | **Prep time:** 7 minutes | **Cook time:** 45 minutes

- 15 oz king crab legs
- 1 tablespoon butter
- 1 cup of water
- 1 teaspoon dried basil

1. Put the crab legs in the Crock Pot.
2. Add basil and water and cook them on High for 45 minutes.

per serving: 133 calories, 20.4g protein, 0g carbohydrates, 4.5g fat, 0g fiber, 67mg cholesterol, 1161mg sodium, 2mg potassium

Pesto Salmon
Yield: 4 servings | **Prep time:** 10 minutes | **Cook time:** 2.5 hours

- 1-pound salmon fillet
- 3 tablespoons pesto sauce
- 1 tablespoon butter
- ¼ cup of water

1. Pour water in the Crock Pot.
2. Add butter and 1 tablespoon of pesto.
3. Add salmon and cook the fish on High for 2.5 hours.

4. Chop the cooked salmon and top with remaining pesto sauce.
per serving: 226 calories, 23.2g protein, 0.8g carbohydrates, 14.8g fat, 0.2g fiber, 60mg cholesterol, 142mg sodium, 436mg potassium

Basil Octopus
Yield: 3 servings | **Prep time:** 10 minutes | **Cook time:** 4 hours

- 12 oz octopus, chopped
- 1 orange, chopped
- 1 teaspoon dried basil
- ½ cup of water
- 1 teaspoon butter

1. Put all ingredients in the Crock Pot.
2. Close the lid and cook the octopus on Low for 4 hours or until it is soft.

per serving: 226 calories, 34.4g protein, 12.2g carbohydrates, 3.7g fat, 1.5g fiber, 112mg cholesterol, 532mg sodium, 827mg potassium

Cilantro Haddock
Yield: 2 servings | **Prep time:** 10 minutes | **Cook time:** 1.5 hour

- 6 oz haddock fillet
- 1 teaspoon dried cilantro
- 1 teaspoon olive oil
- 1 teaspoon lemon juice
- ¼ cup fish stock

1. Heat the olive oil in the skillet well.
2. Then put the haddock fillet and roast it for 1 minute per side.
3. Transfer the fillets in the Crock Pot.
4. Add fish stock, cilantro, and lemon juice.
5. Cook the fish on high for 1.5 hours.

per serving: 121 calories, 21.3g protein, 0.1g carbohydrates, 3.4g fat, 0g fiber, 63mg cholesterol, 120mg sodium, 385mg potassium

Mustard Cod
Yield: 4 servings | **Prep time:** 15 minutes | **Cook time:** 3 hours

- 4 cod fillets
- 4 teaspoons mustard
- 2 tablespoons sesame oil
- ¼ cup of water

1. Mix mustard with sesame oil.
2. Then brush the cod fillets with mustard mixture and transfer in the Crock Pot.
3. Add water and cook the fish on low for 3 hours.

per serving: 166 calories, 20.8g protein, 1.2g carbohydrates, 8.8g fat, 0.5g fiber, 55mg cholesterol, 71mg sodium, 23mg potassium

Garlic Tuna
Yield: 4 servings | **Prep time:** 15 minutes | **Cook time:** 2 hours

- 1-pound tuna fillet
- 1 teaspoon garlic powder
- 1 tablespoon olive oil
- ½ cup of water

1. Sprinkle the tuna fillet with garlic powder.
2. Then pour olive oil in the skillet and heat it well.
3. Add the tuna and roast it for 1 minute per side.

4. Transfer the tuna in the Crock Pot.
5. Add water and cook it on High for 2 hours.
per serving: 444 calories, 23.9g protein, 0.5g carbohydrates, 38.7g fat, 0.1g fiber, 0mg cholesterol, 1mg sodium, 8mg potassium

Cilantro Salmon
Yield: 4 servings | **Prep time:** 15 minutes | **Cook time:** 3 hours
- 12 oz salmon fillet
- 1 teaspoon dried cilantro
- 1 tablespoon butter
- 1 teaspoon ground black pepper
- ½ cup of coconut milk
1. Toss butter in the skillet and melt it.
2. Add salmon fillet and sprinkle it with ground black pepper. Roast the salmon on high heat for 1 minute per side.
3. Then put the fish in the Crock Pot.
4. Add coconut milk and cilantro.
5. Cook the fish on high for 3 hours.
per serving: 208 calories, 17.3g protein, 2g carbohydrates, 15.3g fat, 0.8g fiber, 45mg cholesterol, 63mg sodium, 413mg potassium

Vegan Milk Clams
Yield: 4 servings | **Prep time:** 5 minutes | **Cook time:** 3 hours
- 1 cup organic almond milk
- 1 teaspoon dried parsley
- 1 teaspoon dried dill
- ½ teaspoon salt
- 1-pound clams
1. Put all ingredients in the Crock Pot and gently mix.
2. Close the lid and cook the clams on Low for 3 hours.
per serving: 70 calories, 1g protein, 14.6g carbohydrates, 0.9g fat, 0.5g fiber, 0mg cholesterol, 737mg sodium, 111mg potassium

Seafood Gravy
Yield: 4 servings | **Prep time:** 10 minutes | **Cook time:** 5 hours
- 8 oz shrimps, peeled, chopped
- 1 bell pepper, diced
- 1 onion, diced
- 1 cup cream
- 1 teaspoon butter
- ¼ cup Cheddar cheese, shredded
1. Put all ingredients in the Crock Pot and gently mix with the help of the spoon.
2. Close the lid and cook the meal on low for 5 hours.
3. Carefully mix the meal before serving.
per serving: 163 calories, 15.8g protein, 7.6g carbohydrates, 7.7g fat, 1g fiber, 141mg cholesterol, 210mg sodium, 221mg potassium

Swiss Chard Trout
Yield: 4 servings | **Prep time:** 15 minutes | **Cook time:** 2 hours
- 2 cups swiss chard, chopped
- 9 oz trout fillet, chopped

- 1 cup of water
- 1 teaspoon ground cumin
- ½ teaspoon salt
- 1 tablespoon sunflower oil
1. Sprinkle the chopped fish with salt and ground cumin.
2. Put it in the hot skillet, add sunflower oil, and roast for 2 minutes per side.
3. Then put the roasted fish in the Crock Pot, add all remaining ingredients and close the lid.
4. Cook the trout on High for 2 hours.
per serving: 158 calories, 17.4g protein, 0.9g carbohydrates, 9.1g fat, 0.4g fiber, 47mg cholesterol, 375mg sodium, 374mg potassium

Salmon with Almond Crust
Yield: 2 servings | **Prep time:** 15 minutes | **Cook time:** 2.5 hours
- 8 oz salmon fillet
- 2 tablespoons almond flakes
- 1 teaspoon butter
- 1 teaspoon ground black pepper
- 1 teaspoon salt
- 1 egg, beaten
- ¼ cup of coconut milk
1. Sprinkle the salmon fillet with ground black pepper and salt.
2. Then dip the fish in egg and coat in the almond flakes.
3. Put butter and coconut milk in the Crock Pot.
4. Then add salmon and close the lid.
5. Cook the salmon on High for 2.5 hours.
per serving: 301 calories, 26.6g protein, 3g carbohydrates, 20.9g fat, 1.5g fiber, 137mg cholesterol, 1262mg sodium, 558mg potassium

Turmeric Mackerel
Yield: 4 servings | **Prep time:** 10 minutes | **Cook time:** 2.5 hours
- 1-pound mackerel fillet
- 1 tablespoon ground turmeric
- ½ teaspoon salt
- ¼ teaspoon chili powder
- ½ cup of water
1. Rub the mackerel fillet with ground turmeric and chili powder.
2. Then put it in the Crock Pot.
3. Add water and salt.
4. Close the lid and cook the fish on High for 2.5 hours.
per serving: 304 calories, 27.2g protein, 1.2g carbohydrates, 20.4g fat, 0.4g fiber, 58mg cholesterol, 388mg sodium, 501mg potassium

Mussels and Vegetable Ragout
Yield: 4 servings | **Prep time:** 10 minutes | **Cook time:** 5 hours
- 1 cup potato, chopped
- ½ onion, chopped
- 2 cups of water
- 1 bell pepper, chopped
- 1 teaspoon peppercorns
- 1 cup tomatoes, chopped
- 1 cup mussels

- 1 teaspoon salt
1. Put all ingredients except mussels in the Crock Pot.
2. Close the lid and cook the meal on High for 3 hours.
3. Then add mussels and mix the meal.
4. Close the lid and cook the ragout on Low for 2 hours.

per serving: 71 calories, 5.8g protein, 10.3g carbohydrates, 1.1g fat, 1.8g fiber, 11mg cholesterol, 697mg sodium, 390mg potassium

Arugula and Clams Salad
Yield: 4 servings | **Prep time:** 15 minutes | **Cook time:** 1 hour

- 1 cup clams
- 1 cup of water
- 1 garlic clove, diced
- 2 cups arugula, chopped
- 1 tablespoon lemon juice
- 1 tablespoon olive oil
1. Pour water in the Crock Pot.
2. Add clams and close the lid.
3. Cook the clams on High for 1 hour.
4. Then drain water and put the clams in the salad bowl.
5. Add arugula and garlic.
6. After this, sprinkle the salad with olive oil and lemon juice and carefully mix.

per serving: 64 calories, 0.7g protein, 7.3g carbohydrates, 3.7g fat, 0.4g fiber, 0mg cholesterol, 224mg sodium, 99mg potassium

Cod and Clams Saute
Yield: 2 servings | **Prep time:** 10 minutes | **Cook time:** 4 hours

- 1 cod fillet
- 1 cup clams
- 1 tablespoon fresh parsley, chopped
- 1 garlic clove, diced
- 2 cups tomatoes, chopped
- 1 jalapeno pepper, diced
- 1 tablespoon olive oil
- 1 cup of water
1. Slice the cod fillet and put it in the Crock Pot.
2. Add all remaining ingredients and close the lid.
3. Cook the saute on Low for 4 hours.

per serving: 200 calories, 12.6g protein, 21.3g carbohydrates, 8.2g fat, 2.9g fiber, 28mg cholesterol, 487mg sodium, 567mg potassium

Mashed Potato Fish Casserole
Yield: 4 servings | **Prep time:** 15 minutes | **Cook time:** 5 hours

- 1 cup potatoes, cooked, mashed
- 1 egg, beaten
- ½ cup Monterey Jack cheese, shredded
- 1 cup of coconut milk
- 1 tablespoon avocado oil
- ½ teaspoon ground black pepper
- 7 oz cod fillet, chopped
1. Brush the Crock Pot bottom with avocado oil.
2. Then mix chopped fish with ground black pepper and put in the Crock Pot in one layer.

3. Top it with mashed potato and cheese.
4. Add egg and coconut milk.
5. Close the lid and cook the casserole on Low for 5 hours.

per serving: 283 calories, 16.9g protein, 9.8g carbohydrates, 20.7g fat, 2.4g fiber, 81mg cholesterol, 138mg sodium, 351mg potassium

Sweden Fish Casserole
Yield: 4 servings | **Prep time:** 15 minutes | **Cook time:** 3.5 hours

- 8 oz mackerel fillet, chopped
- 1 cup of water
- 3 tablespoons mayonnaise
- 1 tablespoon sesame oil
- 1 teaspoon ground black pepper
- 2 onions, sliced
- 2 oz Provolone cheese, grated
1. Brush the Crock Pot bottom with sesame oil.
2. Then mix chopped mackerel with onion and put in the Crock Pot.
3. Spread the mayonnaise over the fish.
4. Add grated Provolone cheese, ground black pepper, and water.
5. Close the lid and cook the casserole on High for 3.5 hours.

per serving: 295 calories, 17.9g protein, 8.4g carbohydrates, 21g fat, 1.3g fiber, 55mg cholesterol, 254mg sodium, 335mg potassium

Tomato Fish Casserole
Yield: 2 servings | **Prep time:** 10 minutes | **Cook time:** 6 hours

- 2 cod fillets
- ½ cup tomato juice
- 1 cup bell pepper, chopped
- 1 teaspoon ground cumin
- ½ teaspoon salt
- 1 teaspoon olive oil
- ½ cup spinach, chopped
1. Slice the cod fillets and sprinkle them with olive oil, salt, and ground cumin.
2. Put the fish in the Crock Pot.
3. Top it with bell pepper and spinach.
4. Then add tomato juice and close the lid.
5. Cook the casserole on Low for 6 hours.

per serving: 145 calories, 21.5g protein, 7.8g carbohydrates, 3.8g fat, 1.3g fiber, 55mg cholesterol, 824mg sodium, 312mg potassium

Mozzarella Fish Casserole
Yield: 4 servings | **Prep time:** 10 minutes | **Cook time:** 2.5 hours

- 1 cup Mozzarella, shredded
- 1-pound salmon fillet, chopped
- 1 cup onion, sliced
- 1 teaspoon salt
- ½ cup of water
- 1 teaspoon avocado oil
1. Mix salmon with salt and put it in the Crock Pot.
2. Add avocado oil and water.
3. After this, top the fish with sliced onion and Mozzarella.

4. Close the lid and cook the casserole on High for 2.5 hours.

per serving: 183 calories, 24.3g protein, 3g carbohydrates, 8.4g fat, 0.7g fiber, 54mg cholesterol, 676mg sodium, 482mg potassium

Scallops Casserole

Yield: 4 servings | **Prep time:** 10 minutes | **Cook time:** 3 hours

- 2 potatoes, sliced
- 8 oz tuna, chopped
- 3 oz Parmesan, grated
- ¼ cup fresh cilantro, chopped
- 1 cup of coconut milk
- Cooking spray

1. Spray the Crock Pot bowl with cooking spray from inside.
2. Then put the layer of the sliced potato. Sprinkle it with chopped cilantro.
3. After this, add tuna and Parmesan.
4. Add coconut milk and cook the casserole on High for 3 hours.

per serving: 386 calories, 25.1g protein, 20.9g carbohydrates, 23.6g fat, 3.9g fiber, 33mg cholesterol, 242mg sodium, 785mg potassium

Fish and Mac Casserole

Yield: 6 servings | **Prep time:** 10 minutes | **Cook time:** 2 hours

- ½ cup Cheddar cheese, shredded
- 2 cod fillets, chopped
- 6 oz macaroni, cooked
- 1 teaspoon coconut oil
- 1 teaspoon white pepper
- 1/2 cup cream cheese

1. Put cream cheese in the Crock Pot.
2. Add coconut oil, white pepper, and chopped cod.
3. Cook the fish on high for 1.5 hours.
4. Then add cooked macaroni and Cheddar cheese.
5. Carefully mix the mixture and cook it on High for 30 minutes.

per serving: 248 calories, 14.2g protein, 22g carbohydrates, 11.4g fat, 1g fiber, 49mg cholesterol, 141mg sodium, 100mg potassium

Creamy Onion Casserole

Yield: 6 servings | **Prep time:** 10 minutes | **Cook time:** 3 hours

- 3 white onions, sliced
- 1 cup cream
- 1-pound salmon fillet, chopped
- 1 teaspoon ground coriander
- ¼ cup fresh parsley, chopped
- 2 tablespoons breadcrumbs

1. Sprinkle the salmon fillet with ground coriander and coat in the breadcrumbs.
2. Put the fish in the Crock Pot.
3. Then top it with sliced onion and fresh parsley.
4. Add cream and close the lid.
5. Cook the casserole on High for 3 hours.

per serving: 158 calories, 16g protein, 8.2g carbohydrates, 7.1g fat, 1.4g fiber, 41mg cholesterol, 66mg sodium, 404mg potassium

Salmon and Yam Casserole

Yield: 4 servings | **Prep time:** 10 minutes | **Cook time:** 5 hours

- 1 cup yams, chopped
- 7 oz salmon fillet, sliced
- 1 zucchini, chopped
- 1 oz Monterey Jack cheese, shredded
- ½ cup of water
- 1 teaspoon sesame oil
- 1 teaspoon salt

1. Mix yams with zucchini and put in the Crock Pot.
2. Then mix salt with salmon and sesame oil.
3. Put the fish over the vegetables and top with shredded cheese.
4. Add water and close the lid.
5. Cook the casserole on Low for 5 hours.

per serving: 149 calories, 12.5g protein, 11g carbohydrates, 6.5g fat, 1.9g fiber, 28mg cholesterol, 650mg sodium, 553mg potassium

Shrimps and Carrot Saute

Yield: 4 servings | **Prep time:** 10 minutes | **Cook time:** 6 hours

- 1 cup carrot, diced
- 1-pound shrimps, peeled
- 1 cup tomatoes, chopped
- ½ cup of water
- 1 teaspoon fennel seeds

1. Put all ingredients in the Crock Pot.
2. Gently mix the mixture and close the lid.
3. Cook the saute on Low for 6 hours.

per serving: 156 calories, 26.5g protein, 6.4g carbohydrates, 2.1g fat, 1.4g fiber, 239mg cholesterol, 299mg sodium, 395mg potassium

Baked Cod

Yield: 2 servings | **Prep time:** 10 minutes | **Cook time:** 5 hours

- 2 cod fillets
- 2 teaspoons cream cheese
- 2 tablespoons bread crumbs
- 1 teaspoon salt
- ½ teaspoon cayenne pepper
- 2 oz Mozzarella, shredded

1. Sprinkle the cod fillets with cayenne pepper and salt.
2. Put the fish in the Crock Pot.
3. Then top it with cream cheese, bread crumbs, and Mozzarella.
4. Close the lid and cook the meal for 5 hours on Low.

per serving: 210 calories, 29.2g protein, 6.2g carbohydrates, 7.6g fat, 0.4g fiber, 74mg cholesterol, 1462mg sodium, 26mg potassium

Fish Soufflé

Yield: 4 servings | **Prep time:** 10 minutes | **Cook time:** 7 hours

- 4 eggs, beaten
- 8 oz salmon fillet, chopped
- ¼ cup of coconut milk
- 2 oz Provolone cheese, grated

1. Mix coconut milk with eggs and pour the liquid in the Crock Pot.
2. Add salmon and cheese.
3. Close the lid and cook soufflé for 7 hours on low.
per serving: 222 calories, 20.5g protein, 1.5g carbohydrates, 15.2g fat, 0.3g fiber, 198mg cholesterol, 212mg sodium, 336mg potassium

Butter Tilapia
Yield: 4 servings | **Prep time:** 10 minutes | **Cook time:** 6 hours
- 4 tilapia fillets
- ½ cup butter
- 1 teaspoon dried dill
- ½ teaspoon ground black pepper
1. Sprinkle the tilapia fillets with dried dill and ground black pepper. Put them in the Crock Pot.
2. Add butter.
3. Cook the tilapia on Low for 6 hours.
per serving: 298 calories, 21.3g protein, 0.3g carbohydrates, 24.1g fat, 0.1g fiber, 116mg cholesterol, 204mg sodium, 18mg potassium

Mackerel Bites
Yield: 4 servings | **Prep time:** 12 minutes | **Cook time:** 3 hours
- 1-pound mackerel fillet, chopped
- 1 tablespoon avocado oil
- ½ teaspoon ground paprika
- ½ teaspoon ground turmeric
- 1/3 cup water
1. In the shallow bowl mix ground paprika with ground turmeric.
2. Then sprinkle the mackerel fillet with a spice mixture.
3. Heat the avocado oil in the skillet well.
4. Add fish and roast it for 1 minute per side on high heat.
5. Pour water in the Crock Pot.
6. Add fish and close the lid.
7. Cook the mackerel bites on High for 3 hours.
per serving: 304 calories, 27.2g protein, 0.5g carbohydrates, 20.7g fat, 0.3g fiber, 85mg cholesterol, 95mg sodium, 479mg potassium

Tilapia Fish Balls
Yield: 5 servings | **Prep time:** 15 minutes | **Cook time:** 2.5 hours
- 1-pound tilapia fillet, grinded
- 2 tablespoons breadcrumbs
- 1 egg, beaten
- 1 tablespoon flour
- 1 teaspoon ground cumin
- ½ teaspoon salt
- ½ cup of water
1. In the mixing bowl mix grinded tilapia with breadcrumbs, egg, flour, ground cumin, and salt.
2. Then make the small balls from the mixture and arrange them in the Crock Pot in one layer.
3. Add water and close the lid.
4. Cook the fish balls on High for 2.5 hours.
per serving: 105 calories, 18.6g protein, 3.4g carbohydrates, 1.9g fat, 0.2g fiber, 77mg cholesterol, 298mg sodium, 27mg potassium

Coriander Cod Balls
Yield: 3 servings | **Prep time:** 15 minutes | **Cook time:** 2 hours
- ½ teaspoon minced garlic
- 8 oz cod fillet, grinded
- 1 teaspoon dried cilantro
- 2 tablespoons cornflour
- 1 teaspoon avocado oil
- ¼ cup of water
1. Mix minced garlic with grinded cod, dried cilantro, and cornflour.
2. Make the small balls.
3. After this, heat the avocado oil in the skillet well.
4. Add the fish balls and roast them on high heat for 2 minutes per side.
5. Transfer the fish balls in the Crock Pot.
6. Add water and cook them on High for 2 hours.
per serving: 83 calories, 14.4g protein, 4g carbohydrates, 1.1g fat, 0.4g fiber, 39mg cholesterol, 50mg sodium, 23mg potassium

Mackerel in Wine Sauce
Yield: 4 servings | **Prep time:** 10 minutes | **Cook time:** 3.5 hours
- 1-pound mackerel
- ½ cup white wine
- 1 teaspoon cornflour
- 1 teaspoon cayenne pepper
- 1 tablespoon olive oil
- ½ teaspoon dried rosemary
1. Mix white wine with cornflour and pour it in the Crock Pot.
2. Then rub the fish with cayenne pepper and dried rosemary.
3. Sprinkle the fish with olive oil and put it in the Crock Pot.
4. Close the lid and cook the mackerel on High for 3.5 hours.
per serving: 356 calories, 27.2g protein, 1.6g carbohydrates, 23.8g fat, 0.2g fiber, 85mg cholesterol, 96mg sodium, 496mg potassium

Teriyaki Tilapia
Yield: 4 servings | **Prep time:** 10 minutes | **Cook time:** 5 hours
- 1 teaspoon sesame seeds
- ¼ cup teriyaki sauce
- ¼ cup of water
- 1 tablespoon avocado oil
- 12 oz tilapia fillet, roughly chopped
1. Mix water with teriyaki sauce, sesame seeds, and avocado oil.
2. Pour the liquid in the Crock Pot.
3. Add tilapia fillet and close the lid.
4. Cook the fish on Low for 5 hours.
per serving: 95 calories, 17.1g protein, 3.2g carbohydrates, 1.6g fat, 0.3g fiber, 41mg cholesterol, 721mg sodium, 55mg potassium

Cod in Lemon Sauce
Yield: 4 servings | **Prep time:** 10 minutes | **Cook time:** 2.5 hours
- 4 cod fillets

- 4 tablespoons lemon juice
- 2 tablespoons olive oil
- ½ teaspoon fennel seeds
- ¼ cup of water
1. Put the cod fillets in the Crock Pot.
2. Add water, fennel seeds, and olive oil.
3. Cook the fish on high for 2.5 hours.
4. Then transfer the fish in the bowls and sprinkle with lemon juice.

per serving: 155 calories, 20.2g protein, 0.5g carbohydrates, 8.2g fat, 0.2g fiber, 55mg cholesterol, 74mg sodium, 23mg potassium

Soy Sauce Scallops

Yield: 4 servings | **Prep time:** 5 minutes | **Cook time:** 30 minutes

- ¼ cup of soy sauce
- 1 tablespoon butter
- ½ teaspoon white pepper
- 1-pound scallops
1. Pour soy sauce in the Crock Pot.
2. Add butter and white pepper.
3. After this, add scallops and close the lid.
4. Cook them on High for 30 minutes.

per serving: 134 calories, 20.1g protein, 4.1g carbohydrates, 3.8g fat, 0.2g fiber, 45mg cholesterol, 1102mg sodium, 404mg potassium

Coconut Curry Cod

Yield: 2 servings | **Prep time:** 10 minutes | **Cook time:** 2.5 hours

- 2 cod fillets
- ½ teaspoon curry paste
- 1/3 cup coconut milk
- 1 teaspoon sunflower oil
1. Mix coconut milk with curry paste, add sunflower oil, and transfer the liquid in the Crock Pot.
2. Add cod fillets.
3. Cook the meal on High for 2.5 hours.

per serving: 211 calories, 21g protein, 2.6g carbohydrates, 13.6g fat, 0.9g fiber, 55mg cholesterol, 76mg sodium, 105mg potassium

Dill Cod Sticks

Yield: 4 servings | **Prep time:** 15 minutes | **Cook time:** 1.5 hours

- 4 teaspoons breadcrumbs
- 1 egg, beaten
- 1 tablespoon cream cheese
- ½ teaspoon salt
- 1 teaspoon avocado oil
- ¼ cup of water
- 2 cod fillets
1. Slice the cod and sprinkle it with salt.
2. Then dip the fish in the egg and coat in the breadcrumbs.
3. Heat the avocado oil in the skillet well.
4. Add the fish sticks and roast them for 1 minute per side.
5. Transfer the fish sticks in the Crock Pot.
6. Add all remaining ingredients and close the lid.
7. Cook the cod sticks on High for 1.5 hours.

per serving: 80 calories, 11.9g protein, 1.8g carbohydrates, 2.7g fat, 0.2g fiber, 71mg cholesterol, 365mg sodium, 26mg potassium

Coated Salmon Fillets

Yield: 3 servings | **Prep time:** 10 minutes | **Cook time:** 2.5 hours

- 2 tablespoons coconut flakes
- 8 oz salmon fillet
- 1 egg white, whisked
- 1 teaspoon flour
- ½ teaspoon chili powder
- 1 teaspoon butter
- 1/3 cup water
1. Sprinkle the salmon fillet with chili powder.
2. Then dip it with egg and coat in the flour.
3. Sprinkle with remaining egg mixture and top with coconut flakes.
4. Put the fish in the Crock Pot.
5. Add butter and water.
6. Close the lid and cook the salmon on High for 2.5 hours.

per serving: 133 calories, 16.1g protein, 1.5g carbohydrates, 7.2g fat, 0.5g fiber, 37mg cholesterol, 59mg sodium, 330mg potassium

Cream Cheese Fish Balls

Yield: 4 servings | **Prep time:** 15 minutes | **Cook time:** 2 hours

- 8 oz salmon fillet, minced
- 1 tablespoon cream cheese
- ½ teaspoon dried cilantro
- ¼ teaspoon garlic powder
- 2 tablespoons flour
- ¼ cup fish stock
1. In the mixing bowl mix minced salmon fillet with cream cheese, dried cilantro, garlic powder, and flour.
2. Make the fish balls and put them in the Crock Pot.
3. Add fish stock and close the lid.
4. Cook the meal on High for 2 hours.

per serving: 101 calories, 12g protein, 3.2g carbohydrates, 4.5g fat, 0.1g fiber, 28mg cholesterol, 55mg sodium, 248mg potassium

Taco Mackerel

Yield: 4 servings | **Prep time:** 15 minutes | **Cook time:** 1.5 hours

- 12 oz mackerel fillets
- 1 tablespoon taco seasonings
- 2 tablespoons coconut oil
- 3 tablespoons water
1. Melt the coconut oil in the skillet and heat it well.
2. Meanwhile, rub the mackerel fillets with taco seasonings.
3. Put the fish in the hot coconut oil.
4. Roast it for 2 minutes per side.
5. Then put the roasted fish in the Crock Pot.
6. Add water and cook it on High for 1.5 hours.

per serving: 289 calories, 20.3g protein, 1g carbohydrates, 22g fat, 0g fiber, 64mg cholesterol, 176mg sodium, 341mg potassium

Caribbean Seasoning Fish Balls

Yield: 4 servings | **Prep time:** 15 minutes | **Cook time:** 3 hours

- 1 teaspoon Caribbean seasonings
- ½ teaspoon dried thyme
- 12 oz salmon fillet, chopped
- 1 egg, beaten
- 1 teaspoon sunflower oil
- ¼ cup of water
1. Mix Caribbean seasonings with dried thyme.
2. Then add chopped salmon and carefully mix. Add egg.
3. Pour sunflower oil in the Crock Pot. Add water.
4. Make the fish balls with the help of the spoon and put them in the Crock Pot.
5. Cook the fish balls on High for 3 hours.

per serving: 145 calories, 17.9g protein, 1.7g carbohydrates, 0.1g fat, 0.1g fiber, 78mg cholesterol, 161mg sodium, 343mg potassium

Braised Tilapia with Capers

Yield: 4 servings | **Prep time:** 5 minutes | **Cook time:** 5 hours

- 4 tilapia fillets
- ½ cup of water
- 2 tablespoons sour cream
- ½ teaspoon salt
- ¼ teaspoon chili flakes
- 1 tablespoon capers
1. Put all ingredients in the Crock Pot and close the lid.
2. Cook the tilapia on Low for 5 hours.

per serving: 106 calories, 21.3g protein, 0.4g carbohydrates, 2.3g fat, 0.1g fiber, 58mg cholesterol, 399mg sodium, 10mg potassium

Bacon-Wrapped Salmon

Yield: 2 servings | **Prep time:** 15 minutes | **Cook time:** 6 hours

- 2 salmon fillets
- 1 teaspoon liquid honey
- ¼ teaspoon dried thyme
- 2 bacon slices
- 1 teaspoon sunflower oil
- ¼ cup of water
1. Sprinkle the salmon fillets with dried thyme and wrap in the bacon.
2. Then pour water in the Crock Pot.
3. Add sunflower oil and honey.
4. Then add wrapped salmon and close the lid.
5. Cook the meal on low for 6 hours.

per serving: 370 calories, 41.6g protein, 3.2g carbohydrates, 21.3g fat, 0.1g fiber, 99mg cholesterol, 518mg sodium, 794mg potassium

Fish Pie

Yield: 6 servings | **Prep time:** 15 minutes | **Cook time:** 6 hours

- 1 teaspoon cream cheese
- 1 garlic clove, diced ● ¼ cup fresh dill, chopped
- 1 teaspoon butter, softened
- 1 carrot, diced
- 1 teaspoon sesame oil
- 7 oz tuna, canned, shredded
- 7 oz puff pastry
1. Brush the Crock Pot bottom with sesame oil.
2. Then put the puff pastry inside and flatten it in the shape of the pie crust.
3. After this, mix garlic with cream cheese, dill, butter, carrot, and tuna.
4. Put the tuna mixture over the pie crust and flatten it.
5. Close the lid and cook the pie on Low for 6 hours.

per serving: 268 calories, 11.7g protein, 17.2g carbohydrates, 17g fat, 1g fiber, 13mg cholesterol, 116mg sodium, 232mg potassium

Fish Corners

Yield: 4 servings | **Prep time:** 20 minutes | **Cook time:** 3.5 hours

- 7 oz salmon, canned, shredded
- ¼ onion, diced
- 1 teaspoon dried basil
- 1 egg, beaten
- 1 teaspoon sesame oil
- ¼ teaspoon chili powder
- 4 oz puff pastry
1. Roll up the puff pastry and cut it into squares.
2. After this, mix canned salmon with onion, basil, egg, and chili powder.
3. Put the salmon mixture in the center of every puff pastry square and roll into the shape of corners.
4. Then brush the fish corners with sesame oil and put in the Crock Pot.
5. Cook the meal on High for 3.5 hours.

per serving: 251 calories, 13.2g protein, 13.6g carbohydrates, 16.1g fat, 0.6g fiber, 63mg cholesterol, 110mg sodium, 236mg potassium

Fish Tart

Yield: 6 servings | **Prep time:** 20 minutes | **Cook time:** 4 hours

- 1-pound anchovies
- 2 tablespoons cornflour
- 1 teaspoon ground nutmeg
- 2 eggs, beaten
- 1 oz Parmesan, grated
- 5 oz puff pastry
- Cooking spray
1. Spray the Crock Pot bottom with cooking spray.
2. Then put the puff pastry inside.
3. Flatten it in the shape of the pie crust.
4. After this, mix anchovies with cornflour and ground nutmeg.
5. Put them over the puff pastry in one layer.
6. Then pour the beaten egg over the anchovies.
7. Add parmesan and close the lid.
8. Cook the fish tart on High for 4 hours.

per serving: 336 calories, 27.1g protein, 13g carbohydrates, 19g fat, 0.6g fiber, 122mg cholesterol, 2896mg sodium, 454mg potassium

Cod Sticks in Blankets

Yield: 4 servings | **Prep time:** 15 minutes | **Cook time:** 4 hours

- 4 cod fillets

- 4 oz puff pastry
- 1 teaspoon mayonnaise
- 1 teaspoon ground black pepper
- 1 teaspoon olive oil
1.   Cut the cod fillets into the sticks.
2.   Then sprinkle them with mayonnaise and ground black pepper.
3.   Roll up the puff pastry and cut into strips.
4.   Roll every cod stick in the puff pastry and brush with olive oil.
5.   Put the cod sticks in the Crock Pot in one layer and cook on high for 4 hours.
 per serving: 262 calories, 22.1g protein, 13.4g carbohydrates, 13.g fat, 0.6g fiber, 55mg cholesterol, 150mg sodium, 24mg potassium

Fish Hot Dog Sticks
Yield: 4 servings | **Prep time:** 20 minutes | **Cook time:** 2 hours
- 5 oz salmon fillet, minced
- 2 oz potato, cooked, mashed
- 1 egg, beaten
- 2 tablespoons cornflour
- ½ teaspoon salt
- 1 teaspoon dried parsley
- 1 tablespoon avocado oil
- ¼ cup of water
1.   In the mixing bowl mix minced salmon with mashed potato, egg, cornflour, salt, and dried parsley.
2.   Then make the medium size hot dog sticks and put them in the hot skillet.
3.   Add avocado oil and roast them on high heat for 1 minute per side.
4.   Transfer the hot dog sticks in the Crock Pot.
5.   Add water and close the lid.
6.   Cook the meal on high for 2 hours.
 per serving: 92 calories, 8.9g protein, 5.6g carbohydrates, 3.9g fat, 0.7g fiber, 57mg cholesterol, 324mg sodium, 235mg potassium

Garlic Sardines
Yield: 4 servings | **Prep time:** 10 minutes | **Cook time:** 3 hours
- 1-pound sardines, cleaned
- 1 teaspoon garlic powder
- ½ teaspoon ground black pepper
- ¼ cup cornflour
- 1 tablespoon avocado oil
- ¼ cup of water
1.   Pour water in the Crock Pot.
2.   Add avocado oil.
3.   Then sprinkle the sardines with garlic powder, ground black pepper, and cornflour.
4.   Put the fish in the Crock Pot and close the lid.
5.   Cook the sardines on High for 3 hours.
 per serving: 280 calories, 27.6g protein, 6.5g carbohydrates, 13.7g fat, 0.8g fiber, 161mg cholesterol, 574mg sodium, 495mg potassium

Apple Cider Vinegar Sardines
Yield: 4 servings | **Prep time:** 10 minutes | **Cook time:** 4.5 hours
- 14 oz sardines
- 1 tablespoon butter
- ¼ cup apple cider vinegar
- ½ teaspoon cayenne pepper
- 4 tablespoons coconut cream
1.   Put sardines in the Crock Pot.
2.   Add butter, apple cider vinegar, cayenne pepper, and coconut cream.
3.   Close the lid and cook the meal on Low for 4.5 hours.
 per serving: 270 calories, 24.8g protein, 1.1g carbohydrates, 17.9g fat, 0.4g fiber, 149mg cholesterol,525mg sodium, 450mg potassium

Stuffed Mackerel
Yield: 4 servings | **Prep time:** 15 minutes | **Cook time:** 4.5 hours
- ½ cup yams, diced
- 1-pound mackerel, cleaned, trimmed
- 1 teaspoon dried thyme
- 1 teaspoon salt
- 1 tablespoon sour cream
- 1 teaspoon chili powder
- 1 teaspoon olive oil
1.   Rub the mackerel with dried thyme, salt, and chili powder.
2.   Then fil it with yams and secure the cut.
3.   After this, sprinkle the fish with olive oil and sour cream and wrap in the foil.
4.   Put the fish in the Crock Pot and close the lid.
5.   Cook the fish on high for 4.5 hours.
 per serving: 336 calories, 27.5g protein, 5.3g carbohydrates, 22.2g fat, 1g fiber, 86mg cholesterol, 685mg sodium, 588mg potassium

Marinara Salmon
Yield: 4 servings | **Prep time:** 5 minutes | **Cook time:** 3 hours
- 1-pound salmon fillet, chopped
- ½ cup marinara sauce
- ¼ cup fresh cilantro, chopped
- ¼ cup of water
1.   Put the salmon in the Crock Pot.
2.   Add marinara sauce, cilantro, and water.
3.   Close the lid and cook the fish on High for 3 hours.
 per serving: 177 calories, 22.6g protein, 4.3g carbohydrates, 7.9g fat, 0.8g fiber, 51mg cholesterol, 179mg sodium, 540mg potassium

Salmon Picatta
Yield: 4 servings | **Prep time:** 10 minutes | **Cook time:** 3.5 hours
- 4 salmon fillets
- 1 tablespoon avocado oil
- ½ lemon, sliced
- 1 tablespoon butter
- ¼ cup white wine
- 1 teaspoon capers
- 1 tablespoon flour
- ¼ cup chicken stock
- ½ teaspoon minced garlic
1.   In the mixing bowl mix minced garlic and butter.
2.   Put the mixture in the Crock Pot.
3.   Add chicken stock and flour.

4. Gently whisk the mixture.
5. Add lemon, white wine, and avocado oil.
6. Then add salmon fillets and capers.
7. Close the lid and cook the meal on High for 3.5 hours.
per serving: 288 calories, 35g protein, 3g carbohydrates, 14.4g fat, 0.4g fiber, 86mg cholesterol, 169mg sodium, 725mg potassium

Sweet and Mustard Tilapia
Yield: 4 servings | **Prep time:** 10 minutes | **Cook time:** 4.5 hours
- 16 oz tilapia fillets
- 1 teaspoon brown sugar
- 2 tablespoons mustard
- 1 tablespoon sesame oil
- ¼ cup of water
1. Mix brown sugar with mustard and sesame oil.
2. Carefully rub the tilapia fillets with mustard mixture and transfer them in the Crock Pot.
3. Add water.
4. Cook the tilapia on Low for 4.5 hours.
per serving: 153 calories, 22.5g protein, 2.7g carbohydrates, 6g fat, 0.8g fiber, 55mg cholesterol, 41mg sodium, 39mg potassium

Soy Sauce Catfish
Yield: 4 servings | **Prep time:** 10 minutes | **Cook time:** 5 hours
- 1-pound catfish fillet, chopped
- ¼ cup of soy sauce
- 1 jalapeno pepper, diced
- 1 tablespoon olive oil
- 4 tablespoons fish stock
1. Sprinkle the catfish with olive oil and put in the Crock Pot.
2. Add soy sauce, jalapeno pepper, and fish stock.
3. Close the lid and cook the meal on Low for 5 hours.
per serving: 195 calories, 19g protein, 1.4g carbohydrates, 12.3g fat, 0.2g fiber, 53mg cholesterol, 981mg sodium, 427mg potassium

Peppercorn Sweet and Sour Catfish
Yield: 4 servings | **Prep time:** 10 minutes | **Cook time:** 3 hours
- ¼ cup sour cream
- 1 teaspoon peppercorns
- 12 oz catfish fillet
- ¼ cup fresh dill, chopped
- 1 tablespoon maple syrup
- ¼ cup of water
1. Roughly chop the catfish fillet and put it in the Crock Pot.
2. Sprinkle it with peppercorns, sour cream, dill, and maple syrup.
3. Add water.
4. Cook the fish on high for 3 hours.
per serving: 248 calories, 16.5g protein, 12.8g carbohydrates, 14.5g fat, 1.2g fiber, 75mg cholesterol, 253mg sodium, 426mg potassium

Miso-Poached Cod
Yield: 4 servings | **Prep time:** 10 minutes | **Cook time:** 2.5 hours
- 1 teaspoon miso paste
- ½ cup of water
- ½ teaspoon dried lemongrass
- 4 cod fillets
- 1 teaspoon olive oil
1. Mix miso paste with water, dried lemongrass, and olive oil.
2. Then pour the liquid in the Crock Pot.
3. Add cod fillets.
4. Cook the cod on High for 2.5 hours.
per serving: 103 calories, 20.2g protein, 0.4g carbohydrates, 2.3g fat, 0.1g fiber, 55mg cholesterol, 124mg sodium, 5mg potassium

Pineapple Milkfish
Yield: 4 servings | **Prep time:** 10 minutes | **Cook time:** 3 hours
- 16 oz milkfish fillet, chopped
- ½ cup pineapple, chopped
- 1 cup of coconut milk
- 1 teaspoon white pepper
- ½ teaspoon curry powder
1. Sprinkle the milkfish fillet with curry powder and white pepper.
2. Then put it in the Crock Pot.
3. Top the fish with pineapple and coconut milk.
4. Close the lid and cook the fish on High for 3 hours.
per serving: 304 calories, 19.2g protein, 6.2g carbohydrates, 23g fat, 1.8g fiber, 53mg cholesterol, 70mg sodium, 555mg potassium

Ginger Cod
Yield: 6 servings | **Prep time:** 10 minutes | **Cook time:** 5 hours
- 6 cod fillets
- 1 teaspoon minced ginger
- 1 tablespoon olive oil
- ¼ teaspoon minced garlic
- ¼ cup chicken stock
1. In the mixing bowl mix minced ginger with olive oil and minced garlic.
2. Gently rub the fish fillets with the ginger mixture and put in the Crock Pot.
3. Add chicken stock.
4. Cook the cod on Low for 5 hours.
per serving: 112 calories, 20.1g protein, 0.3g carbohydrates, 3.4g fat, 0g fiber, 55mg cholesterol, 102mg sodium, 5mg potassium

Poached Catfish
Yield: 4 servings | **Prep time:** 10 minutes | **Cook time:** 3.5 hours
- 12 oz catfish fillet
- 1 teaspoon dried rosemary
- 1 cup chicken stock
- 1 teaspoon salt
1. Pour the chicken stock in the Crock Pot.
2. Add salt and dried rosemary.
3. Then add catfish fillet and close the lid.
4. Cook the fish on high for 3.5 hours.

per serving: 213 calories, 20.3g protein, 0.8g carbohydrates, 13.9g fat, 0.1g fiber, 69mg cholesterol, 158mg sodium, 392mg potassium

Catfish Paste
Yield: 6 servings | **Prep time:** 15 minutes | **Cook time:** 4 hours
- 1-pound catfish fillet
- 1 tablespoon butter, softened
- ¼ cup fresh parsley, chopped
- 1 garlic clove, peeled
- 1 cup of water
- 1 oz parmesan, grated
- 1 tablespoon cream cheese
1. Put the catfish fillet in the Crock Pot.
2. Add water and garlic. Cook the ingredients on High for 4 hours.
3. Then drain water and transfer the catfish fillets and garlic in the blender.
4. Add all remaining ingredients and blend the mixture until smooth.
5. Transfer the cooked paste in the ramekins.
per serving: 142 calories, 13.5g protein, 0.5g carbohydrates, 9.3g fat, 0.1g fiber, 46mg cholesterol, 105mg sodium, 262mg potassium

Chili Bigeye Jack (Tuna)
Yield: 4 servings | **Prep time:** 10 minutes | **Cook time:** 3.5 hours
- 9 oz tuna fillet (bigeye jack), roughly chopped
- 1 teaspoon chili powder
- 1 teaspoon curry paste
- ½ cup of coconut milk
- 1 tablespoon sesame oil
1. Mix curry paste and coconut milk and pour the liquid in the Crock Pot.
2. Add tuna fillet and sesame oil.
3. Then add chili powder.
4. Cook the meal on High for 3.5 hours.
per serving: 341 calories, 14.2g protein, 2.4g carbohydrates, 31.2g fat, 0.9g fiber, 0mg cholesterol, 11mg sodium, 91mg potassium

Bigeye Jack Saute
Yield: 4 servings | **Prep time:** 7 minutes | **Cook time:** 6 hours
- 7 oz (bigeye jack) tuna fillet, chopped
- 1 cup tomato, chopped
- 1 teaspoon ground black pepper
- 1 jalapeno pepper, chopped
- ½ cup chicken stock
1. Put all ingredients in the Crock Pot and close the lid.
2. Cook the saute on Low for 6 hours.
per serving: 192 calories, 11g protein, 2.4g carbohydrates, 15.6g fat, 0.8g fiber, 0mg cholesterol, 98mg sodium, 123mg potassium

Creamy Pangasius
Yield: 4 servings | **Prep time:** 10 minutes | **Cook time:** 2.5 hours
- 4 pangasius fillets
- ½ cup cream
- 1 teaspoon cornflour
- 1 tablespoon fish sauce
- 1 teaspoon ground nutmeg
1. Coat the fish fillets in the cornflour and sprinkle with ground nutmeg.
2. Put the fish in the Crock Pot.
3. Add cream and fish sauce.
4. Close the lid and cook the meal on High for 2.5 hours.
per serving: 106 calories, 15.5g protein, 1.8g carbohydrates, 4.9g fat, 0.2g fiber, 26mg cholesterol, 617mg sodium, 28mg potassium

Pangasius Fish Balls
Yield: 4 servings | **Prep time:** 15 minutes | **Cook time:** 2.5 hours
- 10 oz pangasius fillet, minced
- 3 tablespoons breadcrumbs
- 1 teaspoon minced garlic
- ½ teaspoon salt
- 1 tablespoon flour
- 1 tablespoon coconut oil
- ½ cup of water
1. In the mixing bowl mix fish fillet with minced garlic, bread crumbs, salt, and flour.
2. Make the fish balls.
3. Then heat the coconut oil in the skillet well.
4. Add the fish balls and roast them on high heat for 2 minutes per side.
5. Transfer the fish balls in the Crock Pot.
6. Add water and cook them on High for 2.5 hours.
per serving: 107 calories, 10.3g protein, 5.4g carbohydrates, 5.6g fat, 0.3g fiber, 13mg cholesterol, 491mg sodium, 15mg potassium

Coconut Pollock
Yield: 4 servings | **Prep time:** 10 minutes | **Cook time:** 5 hours
- 1-pound Pollock fillet, chopped
- 1 tablespoon coconut flakes
- 1 tablespoon coconut flour
- ½ teaspoon ground nutmeg
- ½ teaspoon salt
- 1 cup coconut cream
- 1 tablespoon sunflower oil
1. Sprinkle the Pollock fillet with coconut flakes, coconut flour, ground nutmeg, and salt.
2. Then transfer the fillets in the Crock Pot.
3. Add coconut cream and sunflower oil.
4. Cook the fish on Low for 5 hours.
per serving: 284 calories, 24g protein, 4.7g carbohydrates, 19.6g fat, 2.1g fiber, 56mg cholesterol, 370mg sodium, 163mg potassium

Pangasius with Crunchy Crust
Yield: 2 servings | **Prep time:** 20 minutes | **Cook time:** 3 hours
- 6 oz pangasius fillet
- 2 tablespoons breadcrumbs
- 1 egg, beaten
- 1 tablespoon flour
- 1/3 cup chicken stock
- 1 teaspoon salt
- 1 teaspoon ground black pepper

1. Sprinkle the fish fillets with ground black pepper and salt.
2. Then mix breadcrumbs with flour. After this, dip the fish fillets in the beaten egg and coat in the flour mixture.
3. Put the fish fillets in the Crock Pot. Add chicken stock and close the lid.
4. Cook the fish on high for 3 hours. Then preheat the skillet well and put the fish fillets inside. Roast them for 2 minutes per side.

per serving: 119 calories, 12.2g protein, 8.8g carbohydrates, 4.3g fat, 0.7g fiber, 92mg cholesterol, 1508mg sodium, 63mg potassium

Tarragon Mahi Mahi
Yield: 4 servings | **Prep time:** 15 minutes | **Cook time:** 2.5 hours
- 1-pound mahi-mahi fillet
- 1 tablespoon dried tarragon
- 1 tablespoon coconut oil
- ½ cup of water

1. Melt the coconut oil in the skillet.
2. Add mahi-mahi fillet and roast it on high heat for 2 minutes per side.
3. Put the fish fillet in the Crock Pot.
4. Add dried tarragon and water.
5. Close the lid and cook the fish on High for 2.5 hours.

per serving: 121 calories, 21.2g protein, 0.2g carbohydrates, 3.4g fat, 0g fiber, 40mg cholesterol, 97mg sodium, 14mg potassium

Taco Mahi Mahi
Yield: 6 servings | **Prep time:** 10 minutes | **Cook time:** 6 hours
- 2-pounds Mahi Mahi fillets
- 1 tablespoon taco seasonings
- 1 teaspoon fish sauce
- 1/3 cup chicken stock
- 1 tablespoon sunflower oil

1. Sprinkle the fish fillets with taco seasonings and fish sauce.
2. Pour sunflower oil in the Crock Pot.
3. Add fish and chicken stock.
4. Close the lid and cook the fish on Low for 6 hours.

per serving: 163 calories, 28.7g protein, 1.4g carbohydrates, 3.8g fat, 0g fiber, 130mg cholesterol, 453mg sodium, 563mg potassium

Chili Perch
Yield: 4 servings | **Prep time:** 10 minutes | **Cook time:** 3 hours
- 1 chili pepper, chopped
- 1 carrot, grated
- 1 onion, diced
- 1 tablespoon coconut oil
- 1 teaspoon salt
- ½ cup chicken stock
- 1-pound perch fillet, chopped

1. Put the chili pepper in the Crock Pot.
2. Add carrot, onion, and coconut oil.
3. Sprinkle the perch fillet with salt and transfer in the Crock Pot.

4. Add chicken stock and close the lid.
5. Cook the perch on High for 3 hours.

per serving: 159 calories, 21.6g protein, 4.3g carbohydrates, 5.6g fat, 1g fiber, 45mg cholesterol, 779mg sodium, 93mg potassium

Tomato Seabass
Yield: 4 servings | **Prep time:** 10 minutes | **Cook time:** 2.5 hours
- 1-pound seabass, cleaned, trimmed
- 1 tablespoon tomato paste
- 1 tablespoon avocado oil
- 1 cup tomatoes, chopped
- ½ cup of water
- 1 teaspoon cayenne pepper

1. Mix water with tomato paste and pour it in the Crock Pot.
2. Add cayenne pepper, seabass, and chopped tomatoes.
3. Close the lid and cook the seabass on High for 2.5 hours.
4. Then transfer the seabass in the serving bowls and sprinkle with avocado oil.

per serving: 157 calories, 11.3g protein, 9.6g carbohydrates, 9.1g fat, 1.9g fiber, 0mg cholesterol, 696mg sodium, 168mg potassium

Mustard Salmon Salad
Yield: 4 servings | **Prep time:** 15 minutes | **Cook time:** 3 hours
- 1 cup lettuce, chopped
- 1 cup spinach, chopped
- 1 tablespoon mustard
- 2 tablespoons plain yogurt
- 1 teaspoon olive oil
- 8 oz salmon fillet
- ¼ cup of water
- 1 teaspoon butter

1. Pour water in the Crock Pot.
2. Add butter and salmon.
3. Close the lid and cook it on High for 3 hours.
4. After this, chop the salmon roughly and put it in the salad bowl.
5. Add chopped spinach and lettuce.
6. In the shallow bowl mix mustard, plain yogurt, and olive oil. Whisk the mixture.
7. Shake the salmon salad and sprinkle with mustard dressing.

per serving: 116 calories, 12.4g protein, 2.2g carbohydrates, 6.6g fat, 0.7g fiber, 28mg cholesterol, 44mg sodium, 316mg potassium

Honey Mahi Mahi
Yield: 4 servings | **Prep time:** 10 minutes | **Cook time:** 2 hours
- 2 tablespoons of liquid honey
- 2 tablespoons butter, softened
- ½ teaspoon white pepper
- 15 oz Mahi Mahi fillet
- 1 tablespoon olive oil
- ½ cup of water

1. Slice the fish fillet and put it in the hot skillet.
2. Add olive oil and roast the fish for 2-3 minutes per side on high heat.

3. After this, transfer the fish in the Crock Pot.
4. Add all remaining ingredients and close the lid.
5. Cook the fish on high for 2 hours.
per serving: 208 calories, 20.2g protein, 8.8g carbohydrates, 10.3g fat, 0.1g fiber, 107mg cholesterol, 178mg sodium, 404mg potassium

Butter Smelt
Yield: 4 servings | **Prep time:** 10 minutes | **Cook time:** 6 hours
- 16 oz smelt fillet
- 1/3 cup butter
- 1 teaspoon dried thyme
- 1 teaspoon salt

1. Sprinkle the fish with dried thyme and salt and put in the Crock Pot.
2. Add butter and close the lid.
3. Cook the smelt on Low for 6 hours.
per serving: 226 calories, 17.2g protein, 0.2g carbohydrates, 17.4g fat, 0.1g fiber, 191mg cholesterol, 750mg sodium, 7mg potassium

Sautéed Smelt
Yield: 4 servings | **Prep time:** 10 minutes | **Cook time:** 4.5 hours
- 1 onion, chopped
- 1 cup bell pepper, chopped
- 1 tablespoon coconut oil
- 1 cup of coconut milk
- 12 oz smelt fillet, chopped
- 1 teaspoon ground nutmeg

1. Put all ingredients in the Crock Pot and gently mix with the help of the spoon.
2. Close the lid and cook the smelt on High for 4.5 hours.
per serving: 296 calories, 21.2g protein, 8.4g carbohydrates, 20.7g fat, 2.4g fiber, 77mg cholesterol, 76mg sodium, 572mg potassium

Smelt in Avocado Oil
Yield: 4 servings | **Prep time:** 10 minutes | **Cook time:** 4 hours
- 12 oz smelt fillet
- 1 teaspoon chili powder
- ¼ teaspoon ground turmeric
- ½ teaspoon smoked paprika
- 4 tablespoons avocado oil

1. Cut the smelt fillet into 4 servings.
2. Then sprinkle every fish fillet with chili powder, ground turmeric, and smoked paprika.
3. Put the fish in the Crock Pot.
4. Add avocado oil and close the lid.
5. Cook the fish on Low for 4 hours.
per serving: 89 calories, 13.1g protein, 1.4g carbohydrates, 3.5g fat, 1g fiber, 112mg cholesterol, 52mg sodium, 66mg potassium

Curry Shrimps
Yield: 4 servings | **Prep time:** 10 minutes | **Cook time:** 45 minutes
- 16 oz shrimps, peeled
- 1 teaspoon curry paste
- ½ cup fish stock

1. Mix the curry paste with fish stock and pour it in the Crock Pot.
2. Add shrimps and cook them on High for 45 minutes.
per serving: 148 calories, 26.6g protein, 2.1g carbohydrates, 2.9g fat, 0g fiber, 239mg cholesterol, 322mg sodium, 234mg potassium

Shrimps Boil
Yield: 2 servings | **Prep time:** 15 minutes | **Cook time:** 45 minutes
- ½ cup of water
- 1 tablespoon piri piri sauce
- 1 tablespoon butter
- 7 oz shrimps, peeled

1. Pour water in the Crock Pot.
2. Add shrimps and cook them on high for 45 minutes.
3. Then drain water and transfer shrimps in the skillet.
4. Add butter and piri piri sauce.
5. Roast the shrimps for 2-3 minutes on medium heat.
per serving: 174 calories, 22.7g protein, 1.8g carbohydrates, 7.8g fat, 0.1g fiber, 224mg cholesterol, 285mg sodium, 170mg potassium

Taco Shrimps
Yield: 4 servings | **Prep time:** 15 minutes | **Cook time:** 40 minutes
- 1-pound shrimps, peeled
- 1 teaspoon taco seasonings
- 3 tablespoons lemon juice
- 1 teaspoon dried thyme
- 1/3 cup water

1. In the mixing bowl mix shrimps with taco seasonings and dried thyme.
2. Put the shrimps in the Crock Pot. Add water.
3. Cook them on High for 40 minutes.
4. Then drain water and sprinkle the cooked shrimps with lemon juice.
per serving: 143 calories, 25.9g protein, 3.1g carbohydrates, 2g fat, 0.1g fiber, 239mg cholesterol, 385mg sodium, 209mg potassium

BBQ Shrimps
Yield: 6 servings | **Prep time:** 10 minutes | **Cook time:** 40 minutes
- 1/3 cup BBQ sauce
- ¼ cup plain yogurt
- 1-pound shrimps, peeled
- 1 tablespoon butter

1. Melt butter and mix it with shrimps.
2. Put the mixture in the Crock Pot.
3. Add plain yogurt and BBQ sauce.
4. Close the lid and cook the meal on High for 40 minutes.
per serving: 135 calories, 17.8g protein, 6.9g carbohydrates, 3.4g fat, 0.1g fiber, 165mg cholesterol, 361mg sodium, 181mg potassium

Hot Sauce Shrimps
Yield: 4 servings | **Prep time:** 25 minutes | **Cook time:** 35 minutes

- 2 tablespoons hot sauce
- 1 tablespoon sunflower oil
- 4 tablespoons lemon juice
- ¼ cup of water
- 1-pound shrimps, peeled

1. Mix shrimps with lemon juice, sunflower oil, and hot sauce. Leave them for 20 minutes to marinate.
2. After this, transfer the shrimps in the Crock Pot. Add water.
3. Cook the shrimps on High for 35 minutes.

per serving: 170 calories, 26g protein, 2.2g carbohydrates, 5.6g fat, 0.1g fiber, 239mg cholesterol, 470mg sodium, 222mg potassium

Vegetarian Mains

Cauliflower Rice

Yield: 6 servings | **Prep time:** 10 minutes | **Cook time:** 2 hours

- 4 cups cauliflower, shredded
- 1 cup vegetable stock
- 1 cup of water
- 1 tablespoon cream cheese
- 1 teaspoon dried oregano

1. Put all ingredients in the Crock Pot.
2. Close the lid and cook the cauliflower rice on High for 2 hours.

per serving: 25 calories, 0.8g protein, 3.9g carbohydrates, 0.8g fat, 1.8g fiber, 2mg cholesterol, 153mg sodium, 211mg potassium

Squash Noodles

Yield: 4 servings | **Prep time:** 15 minutes | **Cook time:** 4 hours

- 1-pound butternut squash, seeded, halved
- 1 tablespoon vegan butter
- 1 teaspoon salt
- ½ teaspoon garlic powder
- 3 cups of water

1. Pour water in the Crock Pot.
2. Add butternut squash and close the lid.
3. Cook the vegetable on high for 4 hours.
4. Then drain water and shred the squash flesh with the help of the fork and transfer in the bowl.
5. Add garlic powder, salt, and butter. Mix the squash noodles.

per serving: 78 calories, 1.2g protein, 13.5g carbohydrates, 3g fat, 2.3g fiber, 8mg cholesterol, 612mg sodium, 406mg potassium

Thyme Tomatoes

Yield: 4 servings | **Prep time:** 10 minutes | **Cook time:** 5 hours

- 1-pound tomatoes, sliced
- 1 tablespoon dried thyme
- 1 teaspoon salt
- 2 tablespoons olive oil
- 1 tablespoon apple cider vinegar
- ½ cup of water

1. Put all ingredients in the Crock Pot and close the lid.
2. Cook the tomatoes on Low for 5 hours.

per serving: 83 calories, 1.1g protein, 4.9g carbohydrates, 7.3g fat, 1.6g fiber, 0mg cholesterol, 588mg sodium, 277mg potassium

Quinoa Dolma

Yield: 6 servings | **Prep time:** 15 minutes | **Cook time:** 3 hours

- 6 sweet peppers, seeded
- 1 cup quinoa, cooked
- ½ cup corn kernels, cooked
- 1 teaspoon chili flakes
- 1 cup of water
- ½ cup tomato juice

1. Mix quinoa with corn kernels, and chili flakes.
2. Fill the sweet peppers with quinoa mixture and put in the Crock Pot.
3. Add water and tomato juice.
4. Close the lid and cook the peppers on High for 3 hours.

per serving: 171 calories, 6.6g protein, 33.7g carbohydrates, 2.3g fat, 4.8g fiber, 0mg cholesterol, 29mg sodium, 641mg potassium

Creamy Puree

Yield: 4 servings | **Prep time:** 10 minutes | **Cook time:** 4 hours

- 2 cups potatoes, chopped
- 3 cups of water
- 1 tablespoon vegan butter
- ¼ cup cream
- 1 teaspoon salt

1. Pour water in the Crock Pot.
2. Add potatoes and salt.
3. Cook the vegetables on high for 4 hours.
4. Then drain water, add butter, and cream.
5. Mash the potatoes until smooth.

per serving: 87 calories, 1.4g protein, 12.3g carbohydrates, 3.8g fat, 1.8g fiber, 10mg cholesterol, 617mg sodium, 314mg potassium

Cauliflower Hash

Yield: 4 servings | **Prep time:** 10 minutes | **Cook time:** 2.5 hours

- 3 cups cauliflower, roughly chopped
- ½ cup potato, chopped
- 3 oz Provolone, grated
- 2 tablespoons chives, chopped
- 1 cup milk
- ½ cup of water
- 1 teaspoon chili powder

1. Pour water and milk in the Crock Pot.
2. Add cauliflower, potato, chives, and chili powder.
3. Close the lid and cook the mixture on high for 2 hours.
4. Then sprinkle the hash with provolone cheese and cook the meal on High for 30 minutes.

per serving: 134 calories, 9.3g protein, 9.5g carbohydrates, 7.1g fat, 2.4g fiber, 20mg cholesterol, 246mg sodium, 348mg potassium

Brussel Sprouts

Yield: 4 servings | **Prep time:** 10 minutes | **Cook time:** 2.5 hours

- 1-pound Brussel sprouts
- 2 oz tofu, chopped, cooked
- 1 teaspoon cayenne pepper
- 2 cups of water
- 1 tablespoon vegan butter

1. Pour water in the Crock Pot.
2. Add Brussel sprouts and cayenne pepper.
3. Cook the vegetables on high for 2.5 hours.
4. Then drain water and mix Brussel sprouts with butter and tofu.
5. Shake the vegetables gently.

per serving: 153 calories, 9.2g protein, 10.8g carbohydrates, 9.3g fat, 4.4g fiber, 23mg cholesterol, 380mg sodium, 532mg potassium

Sauteed Garlic

Yield: 4 servings | **Prep time:** 10 minutes | **Cook time:** 6 hours

- 10 oz garlic cloves, peeled
- 2 tablespoons lemon juice
- 1 teaspoon ground black pepper
- 1 cup of water
- 1 tablespoon vegan butter
- 1 bay leaf

1. Put all ingredients in the Crock Pot.
2. Close the lid and cook the garlic on Low for 6 hours.

per serving: 135 calories, 4.7g protein, 24.1g carbohydrates, 3.3g fat, 1.7g fiber, 8mg cholesterol, 36mg sodium, 303mg potassium

Cheesy Corn

Yield: 5 servings | **Prep time:** 5 minutes | **Cook time:** 5 hours

- 4 cups corn kernels
- ½ cup Cheddar cheese, shredded
- 1 tablespoon vegan butter
- 1 teaspoon ground black pepper
- 1 teaspoon salt
- 2 cups of water

1. Mix corn kernels with ground black pepper, butter, salt, and cheese.
2. Transfer the mixture in the Crock Pot and add water.
3. Close the lid and cook the meal on Low for 5 hours.

per serving: 173 calories, 6.9g protein, 23.6g carbohydrates, 7.5g fat, 3.5g fiber, 18mg cholesterol, 573mg sodium, 351mg potassium

Shredded Cabbage Saute

Yield: 4 servings | **Prep time:** 10 minutes | **Cook time:** 6 hours

- 3 cups white cabbage, shredded
- 1 cup tomato juice
- 1 teaspoon salt
- 1 teaspoon sugar
- 1 teaspoon dried oregano
- 3 tablespoons olive oil
- 1 cup of water

1. Put all ingredients in the Crock Pot.

2. Carefully mix all ingredients with the help of the spoon and close the lid.
3. Cook the cabbage saute for 6 hours on Low.
 per serving: 118 calories, 1.2g protein, 6.9g carbohydrates, 10.6g fat, 1.7g fiber, 0mg cholesterol, 756mg sodium, 235mg potassium

Ranch Broccoli
Yield: 3 servings | **Prep time:** 10 minutes | **Cook time:** 1.5 hours
- 3 cups broccoli
- 1 teaspoon chili flakes
- 2 tablespoons ranch dressing
- 2 cups of water
1. Put the broccoli in the Crock Pot.
2. Add water and close the lid.
3. Cook the broccoli on high for 1.5 hours.
4. Then drain water and transfer the broccoli in the bowl.
5. Sprinkle it with chili flakes and ranch dressing. Shake the meal gently.
 per serving: 34 calories, 2.7g protein, 6.6g carbohydrates, 0.3g fat, 2.4g fiber, 0mg cholesterol, 91mg sodium, 291mg potassium.

Sauteed Spinach
Yield: 3 servings | **Prep time:** 10 minutes | **Cook time:** 1 hour
- 3 cups spinach
- 1 tablespoon vegan butter, softened
- 2 cups of water
- 2 oz Parmesan, grated
- 1 teaspoon pine nuts, crushed
1. Chop the spinach and put it in the Crock Pot.
2. Add water and close the lid.
3. Cook the spinach on High for 1 hour.
4. Then drain water and put the cooked spinach in the bowl.
5. Add pine nuts, Parmesan, and butter.
6. Carefully mix the spinach.
 per serving: 108 calories, 7.1g protein, 1.9g carbohydrates, 8.7g fat, 0.7g fiber, 24mg cholesterol, 231mg sodium, 176mg potassium.

Cheddar Mushrooms
Yield: 4 servings | **Prep time:** 10 minutes | **Cook time:** 6 hours
- 4 cups cremini mushrooms, sliced
- 1 teaspoon dried oregano
- 1 teaspoon ground black pepper
- ½ teaspoon salt
- 1 cup Cheddar cheese, shredded
- 1 cup heavy cream
- 1 cup of water
1. Pour water and heavy cream in the Crock Pot.
2. Add salt, ground black pepper, and dried oregano.
3. Then add sliced mushrooms, and Cheddar cheese.
4. Cook the meal on Low for 6 hours.
5. When the mushrooms are cooked, gently stir them and transfer in the serving plates.

 per serving: 239 calories, 9.6g protein, 4.8g carbohydrates, 20.6g fat, 0.7g fiber, 71mg cholesterol, 484mg sodium, 386mg potassium.

Fragrant Appetizer Peppers
Yield: 2 serving | **Prep time:** 15 minutes | **Cook time:** 1.5 hours
- 4 sweet peppers, seeded
- ¼ cup apple cider vinegar
- 1 red onion, sliced
- 1 teaspoon peppercorns
- ½ teaspoon sugar
- ¼ cup of water
- 1 tablespoon olive oil
1. Slice the sweet peppers roughly and put in the Crock Pot.
2. Add all remaining ingredients and close the lid.
3. Cook the peppers on high for 1.5 hours.
4. Then cool the peppers well and store them in the fridge for up to 6 days.
 per serving: 171 calories, 3.1g protein, 25.1g carbohydrates, 7.7g fat, 4.7g fiber, 0mg cholesterol, 11mg sodium, 564mg potassium.

Paprika Baby Carrot
Yield: 2 servings | **Prep time:** 10 minutes | **Cook time:** 2.5 hours
- 1 tablespoon ground paprika
- 2 cups baby carrot
- 1 teaspoon cumin seeds
- 1 cup of water
- 1 teaspoon vegan butter
1. Pour water in the Crock Pot.
2. Add baby carrot, cumin seeds, and ground paprika.
3. Close the lid and cook the carrot on High for 2.5 hours.
4. Then drain water, add butter, and shake the vegetables.
 per serving: 60 calories, 1.6g protein, 8.6g carbohydrates, 2.7g fat, 4.2g fiber, 5mg cholesterol, 64mg sodium, 220mg potassium.

Butter Asparagus
Yield: 4 servings | **Prep time:** 15 minutes | **Cook time:** 5 hours
- 1-pound asparagus
- 2 tablespoons vegan butter
- 1 teaspoon ground black pepper
- 1 cup vegetable stock
1. Pour the vegetable stock in the Crock Pot.
2. Chop the asparagus roughly and add in the Crock Pot.
3. Close the lid and cook the asparagus for 5 hours on Low.
4. Then drain water and transfer the asparagus in the bowl.
5. Sprinkle it with ground black pepper and butter.
 per serving: 77 calories, 2.8g protein, 4.9g carbohydrates, 6.1g fat, 2.5g fiber, 15mg cholesterol, 234mg sodium, 241mg potassium.

Jalapeno Corn

Yield: 4 servings | **Prep time:** 10 minutes | **Cook time:** 5 hours

- 1 cup heavy cream
- ½ cup Monterey Jack cheese, shredded
- 1-pound corn kernels
- 3 jalapenos, minced
- 1 teaspoon vegan butter
- 1 tablespoon dried dill
1. Pour heavy cream in the Crock Pot.
2. Add Monterey Jack cheese, corn kernels, minced jalapeno, butter, and dried dill.
3. Cook the corn on Low for 5 hours.
per serving: 203 calories, 5.6g protein, 9.3g carbohydrates, 16.9g fat, 1.5g fiber, 56mg cholesterol, 101mg sodium, 187mg potassium.

Garlic Sweet Potato

Yield: 4 servings | **Prep time:** 10 minutes | **Cook time:** 6 hours

- 2-pounds sweet potatoes, chopped
- 1 teaspoon minced garlic
- 2 tablespoons vegan butter
- 1 teaspoon salt
- 3 cups of water
1. Pour water in the Crock Pot. Add sweet potatoes.
2. Then add salt and close the lid.
3. Cook the sweet potato on Low for 6 hours.
4. After this, drain the water and transfer the vegetables in the big bowl.
5. Add minced garlic and butter. Carefully stir the sweet potatoes until butter is melted.
per serving: 320 calories, 3.6g protein, 63.5g carbohydrates, 6.2g fat, 9.3g fiber, 15mg cholesterol, 648mg sodium, 1857mg potassium.

Potato Salad

Yield: 2 servings | **Prep time:** 10 minutes | **Cook time:** 3 hours

- 1 cup potato, chopped
- 1 cup of water
- 1 teaspoon salt
- 2 oz celery stalk, chopped
- 2 oz fresh parsley, chopped
- ¼ onion, diced
- 1 tablespoon mayonnaise
1. Put the potatoes in the Crock Pot.
2. Add water and salt.
3. Cook the potatoes on High for 3 hours.
4. Then drain water and transfer the potatoes in the salad bowl.
5. Add all remaining ingredients and carefully mix the salad.
per serving: 129 calories, 5.5g protein, 12.4g carbohydrates, 6.7g fat, 2.5g fiber, 12mg cholesterol, 1479mg sodium, 465mg potassium.

Sautéed Greens

Yield: 4 servings | **Prep time:** 15 minutes | **Cook time:** 1 hour

- 1 cup spinach, chopped
- 2 cups collard greens, chopped
- 1 cup Swiss chard, chopped
- 2 cups of water
- ½ cup half and half
1. Put spinach, collard greens, and Swiss chard in the Crock Pot.
2. Add water and close the lid.
3. Cook the greens on High for 1 hour.
4. Then drain water and transfer the greens in the bowl.
5. Bring the half and half to boil and pour over greens. Carefully mix the greens.
per serving: 49 calories, 1.8g protein, 3.2g carbohydrates, 3.7g fat, 1.1g fiber, 11mg cholesterol, 45mg sodium, 117mg potassium.

Mashed Turnips

Yield: 6 servings | **Prep time:** 10 minutes | **Cook time:** 7 hours

- 3-pounds turnip, chopped
- 3 cups of water
- 1 tablespoon vegan butter
- 1 tablespoon chives, chopped
- 2 oz Parmesan, grated
1. Put turnips in the Crock Pot.
2. Add water and cook the vegetables on low for 7 hours.
3. Then drain water and mash the turnips.
4. Add chives, butter, and Parmesan.
5. Carefully stir the mixture until butter and Parmesan are melted.
6. Then add chives. Mix the mashed turnips again.
per serving: 162 calories, 8.6g protein, 15.1g carbohydrates, 8.1g fat, 4.1g fiber, 22mg cholesterol, 475mg sodium, 490mg potassium.

Artichoke Dip

Yield: 6 servings | **Prep time:** 10 minutes | **Cook time:** 6 hours

- 2 cups Cheddar cheese, shredded
- 1 cup of coconut milk
- 1-pound artichoke, drained, chopped
- 1 tablespoon Ranch dressing
1. Put all ingredients in the Crock Pot.
2. Mix them gently and close the lid.
3. Cook the artichoke dip on Low for 6 hours.
per serving: 280 calories, 12.8g protein, 10.8g carbohydrates, 22.1g fat, 5g fiber, 40mg cholesterol, 325mg sodium, 422mg potassium.

Sweet Onions

Yield: 4 servings | **Prep time:** 10 minutes | **Cook time:** 4 hours

- 2 cups white onion, sliced
- ½ cup vegan butter
- ¼ cup of water
- 1 teaspoon ground black pepper
- 1 tablespoon maple syrup
- 1 teaspoon lemon juice
1. Put all ingredients in the Crock Pot.
2. Close the lid and cook the onions on low for 4 hours.

per serving: 241 calories, 0.9g protein, 9.1g carbohydrates, 23.1g fat, 1.4g fiber, 61mg cholesterol, 167mg sodium, 109mg potassium.

Swedish Style Beets

Yield: 4 servings | **Prep time:** 3 hours | **Cook time:** 8 hours

- 1-pound beets
- ¼ cup apple cider vinegar
- 1 tablespoon olive oil
- 1 teaspoon salt
- ½ teaspoon sugar
- 3 cups of water
1. Put beets in the Crock Pot.
2. Add water and cook the vegetables for 8 hours on Low.
3. Then drain water and peel the beets.
4. Chop the beets roughly and put in the big bowl.
5. Add all remaining ingredients and leave the beets for 2-3 hours to marinate.

per serving: 85 calories, 1.9g protein, 11.9g carbohydrates, 3.7g fat, 2.3g fiber, 0mg cholesterol, 675mg sodium, 359mg potassium.

Sweet and Tender Squash

Yield: 4 servings | **Prep time:** 15 minutes | **Cook time:** 8 hours

- 2-pound butternut squash, chopped
- 1 tablespoon ground cinnamon
- ½ teaspoon ground ginger
- 1 tablespoon sugar
- ½ cup of water
1. Mix butternut squash with ground cinnamon, ground ginger, and sugar. Leave the vegetables for 10-15 minutes.
2. Then transfer them in the Crock Pot. Add remaining butternut squash juice and water.
3. Close the lid and cook the squash on Low for 8 hours.

per serving: 118 calories, 2.4g protein, 31g carbohydrates, 0.3g fat, 5.5g fiber, 0mg cholesterol, 10mg sodium, 809mg potassium.

Corn Pudding

Yield: 4 servings | **Prep time:** 10 minutes | **Cook time:** 5 hours

- 3 cups corn kernels
- 2 cups heavy cream
- 3 tablespoons muffin mix
- 1 oz Parmesan, grated
1. Mix heavy cream with muffin mix and pour the liquid in the Crock Pot.
2. Add corn kernels and Parmesan. Stir the mixture well.
3. Close the lid and cook the pudding on Low for 5 hours.

per serving: 371 calories, 21.8g protein, 31.4g carbohydrates, 26.3g fat, 3.2g fiber, 87mg cholesterol, 180mg sodium, 378mg potassium.

Marinated Onions

Yield: 4 servings | **Prep time:** 30 minutes | **Cook time:** 330 minutes

- 1 cup of water
- ¼ cup sunflower oil
- 1 bay leaf
- 2 garlic cloves, peeled
- ¼ cup apple cider vinegar
- 1 teaspoon liquid honey
- 4 red onions, sliced
1. Pour water in the Crock Pot.
2. Add the sunflower oil, bay leaf, garlic cloves, and apple cider vinegar.
3. Cook the liquid on High for 30 minutes.
4. Then add onion and liquid honey. Stir the mixture and leave for 30 minutes to marinate.

per serving: 176 calories, 1.3g protein, 12.5g carbohydrates, 13.8g fat, 2.5g fiber, 0mg cholesterol, 7mg sodium, 180mg potassium.

Vanilla Applesauce

Yield: 4 servings | **Prep time:** 10 minutes | **Cook time:** 6 hours

- 4 cups apples, chopped, peeled
- 1 teaspoon vanilla extract
- ½ teaspoon ground cardamom
- 1 cup of water
- 1 tablespoon lemon juice
- 2 tablespoons sugar
1. Put all ingredients in the Crock Pot.
2. Close the lid and cook them on Low for 6 hours.
3. Then blend the mixture with the help of the immersion blender.
4. Transfer the smooth applesauce in the glass cans.

per serving: 143 calories, 0.7g protein, 37.2g carbohydrates, 0.5g fat, 5.5g fiber, 0mg cholesterol, 5mg sodium, 248mg potassium.

Cardamom Pumpkin Wedges

Yield: 4 servings | **Prep time:** 10 minutes | **Cook time:** 6 hours

- 2-pound pumpkin, peeled
- 1 teaspoon ground cardamom
- 2 tablespoons lemon juice
- 1 teaspoon lemon zest, grated
- 2 tablespoons sugar
- 1 cup of water
1. Cut the pumpkin into wedges and place them in the Crock Pot.
2. Add water.
3. Then sprinkle the pumpkin with ground cardamom, lemon juice, lemon zest, and sugar.
4. Close the lid and cook the pumpkin on Low for 6 hours.
5. Serve the pumpkin wedges with sweet liquid from the Crock Pot.

per serving: 103 calories, 2.6g protein, 25g carbohydrates, 0.7g fat, 6.8g fiber, 0mg cholesterol, 15mg sodium, 484mg potassium.

Parmesan Scallops Potatoes

Yield: 5 servings | **Prep time:** 15 minutes | **Cook time:** 7 hours

- 5 potatoes
- 5 teaspoons vegan butter

- 1 teaspoon ground black pepper
- 1 teaspoon garlic powder
- 2 tablespoons flour
- 3 cups of milk
- 3 oz vegan Parmesan, grated
1. Peel and slice the potatoes.
2. Then place the sliced potato in the Crock Pot in one layer.
3. Sprinkle the vegetables with ground black pepper, garlic powder, and butter.
4. After this, mix flour with milk and pour over the potatoes.
5. Then sprinkle the vegetables with Parmesan and close the lid.
6. Cook the meal on Low for 7 hours.

per serving: 323 calories, 14.4g protein, 44.3g carbohydrates, 10.7g fat, 5.4g fiber, 34mg cholesterol, 267mg sodium, 967mg potassium.

Eggplant Salad
Yield: 5 servings | **Prep time:** 10 minutes | **Cook time:** 3 hours

- 4 eggplants, cubed
- 1 teaspoon salt
- 1 teaspoon ground black pepper
- 1 cup of water
- 1 tablespoon sesame oil
- 1 tablespoon apple cider vinegar
- 1 teaspoon sesame seeds
- 2 cups tomatoes, chopped
1. Mix eggplants with salt and ground black pepper and leave for 10 minutes.
2. Then transfer the eggplants in the Crock Pot. Add water and cook them for 3 hours on High.
3. Drain water and cool the eggplants to the room temperature.
4. Add sesame oil, apple cider vinegar, sesame seeds, and tomatoes.
5. Gently shake the salad.

per serving: 152 calories, 5.1g protein, 29g carbohydrates, 4g fat, 16.5g fiber, 0mg cholesterol, 479mg sodium, 1185mg potassium.

Sugar Yams
Yield: 4 servings | **Prep time:** 15 minutes | **Cook time:** 2 hours

- 4 yams, peeled
- 1 cup of water
- 1 tablespoon sugar
- 2 tablespoons vegan butter
1. Cut the yams into halves and put them in the Crock Pot.
2. Add water and cook for 2 hours on high.
3. Then melt the butter in the skillet.
4. Add sugar and heat it until sugar is melted.
5. Then drain water from the yams.
6. Put the yams in the sugar butter and roast for 2 minutes per side.

per serving: 63 calories, 0.1g protein, 3.3g carbohydrates, 5.8g fat, 0g fiber, 15mg cholesterol, 43mg sodium, 9mg potassium.

Zucchini Caviar

Yield: 4 servings | **Prep time:** 10 minutes | **Cook time:** 5 hours

- 4 cups zucchini, grated
- 2 onions, diced
- 2 tablespoons tomato paste
- 1 teaspoon salt
- 1 teaspoon ground black pepper
- 1 cup of water
- 1 teaspoon olive oil
1. Put all ingredients in the Crock Pot.
2. Close the lid and cook the meal on Low for 5 hours.
3. Then carefully stir the caviar and cool it to the room temperature.

per serving: 58 calories, 2.4g protein, 10.8g carbohydrates, 1.5g fat, 2.9g fiber, 0mg cholesterol, 605mg sodium, 465mg potassium.

Cauliflower Stuffing
Yield: 4 servings | **Prep time:** 15 minutes | **Cook time:** 5 hours

- 1-pound cauliflower, chopped
- ½ cup panko breadcrumbs
- 1 cup Mozzarella, shredded
- 1 cup of coconut milk
- 2 tablespoons sour cream
- 1 teaspoon onion powder
1. Put all ingredients in the Crock Pot and carefully mix.
2. Then close the lid and cook the stuffing on low for 5 hours.
3. Cool the stuffing for 10-15 minutes and transfer in the bowls.

per serving: 236 calories, 6.9g protein, 17.8g carbohydrates, 17.2g fat, 5.2g fiber, 6mg cholesterol, 158mg sodium, 516mg potassium.

Shallot Saute
Yield: 2 servings | **Prep time:** 10 minutes | **Cook time:** 2.5 hours

- ½ cup carrot, grated
- 1 cup shallot, sliced
- 1 teaspoon ground turmeric
- ½ teaspoon salt
- 1 teaspoon garlic, diced
- ½ cup milk
1. Put all ingredients in the Crock Pot.
2. Close the lid and cook the saute on High for 2 hours.
3. Then leave the cooked meal for 30 minutes to rest.

per serving: 105 calories, 4.4g protein, 20.3g carbohydrates, 1.5g fat, 0.9g fiber, 5mg cholesterol, 639mg sodium, 424mg potassium.

Creamy White Mushrooms
Yield: 4 servings | **Prep time:** 15 minutes | **Cook time:** 8 hours

- 1-pound white mushrooms, chopped
- 1 cup cream
- 1 teaspoon chili flakes
- 1 teaspoon ground black pepper
- 1 tablespoon dried parsley

1. Put all ingredients in the Crock Pot.
2. Cook the mushrooms on low for 8 hours.
3. When the mushrooms are cooked, transfer them in the serving bowls and cool for 10-15 minutes.
per serving: 65 calories, 4.1g protein, 6g carbohydrates, 3.7g fat, 1.3g fiber, 11mg cholesterol, 27mg sodium, 396mg potassium.

Carrot Strips
Yield: 2 servings | **Prep time:** 20 minutes | **Cook time:** 1 hour
- 2 carrots, peeled
- 2 tablespoons sunflower oil
- 1 teaspoon dried thyme
- ½ teaspoon salt
- ½ cup of water
1. Cut the carrots into the strips.
2. Then heat the sunflower oil in the skillet until hot.
3. Put the carrot strips in the hot oil and roast for 2-3 minutes per side.
4. Pour water in the Crock Pot.
5. Add salt and dried thyme.
6. Then add roasted carrot and cook the meal on High for 1 hour.
per serving: 150 calories, 0.6g protein, 6.3g carbohydrates, 14g fat, 1.7g fiber, 0mg cholesterol, 625mg sodium, 200mg potassium.

Potato Bake
Yield: 3 servings | **Prep time:** 10 minutes | **Cook time:** 7 hours
- 2 cups potatoes, peeled, halved
- 4 oz vegan Provolone cheese, grated
- 1 tablespoon vegan butter, softened
- 1 teaspoon dried dill
- ½ cup vegetable stock
- 1 carrot, diced
1. Grease the Crock Pot bottom with butter and put the halved potato inside.
2. Sprinkle it with dried dill and carrot.
3. Then add vegetable stock and Provolone cheese.
4. Cook the potato bake on low for 7 hours.
per serving: 185 calories, 8.8g protein, 14.1g carbohydrates, 10.6g fat, 2.2g fiber, 27mg cholesterol, 380mg sodium, 404mg potassium.

Chili Dip
Yield: 5 servings | **Prep time:** 10 minutes | **Cook time:** 5 hours
- 5 oz chilies, canned, chopped
- 3 oz Mozzarella, shredded
- 1 tomato, chopped
- ½ cup milk
- 1 teaspoon cornflour
1. Mix milk with cornflour and whisk until smooth. Pour the liquid in the Crock Pot.
2. Then add chilies, Mozzarella, and tomato.
3. Close the lid and cook the dip on low for 5 hours.
per serving: 156 calories, 8.7g protein, 22.5g carbohydrates, 5.2g fat, 8.3g fiber, 11mg cholesterol, 140mg sodium, 575mg potassium.

Thyme Fennel Bulb
Yield: 4 servings | **Prep time:** 15 minutes | **Cook time:** 3 hours
- 16 oz fennel bulb
- 1 tablespoon thyme
- 1 cup of water
- 1 teaspoon salt
- 1 teaspoon peppercorns
1. Chop the fennel bulb roughly and put it in the Crock Pot.
2. Add thyme, water, salt, and peppercorns.
3. Cook the fennel on High for 3 hours.
4. Then drain water, remove peppercorns, and transfer the fennel in the serving plates.
per serving: 38 calories, 1.5g protein, 9g carbohydrates, 0.3g fat, 3.9g fiber, 0mg cholesterol, 643mg sodium, 482mg potassium.

Aromatic Artichokes
Yield: 2 servings | **Prep time:** 15 minutes | **Cook time:** 3 hours
- 4 artichokes, trimmed
- 2 tablespoons lemon juice
- 4 teaspoons olive oil
- 1 teaspoon minced garlic
- 1 teaspoon dried rosemary
- 1 cup of water
1. Mix lemon juice with olive oil, minced garlic, and dried rosemary.
2. Then rub every artichoke with oil mixture and arrange it in the Crock Pot.
3. Add water and close the lid.
4. Cook the artichoke on High for 3 hours.
per serving: 240 calories, 10.8g protein, 35.2g carbohydrates, 10g fat, 17.9g fiber, 0mg cholesterol, 312mg sodium, 1230mg potassium.

Rainbow Carrots
Yield: 4 servings | **Prep time:** 10 minutes | **Cook time:** 3.5 hours
- 2-pound rainbow carrots, sliced
- 1 cup vegetable stock
- 1 cup bell pepper, chopped
- 1 onion, sliced
- 1 teaspoon salt
- 1 teaspoon chili powder
1. Put all ingredients in the Crock Pot.
2. Close the lid and cook the meal on High for 3.5 hours.
3. Then cool the cooked carrots for 5-10 minutes and transfer in the serving bowls.
per serving: 118 calories, 3.5g protein, 26.7g carbohydrates, 0.4g fat, 6.6g fiber, 0mg cholesterol, 954mg sodium, 112mg potassium.

Turmeric Parsnip
Yield: 2 servings | **Prep time:** 10 minutes | **Cook time:** 7 hours
- 10 oz parsnip, chopped
- 1 teaspoon ground turmeric
- 1 teaspoon chili flakes

- ½ teaspoon onion powder
- ½ teaspoon salt
- 1 cup of water
- 1 teaspoon vegan butter
1. Put parsnip in the Crock Pot,
2. Add chili flakes and ground turmeric.
3. Then add onion powder, salt, water, and butter.
4. Close the lid and cook the meal on Low for 7 hours.
 per serving: 129 calories, 1.9g protein, 26.7g carbohydrates, 2.5g fat, 7.2g fiber, 5mg cholesterol, 614mg sodium, 569mg potassium.

Garlic Eggplant Rings
Yield: 6 servings | **Prep time:** 15 minutes | **Cook time:** 40 minutes
- 4 eggplants, sliced
- 2 teaspoons garlic, minced
- 1 teaspoon salt
- 3 tablespoons mayonnaise
- 2 tablespoons coconut oil
- ½ cup of water
1. Mix the eggplants with salt and leave for 10 minutes.
2. Then melt the coconut oil in the skillet.
3. Put the sliced eggplants in the hot coconut oil and roast them for 2 minutes per side.
4. Then transfer the eggplants in the Crock Pot.
5. Add water and cook on High for 30 minutes.
6. Transfer the cooked eggplant rings in the plate and sprinkle with mayonnaise and minced garlic.
 per serving: 160 calories, 3.7 protein, 23.6g carbohydrates, 7.6g fat, 12.9g fiber, 2mg cholesterol, 448mg sodium, 841mg potassium.

Butter Hasselback Potatoes
Yield: 2 servings | **Prep time:** 15 minutes | **Cook time:** 4 hours
- 2 large Russet potatoes
- 1 tablespoon olive oil
- 2 teaspoons vegan butter
- 1 teaspoon onion powder
- ½ cup vegetable stock
1. Cut the potatoes in the shape of Hasselback and place it in the Crock Pot.
2. Sprinkle them with olive oil, butter, and onion powder.
3. Add vegetable stock and close the lid.
4. Cook the potatoes on High for 4 hours or until they are soft.
 per serving: 355 calories, 6.5g protein, 59.1g carbohydrates, 11.3g fat, 8.9g fiber, 10mg cholesterol, 241mg sodium, 1518mg potassium.

Sesame Asparagus
Yield: 4 servings | **Prep time:** 10 minutes | **Cook time:** 3 hours
- 1-pound asparagus
- ½ cup of soy sauce
- ½ cup vegetable stock
- 1 teaspoon sesame seeds
- 1 tablespoon vegan butter
1. Trim the asparagus and put it in the Crock Pot.

2. Add soy sauce and vegetable stock.
3. Then add sesame seeds and butter.
4. Close the lid and cook the meal on High for 3 hours.
 per serving: 71 calories, 4.7g protein, 7.1g carbohydrates, 3.5g fat, 2.7g fiber, 8mg cholesterol, 1915mg sodium, 304mg potassium.

Miso Asparagus
Yield: 2 servings | **Prep time:** 10 minutes | **Cook time:** 2.5 hours
- 1 teaspoon miso paste
- 1 cup of water
- 1 tablespoon fish sauce
- 10 oz asparagus, chopped
- 1 teaspoon avocado oil
1. Mix miso paste with water and pour in the Crock Pot.
2. Add fish sauce, asparagus, and avocado oil.
3. Close the lid and cook the meal on High for 2.5 hours.
 per serving: 40 calories, 3.9g protein, 6.7g carbohydrates, 0.6g fat, 3.2g fiber, 0mg cholesterol, 808mg sodium, 327mg potassium.

Chili Okra
Yield: 6 servings | **Prep time:** 10 minutes | **Cook time:** 7 hours
- 6 cups okra, chopped
- 1 cup tomato juice
- 1 teaspoon salt
- ½ teaspoon chili powder
- ½ teaspoon cayenne pepper
- 1 tablespoon olive oil
- 1 cup vegetable stock
1. Put all ingredients from the list above in the Crock Pot.
2. Mix them gently and cook on Low for 7 hours.
 per serving: 69 calories, 2.4g protein, 9.5g carbohydrates, 2.6g fat, 3.6g fiber, 0mg cholesterol, 514mg sodium, 399mg potassium.

Corn Salad
Yield: 4 servings | **Prep time:** 10 minutes | **Cook time:** 1.5 hours
- 2 cups corn kernels
- 1 cup of water
- 1 teaspoon vegan butter
- 1 cup lettuce, chopped
- 1 cup tomatoes, chopped
- 1 teaspoon chili flakes
- 1 teaspoon salt
- 1 tablespoon sunflower oil
1. Pour water in the Crock Pot, add corn kernels and cook them on high for 1.5 hours.
2. Then drain water and transfer the corn kernels in the salad bowl.
3. Add lettuce, tomatoes, chili flakes, salt, and sunflower oil.
4. Shake the salad gently.
 per serving: 116 calories, 3.1g protein, 16.5g carbohydrates, 5.5g fat, 2.8g fiber, 3mg cholesterol, 604mg sodium, 317mg potassium.

Sweet Potato Puree

Yield: 2 servings | **Prep time:** 15 minutes | **Cook time:** 4 hours

- 2 cups sweet potato, chopped
- 1 cup of water
- ¼ cup half and half
- 1 oz scallions, chopped
- 1 teaspoon salt

1. Put sweet potatoes in the Crock Pot.
2. Add water and salt.
3. Cook them on High for 4 hours.
4. The drain water and transfer the sweet potatoes in the food processor.
5. Add half and half and blend until smooth.
6. Transfer the puree in the bowl, and scallions, and mix carefully.

per serving: 225 calories, 5.2g protein, 43.7g carbohydrates, 3.9g fat, 7g fiber, 11mg cholesterol, 1253mg sodium, 1030mg potassium.

Walnut Kale

Yield: 4 servings | **Prep time:** 10 minutes | **Cook time:** 5 hours

- 5 cups kale, chopped
- 2 oz walnuts, chopped
- 1 cup of coconut milk
- 1 teaspoon vegan butter
- 1 cup of water
- 1 oz vegan Parmesan, grated

1. Put all ingredients in the Crock Pot and gently stir.
2. Then close the lid and cook the kale on Low for 5 hours.

per serving: 298 calories, 9.6g protein, 13.7g carbohydrates, 25.1g fat, 3.5g fiber, 8mg cholesterol, 120mg sodium, 644mg potassium.

Apples Sauté

Yield: 4 servings | **Prep time:** 15 minutes | **Cook time:** 2 hours

- 4 cups apples, chopped
- 1 cup of water
- 1 teaspoon ground cinnamon
- 1 teaspoon sugar

1. Put all ingredients in the Crock Pot.
2. Cook the apple sauté for 2 hours on High.
3. When the meal is cooked, let it cool until warm.

per serving: 121 calories, 0.6g protein, 32.3g carbohydrates, 0.4g fat, 5.7g fiber, 0mg cholesterol, 4mg sodium, 242mg potassium.

Spicy Okra

Yield: 2 servings | **Prep time:** 15 minutes | **Cook time:** 1.5 hours

- 2 cups okra, sliced
- ½ cup vegetable stock
- 1 teaspoon chili powder
- ½ teaspoon ground turmeric
- 1 teaspoon chili flakes
- 1 teaspoon dried oregano
- 1 tablespoon butter

1. Put okra in the Crock Pot.
2. Add vegetable stock, chili powder, ground turmeric, chili flakes, and dried oregano.
3. Cook the okra on High for 1.5 hours.
4. Then add butter and stir the cooked okra well.

per serving: 102 calories, 2.5g protein, 9.2g carbohydrates, 6.4g fat, 4.1g fiber, 15mg cholesterol, 252mg sodium, 358mg potassium.

Beet Salad

Yield: 4 servings | **Prep time:** 10 minutes | **Cook time:** 5 hours

- 2 cups beet, peeled, chopped
- 3 oz goat cheese, crumbled
- 4 cups of water
- 1 tablespoon olive oil
- 1 teaspoon liquid honey
- 3 pecans, chopped

1. Put beets in the Crock Pot.
2. Add water and cook them on high for 5 hours.
3. The drain water and transfer the cooked beets in the bowl.
4. Add olive oil, honey, and pecans. Shake the vegetables well and transfer them to the serving plates.
5. Top every serving with crumbled goat cheese.

per serving: 242 calories, 9.1g protein, 11.9g carbohydrates, 18.7g fat, 2.8g fiber, 22mg cholesterol, 146mg sodium, 316mg potassium.

Pumpkin Hummus

Yield: 6 servings | **Prep time:** 15 minutes | **Cook time:** 4 hours

- 1 cup chickpeas, canned
- 1 tablespoon tahini paste
- 1 cup pumpkin, chopped
- 1 teaspoon harissa
- 2 cups of water
- 2 tablespoons olive oil
- 1 tablespoon lemon juice

1. Pour water in the Crock Pot.
2. Add pumpkin and cook it for 4 hours on High or until the pumpkin is soft.
3. After this, drain water and transfer the pumpkin in the food processor.
4. Add all remaining ingredients and blend the mixture until smooth.
5. Add water from pumpkin if the cooked hummus is very thick.

per serving: 193 calories, 7.4g protein, 24.4g carbohydrates, 8.3g fat, 7.2g fiber, 0mg cholesterol, 26mg sodium, 390mg potassium.

Zucchini Mash

Yield: 2 servings | **Prep time:** 10 minutes | **Cook time:** 45 minutes

- 2 cups zucchini, grated
- 1 tablespoon olive oil
- ¼ cup of water
- ½ teaspoon ground black pepper
- 2 tablespoons sour cream

1. Put all ingredients in the Crock Pot and gently stir.
2. Cook the zucchini mash on High for 45 minutes.

per serving: 105 calories, 1.8g protein, 4.6g carbohydrates, 9.7g fat, 1.4g fiber, 5mg cholesterol, 19mg sodium, 320mg potassium.

Garlic Butter
Yield: 8 servings | **Prep time:** 30 minutes | **Cook time:** 20 minutes
- 1 cup vegan butter
- 1 tablespoon garlic powder
- ¼ cup fresh dill, chopped
1. Put all ingredients in the Crock Pot and cook on High for 20 minutes.
2. Then pour the liquid in the ice cubes molds and refrigerate for 30 minutes or until butter is solid.
per serving: 211 calories, 0.7g protein, 1.6g carbohydrates, 23.1g fat, 0.3g fiber, 61mg cholesterol, 167mg sodium, 68mg potassium.

Green Peas Puree
Yield: 2 servings | **Prep time:** 10 minutes | **Cook time:** 1 hour
- 2 cups green peas, frozen
- 1 tablespoon coconut oil
- 1 teaspoon smoked paprika
- 1 cup vegetable stock
1. Put green peas, smoked paprika, and vegetable stock in the Crock Pot.
2. Cook the ingredients in high for 1 hour.
3. Then drain the liquid and mash the green peas with the help of the potato masher.
4. Add coconut oil and carefully stir the cooked puree.
per serving: 184 calories, 8.4g protein, 21.9g carbohydrates, 7.8g fat, 7.8g fiber, 0mg cholesterol, 389mg sodium, 386mg potassium.

Hot Tofu
Yield: 4 servings | **Prep time:** 10 minutes | **Cook time:** 4 hours
- 1-pound firm tofu, cubed
- 1 tablespoon hot sauce
- ½ cup vegetable stock
- 1 teaspoon miso paste
1. Mix vegetables tock with miso paste and pour in the Crock Pot.
2. Add hot sauce and tofu.
3. Close the lid and cook the meal on Low for 4 hours.
4. Then transfer the tofu and liquid in the serving bowls.
per serving: 83 calories, 9.5g protein, 2.5g carbohydrates, 4.8g fat, 1.2g fiber, 0mg cholesterol, 168mg sodium, 176mg potassium.

Sautéed Radish
Yield: 4 servings | **Prep time:** 10 minutes | **Cook time:** 2 hours
- 4 cups radish, halved
- 2 tablespoons sesame oil
- 1 tablespoon dried dill
- ½ teaspoon salt
- 1 tablespoon vegan butter
- 2 cups of water
1. Put all ingredients except butter in the Crock Pot.
2. Cook the mixture on High for 2 hours.
3. Then drain the liquid and transfer the cooked radish in the big bowl.
4. Add butter and stir the radish well.
per serving: 106 calories, 1g protein, 4.4g carbohydrates, 9.8g fat, 2g fiber, 8mg cholesterol, 362mg sodium, 298mg potassium.

Braised Swiss Chard
Yield: 4 servings | **Prep time:** 10 minutes | **Cook time:** 30 minutes
- 1-pound swiss chard, chopped
- 1 lemon
- 1 teaspoon garlic, diced
- 1 tablespoon sunflower oil
- 1 teaspoon salt
- 2 cups of water
1. Put the swiss chard in the Crock Pot.
2. Cut the lemon into halves and squeeze it over the swiss chard.
3. After this, sprinkle the greens with diced garlic, sunflower oil, salt, and water.
4. Mix the mixture gently with the help of the spoon and close the lid.
5. Cook the greens on High for 30 minutes.
per serving: 58 calories, 2.2g protein, 5.8g carbohydrates, 3.9g fat, 2.3g fiber, 0mg cholesterol, 828mg sodium, 455mg potassium.

Braised Sesame Spinach
Yield: 4 servings | **Prep time:** 10 minutes | **Cook time:** 35 minutes
- 1 tablespoon sesame seeds
- ¼ cup of soy sauce
- 2 tablespoons sesame oil
- 4 cups spinach, chopped
- 1 cup of water
1. Pour water in the Crock Pot.
2. Add spinach and cook it on High for 35 minutes.
3. After this, drain water and transfer the spinach in the big bowl.
4. Add soy sauce, sesame oil, and sesame seeds.
5. Carefully mix the spinach and transfer in the serving plates/bowls.
per serving: 88 calories, 2.3g protein, 2.8g carbohydrates, 8.1g fat, 1.1g fiber, 2.8mg cholesterol, 924mg sodium, 213mg potassium.

Collard Greens Saute
Yield: 4 servings | **Prep time:** 15 minutes | **Cook time:** 5 hours
- 1 cup potato, chopped
- 8 oz collard greens, chopped
- 1 cup tomatoes, chopped
- 1 cup of water
- 2 tablespoons coconut oil
- 1 teaspoon dried thyme
- 1 teaspoon salt
1. Put coconut oil in the Crock Pot.
2. Then mix chopped potato with dried thyme and salt.

3.   Put the potato in the Crock Pot and flatten it in one layer.
4.   Add tomatoes, collard greens.
5.   After this, add water and close the lid.
6.   Cook the saute on Low for 5 hours.
 per serving: 97 calories, 2.1g protein, 8.3g carbohydrates, 7.3g fat, 2.9g fiber, 0mg cholesterol, 596mg sodium, 188mg potassium.

Garam Masala Potato Bake
Yield: 2 servings | **Prep time:** 15 minutes | **Cook time:** 6 hours
- 1 cup potatoes, chopped
- 1 teaspoon garam masala
- 3 eggs, beaten
- ½ cup vegan mozzarella, shredded
- 1 tablespoon vegan butter
- 2 tablespoons coconut cream

1.   Mix potatoes with garam masala.
2.   Then put them in the Crock Pot.
3.   Add vegan butter and mozzarella.
4.   After this, mix coconut cream with eggs and pour the liquid over the mozzarella.
5.   Close the lid and cook the meal on Low for 6 hours.
 per serving: 199 calories, 12.1g protein, 16.8g carbohydrates, 9.4g fat, 1.9g fiber, 252mg cholesterol, 156mg sodium, 398mg potassium.

Zucchini Latkes
Yield: 4 servings | **Prep time:** 10 minutes | **Cook time:** 40 minutes
- 2 large zucchinis, grated
- 1 onion, minced
- 1 egg, beaten
- 2 tablespoons flour
- 1 teaspoon ground black pepper
- 1 oz vegan parmesan, grated
- 1 tablespoon olive oil
- ½ cup of water

1.   In the mixing bowl mix grated zucchini, minced onion, egg, flour, ground black pepper, and vegan parmesan.
2.   After this, heat the olive oil in the skillet well.
3.   Make the small latkes from the zucchini mixture and transfer in the hot oil.
4.   Roast the zucchini latkes for 2 minutes per side on high heat.
5.   Then transfer the latkes in the Crock Pot.
6.   Add water and close the lid.
7.   Cook the meal on High for 40 minutes.
 per serving: 121 calories, 6.4g protein, 11.6g carbohydrates, 6.5g fat, 2.6g fiber, 46mg cholesterol, 100mg sodium, 489mg potassium.

Broccoli Fritters
Yield: 4 servings | **Prep time:** 10 minutes | **Cook time:** 40 minutes
- 2 cups broccoli, shredded
- 1 teaspoon chili flakes
- 1 teaspoon salt
- 2 tablespoons semolina
- 1 egg, beaten
- 1 tablespoon cornflour
- 1 tablespoon sunflower oil
- ¼ cup coconut cream

1.   In the mixing bowl mix shredded broccoli, chili flakes, salt, semolina, egg, and cornflour.
2.   Make the small fritters from the broccoli mixture.
3.   Then pour sunflower in the Crock Pot.
4.   Out the fritters in the Crock Pot in one layer.
5.   Add coconut cream.
6.   Cook the fritters on High for 40 minutes.
 per serving: 97 calories, 3.6g protein, 8.8g carbohydrates, 5.7g fat, 1.5g fiber, 44mg cholesterol, 617mg sodium, 181mg potassium.

Yam Fritters
Yield: 1 serving | **Prep time:** 15 minutes | **Cook time:** 4 hours
- 1 yam, grated, boiled
- 1 teaspoon dried parsley
- ¼ teaspoon chili powder
- ¼ teaspoon salt
- 1 egg, beaten
- 1 teaspoon flour
- 5 tablespoons coconut cream
- Cooking spray

1.   In the mixing bowl mix grated yams, dried parsley, chili powder, salt, egg, and flour.
2.   Make the fritters from the yam mixture.
3.   After this, spray the Crock Pot bottom with cooking spray.
4.   Put the fritters inside in one layer.
5.   Add coconut cream and cook the meal on Low for 4 hours.
 per serving: 115 calories, 6.4g protein, 4.9g carbohydrates, 7.9g fat, 0.4g fiber, 175mg cholesterol, 670mg sodium, 110mg potassium.

Curry Couscous
Yield: 4 servings | **Prep time:** 5 minutes | **Cook time:** 20 minutes
- 1 cup of water
- 1 cup couscous
- ½ cup coconut cream
- 1 teaspoon salt

1.   Put all ingredients in the Crock Pot and close the lid.
2.   Cook the couscous on High for 20 minutes.
 per serving: 182 calories, 5.8g protein, 34.4g carbohydrates, 2g fat, 2.2g fiber, 6mg cholesterol, 597mg sodium, 84mg potassium.

Lentils Fritters
Yield: 6 servings | **Prep time:** 20 minutes | **Cook time:** 1.5 hours
- 1 cup red lentils, cooked
- 1 teaspoon fresh cilantro, chopped
- 1 teaspoon scallions, chopped
- 1 tablespoon flour
- ½ carrot, grated
- 1 teaspoon flax meal
- 1 tablespoon coconut oil
- ¼ cup of water

1.   Pour water in the Crock Pot.
2.   Add coconut oil.

3. After this, in the mixing bowl mix all remaining ingredients. Make the small fritters and freeze them for 15-20 minutes in the freezer.
4. Put the fritters in the Crock Pot and close the lid.
5. Cook them on High for 1.5 hours.
per serving: 141 calories, 8.5g protein, 20.9g carbohydrates, 2.8g fat, 10g fiber, 0mg cholesterol, 6mg sodium, 328mg potassium.

Fragrant Jackfruit
Yield: 4 servings | **Prep time:** 15 minutes | **Cook time:** 2 hours
- 1-pound jackfruit, canned, chopped
- 1 teaspoon tomato paste
- 1 teaspoon taco seasoning
- 1 onion, diced
- ½ cup coconut cream
- 1 teaspoon chili powder
1. In the mixing bowl mix taco seasoning, chili powder, tomato paste, and coconut cream.
2. Put the jackfruit and diced onion in the Crock Pot.
3. Pour the tomato mixture over the vegetables and gently mix them.
4. Close the lid and cook the meal on High for 2 hours.
per serving: 145 calories, 2.4g protein, 32.4g carbohydrates, 2.2g fat, 2.7g fiber, 6mg cholesterol, 127mg sodium, 421mg potassium.

Mushroom Saute
Yield: 4 servings | **Prep time:** 15 minutes | **Cook time:** 2.5 hours
- 2 cups cremini mushrooms, sliced
- 1 white onion, sliced
- ½ cup fresh dill, chopped
- 1 cup coconut cream
- 1 teaspoon ground black pepper
- ¼ cup vegan Cheddar cheese, shredded
- 1 tablespoon coconut oil
1. Toss the coconut oil in the skillet and melt it.
2. Add mushrooms and onion.
3. Roast the vegetables on medium heat for 5 minutes.
4. Then transfer them in the Crock Pot.
5. Add all remaining ingredients and carefully mix.
6. Cook the mushroom saute on High for 2.5 hours.
per serving: 134 calories, 4.7g protein, 9.7g carbohydrates, 9.4g fat, 1.8g fiber, 19mg cholesterol, 79mg sodium, 436mg potassium.

Tarragon Pumpkin Bowl
Yield: 2 servings | **Prep time:** 10 minutes | **Cook time:** 4 hours
- 2 cups pumpkin, chopped
- 1 teaspoon dried tarragon
- 1 tablespoon coconut oil
- 1 cup of water
- 1 teaspoon salt
1. Put all ingredients in the Crock Pot. Gently mix them.

2. Close the lid and cook pumpkin on High for 4 hours.
per serving: 143 calories, 2.8g protein, 20g carbohydrates, 7.5g fat, 7.1g fiber, 0mg cholesterol, 1179mg sodium, 515mg potassium.

Coconut Milk Lentils Bowl
Yield: 5 servings | **Prep time:** 10 minutes | **Cook time:** 9 hours
- 2 cups brown lentils
- 3 cups of coconut milk
- 3 cups of water
- 1 teaspoon ground nutmeg
- 1 teaspoon salt
1. Mix the brown lentils with salt and ground nutmeg and put in the Crock Pot.
2. Add coconut milk and water.
3. Close the lid and cook the lentils on Low for 9 hours.
per serving: 364 calories, 5.3g protein, 12.1g carbohydrates, 34.7g fat, 4.9g fiber, 0mg cholesterol, 491mg sodium, 382mg potassium.

Egg Cauliflower
Yield: 2 servings | **Prep time:** 10 minutes | **Cook time:** 4 hours
- 2 cups cauliflower, shredded
- 4 eggs, beaten
- 1 tablespoon vegan butter
- ½ teaspoon salt
1. Mix eggs with salt.
2. Put the shredded cauliflower in the Crock Pot.
3. Add eggs and vegan butter. Gently mix the mixture.
4. Close the lid and cook the meal on low for 4 hours. Stir the cauliflower with the help of the fork every 1 hour.
per serving: 176 calories, 13.5g protein, 9.9g carbohydrates, 9.7g fat, 2.6g fiber, 372mg cholesterol, 746mg sodium, 421mg potassium.

Tofu and Cauliflower Bowl
Yield: 3 servings | **Prep time:** 10 minutes | **Cook time:** 2.15 hours
- 5 oz firm tofu, chopped
- 1 teaspoon curry paste
- ¼ cup of coconut milk
- 1 teaspoon dried basil
- 1 tablespoon sunflower oil
- 2 cups cauliflower, chopped
- 1 cup of water
1. Put cauliflower in the Crock Pot.
2. Add water and cook it on High for 2 hours.
3. Meanwhile, mix curry paste with coconut milk, dried basil, and sunflower oil.
4. Then add tofu and carefully mix the mixture. Leave it for 30 minutes.
5. When the cauliflower is cooked, drain water.
6. Add tofu mixture and shake the meal well. Cook it on High for 15 minutes.
per serving: 148 calories, 5.7g protein, 5.9g carbohydrates, 12.5g fat, 2.5g fiber, 0mg cholesterol, 31mg sodium, 326mg potassium.

Cream Zucchini Pasta

Yield: 2 servings | **Prep time:** 10 minutes | **Cook time:** 2 hours

- 2 large zucchinis, trimmed
- 1 cup coconut cream
- 1 teaspoon white pepper
- 2 oz vegan Parmesan, grated

1. Make the strips from zucchini with the help of a spiralizer and put in the Crock Pot.
2. Add white pepper and coconut cream.
3. Then top the zucchini with grated vegan Parmesan and close the lid.
4. Cook the meal on low for 2 hours.

per serving: 223 calories, 14.1g protein, 16.3g carbohydrates, 13.4g fat, 3.8g fiber, 43mg cholesterol, 335mg sodium, 904mg potassium.

Tofu Curry

Yield: 4 servings | **Prep time:** 10 minutes | **Cook time:** 3 hours

- 1 cup chickpeas, cooked
- 8 oz firm tofu, chopped
- 1 teaspoon curry powder
- ½ cup of coconut milk
- 1 teaspoon ground coriander
- 1 cup vegetable stock
- 1 red onion, diced

1. In the mixing bowl mix curry powder, coconut milk, ground coriander, and red onion.
2. Mix the curry mixture with tofu.
3. Then pour the vegetable stock in the Crock Pot.
4. Add chickpeas, tofu, and all remaining curry mixture.
5. Close the lid and cook the meal on Low for 3 hours. Don't stir the cooked meal.

per serving: 306 calories, 15.3g protein, 36.3g carbohydrates, 13.1g fat, 10.6g fiber, 0mg cholesterol, 205mg sodium, 649mg potassium.

Beans Bake

Yield: 4 servings | **Prep time:** 10 minutes | **Cook time:** 5 hours

- 1-pound green beans
- 1 tablespoon olive oil
- 1 teaspoon salt
- ½ teaspoon ground black pepper
- 2 tablespoons breadcrumbs
- 4 eggs, beaten

1. Chop the green beans roughly and sprinkle them with salt and ground black pepper.
2. Then put them in the Crock Pot.
3. Sprinkle the vegetables with breadcrumbs and eggs.
4. Close the lid and cook the beans bake on Low for 5 hours.

per serving: 142 calories, 8.1g protein, 11g carbohydrates, 8.2g fat, 4.1g fiber, 164mg cholesterol, 675mg sodium, 306mg potassium.

Pumpkin Chili

Yield: 6 servings | **Prep time:** 10 minutes | **Cook time:** 1.5 hours

- ½ cup red kidney beans, canned
- 1 cup pumpkin puree
- ½ cup bell pepper, chopped
- 1 onion, chopped
- ½ cup tomato juice
- 1 teaspoon chili powder
- ½ cup of water
- 1 cup lentils, cooked

1. Put all ingredients in the Crock Pot and carefully mix.
2. Close the lid and cook chili on High for 1.5 hours.

per serving: 194 calories, 12.7g protein, 35.5g carbohydrates, 0.7g fat, 14g fiber, 0mg cholesterol, 66mg sodium, 698mg potassium.

Sweet Pineapple Tofu

Yield: 2 servings | **Prep time:** 15 minutes | **Cook time:** 15 minutes

- 1/3 cup pineapple juice
- 1 teaspoon brown sugar
- 1 teaspoon ground cinnamon
- ¼ teaspoon ground cardamom
- 7 oz firm tofu, chopped
- 1 teaspoon olive oil

1. Put tofu in the mixing bowl.
2. Then sprinkle it with pineapple juice, brown sugar, ground cinnamon, cardamom, and olive oil. Carefully mix the tofu and leave it for 10-15 minutes.
3. Then transfer the tofu mixture in the Crock Pot and close the lid.
4. Cook it on High for 15 minutes.

per serving: 121 calories, 8.4g protein, 9.6g carbohydrates, 6.6g fat, 1.7g fiber, 0mg cholesterol, 13mg sodium, 211mg potassium.

Peach Tofu Crumble

Yield: 4 servings | **Prep time:** 10 minutes | **Cook time:** 2 hours

- 4 peaches, pitted, halved
- 5 oz firm tofu, crumbled
- ½ cup coconut cream
- 1 teaspoon brown sugar
- 1 teaspoon vanilla extract
- 1 teaspoon vegan butter, melted
- 4 tablespoons bread crumbs

1. Brush the ramekins with vegan butter.
2. Then mix tofu with brown sugar and vanilla extract.
3. Put ½ part of tofu in ramekins and top them with peaches.
4. After this, add remaining tofu.
5. Sprinkle it with coconut cream and breadcrumbs.
6. Cover the ramekins with foil and transfer in the Crock Pot.
7. Cook the meal on High for 2 hours.

per serving: 148 calories, 5.6g protein, 23.2g carbohydrates, 4.3g fat, 3g fiber, 6mg cholesterol, 69mg sodium, 364mg potassium.

Rainbow Bake

Yield: 4 servings | **Prep time:** 15 minutes | **Cook time:** 6 hours

- 1 zucchini, sliced

- 1 tomato, sliced
- 1 eggplant, sliced
- 1 red onion, sliced
- 1 tablespoon coconut oil
- 1 teaspoon salt
- 1 teaspoon dried parsley
- 1 teaspoon chili powder
- 1 cup of water

1. Carefully grease the Crock Pot bowl with coconut oil.
2. Then put zucchini, tomato, eggplant, and onion in the Crock Pot one-by-one.
3. Sprinkle the vegetables with salt, dried parsley, and chili powder.
4. Add water and close the lid.
5. Cook the meal on Low for 6 hours.

per serving: 82 calories, 2.2g protein, 11.9g carbohydrates, 3.9g fat, 5.6g fiber, 0mg cholesterol, 597mg sodium, 482mg potassium.

Eggplant Casserole
Yield: 4 servings | **Prep time:** 15 minutes | **Cook time:** 6 hours

- 1 teaspoon minced garlic
- 2 cups eggplants, chopped
- 2 tablespoons sunflower oil
- 1 teaspoon salt
- ½ cup potato, diced
- 1 cup of water
- 1 cup vegan Cheddar cheese, shredded

1. Brush the Crock Pot bottom with sunflower oil.
2. The mix eggplants with minced garlic and salt.
3. Put the vegetables in the Crock Pot.
4. Add potatoes and water.
5. After this, top the vegetables with vegan Cheddar cheese and close the lid.
6. Cook the casserole on Low for 6 hours.

per serving: 194 calories, 7.7g protein, 4.6g carbohydrates, 16.4g fat, 1.7g fiber, 30mg cholesterol, 760mg sodium, 165mg potassium.

Quinoa Fritters
Yield: 4 servings | **Prep time:** 15 minutes | **Cook time:** 1 hour

- 1 sweet potato, peeled, boiled, grated
- ½ cup quinoa, cooked
- 1 teaspoon chili powder
- 1 teaspoon salt
- 2 eggs, beaten
- 3 tablespoons cornflour
- 1 tablespoon coconut oil, melted

1. In the mixing bowl mix grated sweet potato, quinoa, chili powder, salt, cornflour, and eggs.
2. Make the small fritters and put them in the Crock Pot.
3. Add coconut oil and close the lid.
4. Cook the fritters on High for 1 hour.

per serving: 187 calories, 6.8g protein, 24.3g carbohydrates, 7.3g fat, 3.1g fiber, 82mg cholesterol, 630mg sodium, 314mg potassium.

Pinto Beans Balls
Yield: 4 servings | **Prep time:** 15 minutes | **Cook time:** 3 hours

- ½ cup pinto beans, cooked
- 1 egg, beaten
- 1 teaspoon garam masala
- 1 onion, diced, roasted
- 2 tablespoons flour
- 1 teaspoon tomato paste
- 1 tablespoon coconut oil

1. Mash the pinto beans with the help of the potato masher.
2. Then mix them with egg, garam masala, roasted onion, flour, and tomato paste.
3. Make the small balls from the mixture and put them in the Crock Pot.
4. Add coconut oil.
5. Cook the pinto beans balls for 3 hours on Low.

per serving: 155 calories, 7.3g protein, 21g carbohydrates, 4.9g fat, 4.5g fiber, 41mg cholesterol, 22mg sodium, 409mg potassium.

Vegan Pepper Bowl
Yield: 4 servings | **Prep time:** 10 minutes | **Cook time:** 3.5 hours

- 2 cups bell pepper, sliced
- 1 tablespoon olive oil
- 1 tablespoon apple cider vinegar
- 4 tablespoons water
- 5 oz tofu, chopped
- ½ cup of coconut milk
- 1 teaspoon curry powder

1. Put the sliced bell peppers in the Crock Pot.
2. Sprinkle them with olive oil, apple cider vinegar, and water.
3. Close the lid and cook the vegetables on low for 3 hours.
4. Meanwhile, mix curry powder with coconut milk. Put the tofu in the curry mixture and leave for 15 minutes.
5. Add the tofu and all remaining curry mixture in the Crock Pot. Gently mix it and cook for 30 minutes on low.

per serving: 145 calories, 4.3g protein, 7.1g carbohydrates, 12.4g fat, 2g fiber, 0mg cholesterol, 11mg sodium, 254mg potassium.

Braised Root Vegetables
Yield: 4 servings | **Prep time:** 15 minutes | **Cook time:** 8 hours

- 1 cup beets, chopped
- 1 cup carrot, chopped
- 1 teaspoon raisins
- 2 cups vegetable stock
- 1 teaspoon salt
- 1 teaspoon onion powder

1. Put all ingredients in the Crock Pot.
2. Close the lid and cook them on Low for 8 hours.

per serving: 39 calories, 1g protein, 9g carbohydrates, 1.1g fat, 1.6g fiber, 0mg cholesterol, 993mg sodium, 229mg potassium.

Corn Fritters
Yield: 4 servings | **Prep time:** 15 minutes | **Cook time:** 3 hours

- 1 cup mashed potato
- 1/3 cup corn kernels, cooked

- 1 egg, beaten
- 2 tablespoons flour
- 1 teaspoon salt
- 1 teaspoon ground turmeric
- ½ teaspoon chili powder
- 2 tablespoons coconut oil

1. Put the coconut oil in the Crock Pot and melt it on low for 15 minutes.
2. Meanwhile, mix mashed potato with corn kernels, egg, flour, salt, ground turmeric, and chili powder.
3. Make the medium size fritters and put them in the Crock Pot.
4. Cook them on Low for 3 hours.

per serving: 162 calories, 3.3g protein, 14.9g carbohydrates, 10.4g fat, 1.5g fiber, 41mg cholesterol, 777mg sodium, 246mg potassium.

Bulgur Sauté

Yield: 4 servings | **Prep time:** 10 minutes | **Cook time:** 4 hours

- 1 cup bell pepper, chopped
- 1 white onion, diced
- 2 tablespoons tomato paste
- 1 cup bulgur
- 3 cups vegetable stock
- 1 tablespoon olive oil
- 1 teaspoon salt
- 1 teaspoon chili flakes

1. Put all ingredients in the Crock Pot and close the lid.
2. Cook the meal on low doe 4 hours or until the bulgur is tender.

per serving: 181 calories, 5.6g protein, 33.8g carbohydrates, 4.2g fat, 8g fiber, 0mg cholesterol, 747mg sodium, 322mg potassium.

Tomato Okra

Yield: 2 servings | **Prep time:** 10 minutes | **Cook time:** 6 hours

- 2 cups okra, sliced
- 1 teaspoon chili powder
- 1 teaspoon salt
- 1 cup tomato juice
- ¼ cup fresh parsley, chopped

1. Put all ingredients in the Crock Pot and carefully mix.
2. Close the lid and cook the okra on Low for 6 hours.

per serving: 67 calories, 3.2g protein, 13.8g carbohydrates, 0.5g fat, 4.4g fiber, 0mg cholesterol, 1514mg sodium, 644mg potassium.

Stuffed Okra

Yield: 4 servings | **Prep time:** 15 minutes | **Cook time:** 5 hours

- 1-pound okra
- 1 cup cauliflower, shredded
- 1 teaspoon curry powder
- 1 teaspoon tomato paste
- 1 teaspoon dried dill
- 1/3 cup coconut milk
- 1 tablespoon coconut oil

1. Make the cuts in the okra and remove seeds.

2. Then mix shredded cauliflower with curry powder, tomato paste, and dried dill.
3. Fill every okra with cauliflower mixture and put in the Crock Pot.
4. Add coconut oil and coconut milk in the Crock Pot and close the lid.
5. Cook the okra on Low for 5 hours.

per serving: 130 calories, 3.3g protein, 11.6g carbohydrates, 8.5g fat, 5g fiber, 0mg cholesterol, 21mg sodium, 497mg potassium.

Garlic Asparagus

Yield: 5 servings | **Prep time:** 10 minutes | **Cook time:** 6 hours

- 1-pound asparagus, trimmed
- 1 teaspoon salt
- 1 teaspoon garlic powder
- 1 tablespoon vegan butter
- 1 ½ cup vegetable stock

1. Chop the asparagus roughly and sprinkle with salt and garlic powder.
2. Put the vegetables in the Crock Pot.
3. Add vegan butter and vegetable stock. Close the lid.
4. Cook the asparagus on Low for 6 hours.

per serving: 33 calories, 2.3g protein, 6.1g carbohydrates, 1g fat, 2g fiber, 0mg cholesterol, 687mg sodium, 190mg potassium.

Coconut Cauliflower Florets

Yield: 4 servings | **Prep time:** 10 minutes | **Cook time:** 4 hours

- 2 cups cauliflower, florets
- 1 cup of coconut milk
- 1 tablespoon coconut flakes
- 1 teaspoon salt
- 1 teaspoon ground turmeric

1. Sprinkle the cauliflower florets with ground turmeric and salt, and transfer in the Crock Pot.
2. Add coconut flakes and coconut milk.
3. Close the lid and cook the meal on Low for 4 hours.
4. Carefully mix the cauliflower before serving.

per serving: 157 calories, 24.g protein, 6.5g carbohydrates, 14.8g fat, 2.8g fiber, 0mg cholesterol, 606mg sodium, 328mg potassium.

Saag Aloo

Yield: 6 servings | **Prep time:** 10 minutes | **Cook time:** 6 hours

- 1 yellow onion, chopped
- 1 cup potatoes, chopped
- 3 garlic cloves, diced
- 1 chili pepper, chopped
- 1 teaspoon ground cumin
- 1 teaspoon garam masala
- 2 cups of water
- 1 cup tomatoes, chopped
- 1 cup spinach, chopped

1. Put onion, potatoes, and chili pepper in the Crock Pot.
2. Add tomatoes and spinach.
3. After this, add sprinkle the ingredients with garam masala, ground cumin, and garlic.

4.   Add water and close the lid.
5.   Cook the meal on Low for 6 hours.
per serving: 35 calories, 1.2g protein, 7.g car7bohydrates, 0.2g fat, 1.6g fiber, 0mg cholesterol, 12mg sodium, 242mg potassium.

Sweet Potato and Lentils Pate
Yield: 4 servings | **Prep time:** 10 minutes | **Cook time:** 6 hours
- 1 cup sweet potato, chopped
- ½ cup red lentils
- 2.5 cups water
- 1 tablespoon soy milk
- 1 teaspoon cayenne pepper
- ½ teaspoon salt
1.   Put all ingredients in the Crock Pot.
2.   Close the lid and cook the mixture on low for 6 hours.
3.   When the ingredients are cooked, transfer them in the blender and blend until smooth.
4.   Put the cooked pate in the bowl and store it in the fridge for up to 4 days.
per serving: 140 calories, 7.4g protein, 25.1g carbohydrates, 1.3g fat, 9.1g fiber, 3mg cholesterol, 322mg sodium, 488mg potassium.

Sautéed Endives
Yield: 4 servings | **Prep time:** 10 minutes | **Cook time:** 40 minutes
- 1-pound endives, roughly chopped
- ½ cup of water
- 1 tablespoon avocado oil
- 1 teaspoon garlic, diced
- 2 tablespoons coconut cream
1.   Pour water in the Crock Pot.
2.   Add endives and garlic.
3.   Close the lid and cook them on High for 30 minutes.
4.   Then add coconut cream and avocado oil.
5.   Cook the endives for 10 minutes more.
per serving: 42 calories, 1.9g protein, 4.4g carbohydrates, 2.4g fat, 3.7g fiber, 6mg cholesterol, 41mg sodium, 376mg potassium.

Mung Beans Salad
Yield: 4 servings | **Prep time:** 10 minutes | **Cook time:** 3 hours
- ½ avocado, chopped
- 1 cup cherry tomatoes, halved
- ½ cup corn kernels, cooked
- 1 cup mung beans
- 3 cups of water
- 1 tablespoon lemon juice
- 1 tablespoon avocado oil
1.   Put mung beans in the Crock Pot.
2.   Add water and cook them on High for 3 hours.
3.   Then drain water and transfer the mung beans in the salad bowl.
4.   Add avocado, cherry tomatoes, corn kernels, and shake well.
5.   Then sprinkle the salad with avocado oil and lemon juice.

per serving: 287 calories, 13.9g protein, 40g carbohydrates, 9.4g fat, 11.2g fiber, 0mg cholesterol, 20mg sodium, 932mg potassium.

Onion Balls
Yield: 4 servings | **Prep time:** 25 minutes | **Cook time:** 2 hours
- ½ cup red lentils, cooked
- ½ cup onion, minced
- 1 teaspoon ground black pepper
- ¼ cup flax meal
- 1 teaspoon cornflour
- ½ teaspoon salt
- ½ cup of water
- ½ cup ketchup
1.   In the mixing bowl mix red lentils with minced onion, ground black pepper, flax meal, cornflour, and salt.
2.   Make the balls from the onion mixture and freeze them in the freezer for 20 minutes.
3.   After this, mix water and ketchup in the Crock Pot.
4.   Add frozen balls and close the lid.
5.   Cook the meal on High for 2 hours.
per serving: 153 calories, 8.5g protein, 26.1g carbohydrates, 2.9g fat, 9.9g fiber, 0mg cholesterol, 628mg sodium, 430mg potassium.

Vegan Kofte
Yield: 4 servings | **Prep time:** 15 minutes | **Cook time:** 4 hours
- 2 eggplants, peeled, boiled
- 1 teaspoon minced garlic
- 1 teaspoon ground cumin
- ¼ teaspoon minced ginger
- ½ cup chickpeas, canned
- 3 tablespoons breadcrumbs
- 1/3 cup water
- 1 tablespoon coconut oil
1.   Blend the eggplants until smooth.
2.   Add minced garlic, ground cumin, minced ginger, chickpeas, and blend the mixture until smooth.
3.   Transfer it in the mixing bowl. Add breadcrumbs.
4.   Make the small koftes and put them in the Crock Pot.
5.   Add coconut oil and close the lid.
6.   Cook the meal on Low for 4 hours.
per serving: 212 calories, 8.3g protein, 35.5g carbohydrates, 5.8g fat, 14.3g fiber, 0mg cholesterol, 50mg sodium, 870mg potassium.

Tofu Kebabs
Yield: 4 servings | **Prep time:** 15 minutes | **Cook time:** 2 hours
- 2 tablespoons lemon juice
- 1 teaspoon ground turmeric
- 2 tablespoons coconut cream
- 1 teaspoon chili powder
- ¼ cup of water
- 1 teaspoon avocado oil
- 1-pound tofu, cubed
1.   Pour water in the Crock Pot.

2. After this, in the mixing bowl mix lemon juice, ground turmeric, coconut cream, chili powder, and avocado oil.
3. Coat every tofu cube in the coconut cream mixture and string on the wooden skewers. Place them in the Crock Pot.
4. Cook the tofu kebabs on Low for 2 hours.
 per serving: 104 calories, 9.7g protein, 3.3g carbohydrates, 6.9g fat, 1.6g fiber, 0mg cholesterol, 24mg sodium, 227mg potassium.

Carrot and Lentils Sauté
Yield: 4 servings | **Prep time:** 7 minutes | **Cook time:** 5 hours
- 1 cup red lentils
- 1 cup carrot, diced
- 1 cup fresh parsley, chopped
- 4 cups vegetable stock
- 1 teaspoon cayenne pepper
- 1 teaspoon salt
- 1 tablespoon tomato paste

1. Put all ingredients in the Crock Pot and gently stir.
2. Close the lid and cook the meal on low for 5 hours.
 per serving: 201 calories, 13.3g protein, 35.5g carbohydrates, 2.7g fat, 16.1g fiber, 0mg cholesterol, 1336mg sodium, 679mg potassium.

Cashew and Tofu Casserole
Yield: 4 servings | **Prep time:** 15 minutes | **Cook time:** 3.5 hours
- 1 oz cashews, crushed
- 6 oz firm tofu, chopped
- 1 cup broccoli, chopped
- 1 red onion, sliced
- 1 tablespoon avocado oil
- ¼ cup of soy sauce
- ¼ cup maple syrup
- 1 tablespoon cornstarch
- ½ cup of water
- 1 teaspoon garlic powder

1. Pour the avocado oil in the Crock Pot.
2. Then sprinkle the broccoli with garlic powder and put it in the Crock Pot.
3. Add cornstarch.
4. After this, add maple syrup, soy sauce, onion, and tofu.
5. Add cashews and water.
6. Close the lid and cook the casserole on Low for 3.5 hours.
 per serving: 164 calories, 6.7g protein, 24g carbohydrates, 5.7g fat, 2.1g fiber, 0mg cholesterol, 917mg sodium, 309mg potassium.

Teriyaki Kale
Yield: 6 servings | **Prep time:** 10 minutes | **Cook time:** 30 minutes
- 5 cups kale, roughly chopped
- 1/2 cup teriyaki sauce
- 1 teaspoon sesame seeds
- 1 cup of water
- 1 teaspoon garlic powder
- 2 tablespoons coconut oil

1. Melt the coconut oil and mix it with garlic powder, water, sesame seeds, and teriyaki sauce.
2. Pour the liquid in the Crock Pot.
3. Add kale and close the lid.
4. Cook the kale on High for 30 minutes.
5. Serve the kale with a small amount of teriyaki liquid.
 per serving: 92 calories, 3.3g protein, 10g carbohydrates, 4.8g fat, 1g fiber, 0mg cholesterol, 945mg sodium, 336mg potassium.

Potato Balls
Yield: 6 servings | **Prep time:** 15 minutes | **Cook time:** 1.5 hours
- 2 cups mashed potato
- 1 tablespoon coconut cream
- 3 tablespoons breadcrumbs
- 1 teaspoon dried dill
- 2 oz scallions, diced
- 1 egg, beaten
- 2 tablespoons flour
- ½ cup of coconut milk

1. In the mixing bowl mix mashed potato with coconut cream, breadcrumbs, dried dill, scallions, egg, and flour.
2. Make the potato balls and put them in the Crock Pot.
3. Add coconut milk and cook the meal on High for 1.5 hours.
 per serving: 132 calories, 3.4g protein, 17.5g carbohydrates, 5.5g fat, 1.6g fiber, 28mg cholesterol, 273mg sodium, 287mg potassium.

Split Pea Paste
Yield: 4 servings | **Prep time:** 15 minutes | **Cook time:** 2 hours
- 2 cups split peas
- 2 cups of water
- 1 tablespoon coconut oil
- 1 teaspoon salt
- 1 teaspoon ground black pepper

1. Pour water in the Crock Pot.
2. Add split peas and close the lid.
3. Cook them for 2 hours on high or until they are soft.
4. Then drain water and transfer the split peas in the food processor.
5. Add coconut oil, salt, and ground black pepper.
6. Blend the mixture until smooth.
 per serving: 367 calories, 24.2g protein, 59.8g carbohydrates, 4.6g fat, 25.3g fiber, 0mg cholesterol, 600mg sodium, 974mg potassium.

Marinated Poached Aubergines
Yield: 6 servings | **Prep time:** 15 minutes | **Cook time:** 4 hours
- ½ cup apple cider vinegar
- 1-pound eggplants, chopped
- 1 cup of water
- ¼ cup avocado oil
- 3 garlic cloves, diced
- 1 teaspoon salt
- 1 teaspoon sugar

1. Put all ingredients in the Crock Pot.

2. Cook the meal on Low for 4 hours.
3. Cool the cooked aubergines well.
per serving: 40 calories, 1g protein, 6.3g carbohydrates, 1.3g fat, 3.1g fiber, 0mg cholesterol, 392mg sodium, 224mg potassium.

Mushroom Risotto
Yield: 4 servings | **Prep time:** 10 minutes | **Cook time:** 6 hours
- ½ cup Arborio rice
- 2 cups brown mushrooms, chopped
- 1 yellow onion, diced
- 2 tablespoons avocado oil
- 1 teaspoon salt
- 1 teaspoon ground black pepper
- 4 cups vegetable stock
1. Pour the vegetable stock in the Crock Pot.
2. Add ground black pepper and salt.
3. After this, add avocado oil, diced onion, mushrooms, and Arborio rice.
4. Close the lid and cook the risotto on Low for 6 hours.
per serving: 127 calories, 2.9g protein, 25.7g carbohydrates, 3.1g fat, 1.9g fiber, 0mg cholesterol, 1307mg sodium, 248mg potassium.

Cauliflower Curry
Yield: 4 servings | **Prep time:** 10 minutes | **Cook time:** 2 hours
- 4 cups cauliflower
- 1 tablespoon curry paste
- 2 cups of coconut milk
1. In the mixing bowl mix coconut milk with curry paste until smooth.
2. Put cauliflower in the Crock Pot.
3. Pour the curry liquid over the cauliflower and close the lid.
4. Cook the meal on High for 2 hours.
per serving: 236 calories, 4.9g protein, 13g carbohydrates, 30.9g fat, 5.1g fiber, 0mg cholesterol, 48mg sodium, 619mg potassium.

Tender Stuffing
Yield: 4 servings | **Prep time:** 10 minutes | **Cook time:** 4 hours
- 8 oz celery stalks, chopped
- ¼ cup breadcrumbs
- 1 white onion, diced
- 1 teaspoon dried sage
- 2 tablespoons coconut oil
- ½ cup tomatoes, chopped
- 1 cup of coconut milk
1. Put all ingredients in the Crock Pot and gently mix.
2. Then close the lid and cook the stuffing on Low for 4 hours.
per serving: 248 calories, 3.2g protein, 13.4g carbohydrates, 21.7g fat, 3.5g fiber, 0mg cholesterol, 106mg sodium, 414mg potassium.

Soft Sweet Potato Halves
Yield: 4 servings | **Prep time:** 10 minutes | **Cook time:** 5 hours
- 4 sweet potatoes, halved
- 4 teaspoons coconut oil
- 1 teaspoon dried thyme
- ½ teaspoon dried oregano
- 1 teaspoon salt
- ¼ cup of water
1. Pour water in the Crock Pot.
2. Then rub the sweet potato halves with dried thyme, oregano, and salt.
3. Put the sweet potato halves in the Crock Pot.
4. Top every sweet potato halves with coconut oil and close the lid.
5. Cook the sweet potato halves for 5 hours on Low.
per serving: 42 calories, 0.1g protein, 0.6g carbohydrates, 4.6g fat, 0.2g fiber, 0mg cholesterol, 582mg sodium, 14mg potassium.

Parsnip Balls
Yield: 4 servings | **Prep time:** 20 minutes | **Cook time:** 3 hours
- 8 oz parsnip, peeled, grated
- 1 tablespoon coconut cream
- 1/3 cup coconut flour
- 1 tablespoon coconut oil
- 1 carrot, boiled, peeled, mashed
- 1 teaspoon salt
- 1 teaspoon chili powder
1. In the mixing bowl mix grated parsnip, coconut cream, coconut flour, mashed carrot, salt, and chili powder.
2. With the help of the scooper make the small balls and freeze them for 10-15 minutes.
3. Then put coconut oil in the Crock Pot.
4. Add frozen parsnip balls and cook them on Low for 3 hours.
per serving: 129 calories, 2.3g protein, 18.9g carbohydrates, 5.6g fat, 7.5g fiber, 0mg cholesterol, 605mg sodium, 284mg potassium.

Vegetable Korma
Yield: 6 servings | **Prep time:** 10 minutes | **Cook time:** 6 hours
- 1 cup tomatoes, chopped
- 1 cup potatoes, chopped
- 1 cup green peas, frozen
- 1 teaspoon curry powder
- 1 teaspoon garam masala
- 6 oz green beans, chopped
- 2 cups of water
- 1 cup coconut cream
1. Put all ingredients in the Crock Pot and gently stir with the help of the spoon.
2. Close the lid and cook korma on Low for 6 hours.
per serving: 144 calories, 3.5g protein, 13g carbohydrates, 9.8g fat, 4.1g fiber, 0mg cholesterol, 15mg sodium, 402mg potassium.

Tofu Tikka Masala
Yield: 4 servings | **Prep time:** 15 minutes | **Cook time:** 2 hours
- 1-pound tofu, cubed
- 1 teaspoon ground cumin
- 1 teaspoon garam masala

- ½ cup coconut cream
- 1 teaspoon minced garlic
- 1 teaspoon minced ginger
- 1 tablespoon lemon juice
- 1 tablespoon avocado oil
1. In the mixing bowl mix avocado oil, lemon juice, minced ginger, garlic, coconut cream, garam masala, and ground cumin.
2. Then add tofu and carefully mix the mixture.
3. Leave it for 10 minutes and then transfer in the Crock Pot.
4. Close the lid and cook the meal on Low for 2 hours.

per serving: 159 calories, 10.2g protein, 4.6g carbohydrates, 12.5g fat, 2g fiber, 0mg cholesterol, 21mg sodium, 281mg potassium.

Beet and Capers Salad
Yield: 4 servings | **Prep time:** 10 minutes | **Cook time:** 4 hours
- 2 teaspoons capers
- 1 cup lettuce, chopped
- 2 oz walnuts, chopped
- 1 tablespoon lemon juice
- 1 tablespoon sunflower oil
- 1 teaspoon flax seeds
- 3 cups of water
- 2 cups beets, peeled
1. Pour water in the Crock Pot and add beets. Cook them on High for 4 hours.
2. Then drain water, cool the beets and chop.
3. Put the chopped beets in the salad bowl.
4. Add capers, lettuce, walnuts, lemon juice, sunflower oil, and flax seeds.
5. Carefully mix the salad.

per serving: 162 calories, 5.1g protein, 10.6g carbohydrates, 12.3g fat, 3g fiber, 0mg cholesterol, 115mg sodium, 365mg potassium.

Dill Brussel Sprouts
Yield: 4 servings | **Prep time:** 20 minutes | **Cook time:** 2 hours
- 4 cups Brussel sprouts, halved
- 2 tablespoons avocado oil
- 1 tablespoon dried dill
- ½ teaspoon salt
- 1 tablespoon vegan butter
- 2 cups of water
1. Pour water in the Crock Pot. Add Brussel sprouts.
2. Then close the lid and cook the vegetables on high for 2 hours.
3. After this, drain water and transfer the vegetables in the hot skillet.
4. Sprinkle them with avocado oil, dried dill, salt, and vegan butter.
5. Roast Brussel sprouts for 3-4 minutes on high heat.

per serving: 106 calories, 1g protein, 4.4g carbohydrates, 9.8g fat, 2g fiber, 8mg cholesterol, 362mg sodium, 298mg potassium.

Oat Fritters
Yield: 4 servings | **Prep time:** 15 minutes | **Cook time:** 2 hours
- 1 cup rolled oats
- ¼ teaspoon ground paprika
- 1 teaspoon salt
- 2 sweet potatoes, peeled, boiled
- 1 tablespoon coconut oil
- 2 tablespoons coconut cream
1. In the mixing bowl mix rolled oats, ground paprika, salt, and potatoes.
2. When the mixture is homogenous, make the fritters and transfer them in the Crock Pot.
3. Add coconut cream and coconut oil.
4. Cook the fritters in High for 1 hour.
5. Then flip the fritters on another side and cook them for 1 hour more.

per serving: 125 calories, 2.9g protein, 14.5g carbohydrates, 6.5g fat, 2.3g fiber, 0mg cholesterol, 584mg sodium, 101mg potassium.

Avocado Saute
Yield: 4 servings | **Prep time:** 10 minutes | **Cook time:** 6.5 hours
- 1 cup chickpeas
- 4 cups of water
- ½ cup tomato juice
- 1 tablespoon tomato paste
- ½ cup fresh parsley, chopped
- ½ cup coconut cream
- 1 avocado, peeled, pitted, chopped
1. Pour water in the Crock Pot. Add chickpeas and tomato juice. Cook the ingredients on low for 6 hours.
2. Then add tomato paste, fresh parsley, and coconut cream. Cook the meal on High for 30 minutes.
3. Transfer the cooked meal in the bowls and top with avocado.

per serving: 365 calories, 11.9g protein, 38.8g carbohydrates, 20.1g fat, 13.3g fiber, 0mg cholesterol, 116mg sodium, 914mg potassium.

Light Chana Masala
Yield: 4 servings | **Prep time:** 10 minutes | **Cook time:** 8 hours
- 1 teaspoon ginger, peeled, minced
- 1 teaspoon minced garlic
- ¼ cup fresh cilantro, chopped
- 1 jalapeno, chopped
- 1 cup tomatoes, pureed
- 1 cup chickpeas
- 4 cups of water
1. Put all ingredients in the Crock Pot and close the lid.
2. Cook the meal on Low for 8 hours.

per serving: 194 calories, 10.2g protein, 32.9g carbohydrates, 3.2g fat, 9.4g fiber, 0mg cholesterol, 22mg sodium, 568mg potassium.

Quinoa Casserole
Yield: 6 servings | **Prep time:** 10 minutes | **Cook time:** 3 hours
- 1 teaspoon nutritional yeast
- 1 cup quinoa
- 1 cup bell pepper, chopped

- 1 teaspoon smoked paprika
- 1 cup broccoli florets, chopped
- 1 cup cashew cream
- 1 teaspoon chili flakes
- 3 cups of water

1. Mix quinoa with nutritional yeast and put in the Crock Pot.
2. Add bell pepper, smoked paprika, broccoli florets, and chili flakes.
3. Add cashew cream and water.
4. Close the lid and cook the casserole for 3 hours on high.

per serving: 121 calories, 4.9g protein, 23.1g carbohydrates, 2.1g fat, 2.9g fiber, 0mg cholesterol, 13mg sodium, 268mg potassium.

Mushroom Bourguignon
Yield: 3 servings | **Prep time:** 10 minutes | **Cook time:** 7 hours

- ½ cup mushrooms, chopped
- ¼ cup onion, chopped
- ¼ cup carrot, diced
- ½ cup green peas, frozen
- 1 teaspoon dried thyme
- 1 teaspoon salt
- 2 tablespoons tomato paste
- 3 cups vegetable stock

1. Mix vegetable stock with tomato paste and pour liquid in the Crock Pot.
2. Add all remaining ingredients and close the lid.
3. Cook the meal on Low for 7 hours.

per serving: 45 calories, 2.8g protein, 8.8g carbohydrates, 0.3g fat, 2.9g fiber, 0mg cholesterol, 844mg sodium, 250mg potassium.

Sweet Potato Curry
Yield: 4 servings | **Prep time:** 10 minutes | **Cook time:** 3.5 hours

- 2 cups sweet potatoes, chopped
- 1 cup spinach, chopped
- ½ onion, diced
- 1 teaspoon garlic, minced
- 1 teaspoon curry powder
- ½ teaspoon ground turmeric
- 1 tablespoon coconut oil
- 1 cup of coconut milk

1. In the mixing bowl mix coconut milk, ground turmeric, curry powder, garlic, and pour it in the Crock Pot.
2. Add sweet potatoes, onion, and coconut oil.
3. Close the lid and cook the ingredients on High for 3 hours.
4. Then add spinach, carefully mix the mixture and cook it for 30 minutes on High.

per serving: 267 calories, 3g protein, 26.5g carbohydrates, 18g fat, 5.1g fiber, 0mg cholesterol, 23mg sodium, 849mg potassium.

Masala Eggplants
Yield: 2 servings | **Prep time:** 20 minutes | **Cook time:** 2 hours

- ½ cup coconut cream
- ½ cup of water
- 1 teaspoon garam masala
- 2 eggplants, chopped
- 1 teaspoon salt

1. Sprinkle the eggplants with salt and leave for 10 minutes.
2. Then drain eggplant juice and transfer the vegetables in the Crock Pot.
3. Add garam masala, water, and coconut cream.
4. Cook the meal on High for 2 hours.

per serving: 275 calories, 6.8g protein, 35.5g carbohydrates, 15.3g fat, 20.7g fiber, 0mg cholesterol, 1186mg sodium, 1414mg potassium.

Baked Onions
Yield: 4 servings | **Prep time:** 15 minutes | **Cook time:** 2 hours

- 4 onions, peeled
- 1 tablespoon coconut oil
- 1 teaspoon salt
- 1 teaspoon brown sugar
- 1 cup coconut cream

1. Put coconut oil in the Crock Pot.
2. Then make the small cuts in the onions with the help of the knife and put in the Crock Pot in one layer.
3. Sprinkle the vegetables with salt, and brown sugar.
4. Add coconut cream and close the lid.
5. Cook the onions on High for 2 hours.

per serving: 214 calories, 2.6g protein, 14.3g carbohydrates, 17.8g fat, 3.7g fiber, 0mg cholesterol, 595mg sodium, 320mg potassium.

Curry Paneer
Yield: 2 servings | **Prep time:** 10 minutes | **Cook time:** 2 hours

- 6 oz paneer, cubed
- 1 teaspoon garam masala
- ½ cup coconut cream
- 1 chili pepper, chopped
- 1 teaspoon olive oil
- ½ onion, diced
- 1 teaspoon garlic paste

1. In the mixing bowl mix diced onion, garlic paste, olive oil, chili pepper, coconut cream, and garam masala.
2. Then mix the mixture with cubed paneer and put in the Crock Pot.
3. Cook it on Low for 2 hours.

per serving: 309 calories, 7.1g protein, 22.5g carbohydrates, 22.4g fat, 3.5g fiber, 2mg cholesterol, 415mg sodium, 208mg potassium.

Arugula and Halloumi Salad
Yield: 4 servings | **Prep time:** 15 minutes | **Cook time:** 30 minutes

- 1 tablespoon coconut oil
- 1 teaspoon smoked paprika
- ½ teaspoon ground turmeric
- ½ teaspoon garlic powder
- 2 cups arugula, chopped
- 1 cup cherry tomatoes
- 1 tablespoon olive oil
- 6 oz halloumi

1. Slice the halloumi and sprinkle with melted coconut oil.
2. Put the cheese in the Crock Pot in one layer and cook on high for 15 minutes per side.
3. Meanwhile, mix arugula with cherry tomatoes in the salad bowl.
4. Add cooked halloumi, smoked paprika, ground turmeric, garlic powder, and olive oil.
5. Shake the salad gently.
per serving: 210 calories, 9.9g protein, 4.4g carbohydrates, 17.8g fat, 1g fiber, 29mg cholesterol, 430mg sodium, 167mg potassium.

Marinated Jalapeno Rings
Yield: 4 servings | **Prep time:** 40 minutes | **Cook time:** 1 hour
- 1 cup of water
- ¼ cup apple cider vinegar
- 1 teaspoon peppercorns
- 1 garlic clove, crushed
- 3 tablespoons sunflower oil
- 5 oz jalapeno, sliced
1. Put the sliced jalapeno in the plastic vessel (layer by layer).
2. Then put peppercorns in the Crock Pot.
3. Add the garlic clove, sunflower oil, and apple cider vinegar.
4. Close the lid and cook the liquid on High for 1 hour.
5. After this, cool the liquid to the room temperature and pour it over the jalapenos.
6. Close the plastic vessel and leave it in the fridge for 30-40 minutes before serving.
per serving: 109 calories, 0.6g protein, 2.8g carbohydrates, 10.7g fat, 1.2g fiber, 0mg cholesterol, 3mg sodium, 97mg potassium.

Hot Sauce Oysters Mushrooms
Yield: 4 servings | **Prep time:** 15 minutes | **Cook time:** 2 hours
- 2 tablespoons hot sauce
- 2 cups oysters mushrooms, sliced
- ½ cup of water
- 1 tablespoon avocado oil
- 1 teaspoon dried dill
- 1 teaspoon salt
1. Mix sliced oysters with avocado oil, dried dill, and salt.
2. Put them in the Crock Pot.
3. Add water and cook the mushrooms on High for 2 hours.
4. After this, drain the mushrooms and mix them with hot sauce.
per serving: 15 calories, 1.1g protein, 2.2g carbohydrates, 0.6g fat, 0.9g fiber, 0mg cholesterol, 778mg sodium, 149mg potassium.

Buffalo Cremini Mushrooms
Yield: 4 servings | **Prep time:** 10 minutes | **Cook time:** 6 hours
- 3 cups cremini mushrooms, trimmed
- 2 oz buffalo sauce
- ½ cup of water
- 2 tablespoons coconut oil

1. Pour water in the Crock Pot.
2. Melt the coconut oil in the skillet.
3. Add mushrooms and roast them for 3-4 minutes per side. Transfer the roasted mushrooms in the Crock Pot.
4. Cook them on Low for 4 hours.
5. Then add buffalo sauce and carefully mix.
6. Cook the mushrooms for 2 hours on low.
per serving: 79 calories, 1.4g protein, 3.2g carbohydrates, 6.9g fat, 0.8g fiber, 0mg cholesterol, 458mg sodium, 242mg potassium.

Aromatic Marinated Mushrooms
Yield: 4 servings | **Prep time:** 20 minutes | **Cook time:** 5 hours
- 1 teaspoon dried rosemary
- 1 teaspoon dried thyme
- 1 teaspoon onion powder
- 2 cups of water
- 4 cups mushrooms, roughly chopped
- 1 teaspoon salt
- 1 teaspoon sugar
- ½ cup apple cider vinegar
1. Pour water in the Crock Pot.
2. Add all remaining ingredients and carefully mix.
3. Cook the mushrooms on Low for 5 hours.
4. After this, transfer the mushrooms with liquid in the glass cans and cool well.
5. Store the mushrooms in the fridge for up to 4 days.
per serving: 29 calories, 2.3g protein, 4.4g carbohydrates, 0.3g fat, 1g fiber, 0mg cholesterol, 591mg sodium, 256mg potassium.

Mushroom Steaks
Yield: 4 servings | **Prep time:** 10 minutes | **Cook time:** 2 hours
- 4 Portobello mushrooms
- 1 tablespoon avocado oil
- 1 tablespoon lemon juice
- 2 tablespoons coconut cream
- ½ teaspoon ground black pepper
1. Slice Portobello mushrooms into steaks and sprinkle with avocado oil, lemon juice, coconut cream, and ground black pepper.
2. Then arrange the mushroom steaks in the Crock Pot in one layer (you will need to cook all mushroom steaks by 2 times).
3. Cook the meal on High for 1 hour.
per serving: 43 calories, 3.3g protein, 3.9g carbohydrates, 2.3g fat, 1.4g fiber, 0mg cholesterol, 2mg sodium, 339mg potassium.

Herbed Mushrooms
Yield: 4 servings | **Prep time:** 35 minutes | **Cook time:** 4.5 hours
- 1-pound cremini mushrooms
- 1 teaspoon cumin seeds
- 1 teaspoon coriander seeds
- 1 teaspoon fennel seeds
- 2 cups of water
- 3 tablespoons sesame oil
- 1 teaspoon salt

● 3 tablespoons lime juice
1.   Pour water in the Crock Pot. Add mushrooms.
2.   Close the lid and cook them on High for 4.5 hours.
3.   Then drain water and transfer mushrooms in the big bowl.
4.   Sprinkle them with cumin seeds, coriander seeds, fennel seeds, sesame oil, salt, and lime juice.
5.   Carefully mix the mushrooms and leave them to marinate for 30 minutes.

per serving: 125 calories, 3g protein, 5.4g carbohydrates, 10.5g fat, 1g fiber, 0mg cholesterol, 594mg sodium, 531mg potassium.

Paprika Okra

Yield: 4 servings | **Prep time:** 10 minutes | **Cook time:** 40 minutes

● 4 cups okra, sliced
● 1 tablespoon smoked paprika
● 1 teaspoon salt
● 2 tablespoons coconut oil
● 1 cup organic almond milk
1.   Pour almond milk in the Crock Pot.
2.   Add coconut oil, salt, and smoked paprika.
3.   Then add sliced okra and gently mix the ingredients.
4.   Cook the okra on High for 40 minutes. Then cooked okra should be tender but not soft.

per serving: 119 calories, 2.4g protein, 10.4g carbohydrates, 7.8g fat, 3.9g fiber, 0mg cholesterol, 624mg sodium, 340mg potassium.

Okra Curry

Yield: 4 servings | **Prep time:** 10 minutes | **Cook time:** 2.5 hours

● 1 cup potatoes, chopped
● 1 cup okra, chopped
● 1 cup tomatoes, chopped
● 1 teaspoon curry powder
● 1 teaspoon dried dill
● 1 cup coconut cream
● 1 cup of water
1.   Pour water in the Crock Pot.
2.   Add coconut cream, potatoes, tomatoes, curry powder, and dried dill.
3.   Cook the ingredients on High for 2 hours.
4.   Then add okra and carefully mix the meal.
5.   Cook it for 30 minutes on High.

per serving: 184 calories, 3g protein, 13.3g carbohydrates, 14.6g fat, 3.8g fiber, 0mg cholesterol, 18mg sodium, 508mg potassium.

Dessert

Cocoa Cake

Yield: 8 servings | **Prep time:** 10 minutes | **Cook time:** 2 hours

- 1 cup milk
- 1 cup of sugar
- ½ cup of cocoa powder
- 1 teaspoon baking soda
- 1 tablespoon lemon juice
- 1 teaspoon vanilla extract
- 2 cups flour
- 3 tablespoons sunflower oil

1. Line the bottom of the Crock Pot with baking paper.
2. In the food processor mix all ingredients and blend until smooth.
3. Pour the liquid dough in the Crock Pot, flatten the surface of the dough well with the help of the spatula and close the lid.
4. Cook the cake on High for 2 hours.
5. Then cool the pie well ad cut it into servings.

per serving: 283 calories, 5.2g protein, 53.4g carbohydrates, 6.9g fat, 2.5g fiber, 3mg cholesterol, 175mg sodium, 189mg potassium.

Apple Cobbler

Yield: 2 servings | **Prep time:** 10 minutes | **Cook time:** 2 hours

- 1 cup apples, diced
- 1 teaspoon ground cinnamon
- ½ cup flour
- 2 tablespoons coconut oil
- ½ cup cream

1. Mix flour with sugar and coconut oil and knead the dough.
2. Then mix apples with ground cinnamon and place it in the Crock Pot in one layer.
3. Grate the dough over the apples and add cream.
4. Close the lid and cook the cobbler on High for 2 hours.

per serving: 330 calories, 4.1g protein, 42.1g carbohydrates, 17.5g fat, 4.2g fiber, 11mg cholesterol, 21mg sodium, 180mg potassium.

Cinnamon Giant Cookie

Yield: 6 servings | **Prep time:** 15 minutes | **Cook time:** 4 hours

- 5 tablespoons coconut oil
- 1 tablespoon ground ginger
- ½ teaspoon ground cinnamon
- 5 tablespoons sugar
- 1 cup flour
- 1 egg, beaten
- 1 teaspoon baking powder
- ½ cup half and half

1. Put all ingredients in the food processor.
2. Blend the mixture until you get a smooth dough.
3. Then line the bottom of the Crock Pot with baking paper and put the dough inside.
4. Flatten it in the shape of a cookie.
5. Cook the cookie on Low for 4 hours.
6. Then cool the cookie and cut it into servings.

per serving: 252 calories, 3.8g protein, 28g carbohydrates, 14.6g fat, 0.8g fiber, 35mg cholesterol, 20mg sodium, 155mg potassium.

Easy Monkey Rolls

Yield: 8 servings | **Prep time:** 15 minutes | **Cook time:** 3 hours

- 1 tablespoon liquid honey
- 1 tablespoon sugar
- 2 eggs, beaten
- 1-pound cinnamon rolls, dough
- 2 tablespoons butter, melted

1. Cut the cinnamon roll dough on 8 servings.
2. Then line the bottom of the Crock Pot with baking paper and put the rolls inside.
3. In the bowl mix sugar, egg, liquid honey, and butter. Whisk the mixture.
4. Pour the egg mixture over the cinnamon roll dough and flatten well.
5. Close the lid and cook the meal on High for 3 hours.

per serving: 266 calories, 4.9g protein, 32.6g carbohydrates, 13.3g fat, 1.4g fiber, 86mg cholesterol, 253mg sodium, 80mg potassium.

Nuts Brownies

Yield: 6 servings | **Prep time:** 15 minutes | **Cook time:** 2.5 hours

- 3 tablespoons cocoa powder
- 1 tablespoon apple cider vinegar
- 1 teaspoon baking powder
- 3 oz nuts, chopped
- 1 cup flour
- 4 eggs, beaten
- ½ cup skim milk
- ½ cup of sugar

1. Mix cocoa powder with flour and sugar.
2. Add apple cider vinegar, baking powder, and skim milk.
3. Mix the mixture until you get the smooth batter.
4. Then add nuts and carefully mix the batter.
5. Put the baking paper at the bottom of the Crock Pot.
6. Add chocolate batter and close the lid.
7. Cook the brownies on High for 2.5 hours.
8. Then cool the dessert well and cut into bars.

per serving: 279 calories, 9.5g protein, 39.3g carbohydrates, 10.8g fat, 2.7g fiber, 110mg cholesterol, 149mg sodium, 331mg potassium.

Raspberry Muffins

Yield: 6 servings | **Prep time:** 15 minutes | **Cook time:** 5 hours

- 1 teaspoon baking powder
- ¼ cup of sugar
- ½ cup raspberries
- 1 egg, beaten
- ½ cup flour
- 1/3 cup heavy cream
- 2 tablespoon butter, melted

1. Put all ingredients except raspberries in the food processor.
2. Blend the mixture until smooth.
3. Then add raspberries and carefully stir the batter with the help of the spoon.
4. Fill the ½ part of every muffin mold with batter and transfer them in the Crock Pot.
5. Close the lid and cook the muffins on Low 5 hours.

per serving: 143 calories, 2.3g protein, 18.1g carbohydrates, 7.2g fat, 1g fiber, 47mg cholesterol, 41mg sodium, 126mg potassium.

Apricot Spoon Cake
Yield: 10 servings | **Prep time:** 15 minutes | **Cook time:** 2.5 hours

- 2 cups cake mix
- 1 cup milk
- 1 cup apricots, canned, pitted, chopped, with juice
- 2 eggs, beaten
- 1 tablespoon sunflower oil

1. Mix milk with cake mix and egg.
2. Then sunflower oil and blend the mixture until smooth.
3. Then place the baking paper in the Crock Pot.
4. Pour the cake mix batter in the Crock Pot, flatten it gently, and close the lid.
5. Cook the cake on High for 2.5 hours.
6. Then transfer the cooked cake in the plate and top with apricots and apricot juice.
7. Leave the cake until it is warm and cut into servings.

per serving: 268 calories, 4.5g protein, 43.8g carbohydrates, 8.6g fat, 0.8g fiber, 35mg cholesterol, 372mg sodium, 127mg potassium.

Orange Curd
Yield: 6 servings | **Prep time:** 15 minutes | **Cook time:** 7 hours

- 2 cups orange juice
- 1 tablespoon orange zest, grated
- 4 egg yolks
- 1 cup of sugar
- 1 tablespoon cornflour
- 1 teaspoon vanilla extract

1. Whisk the egg yolks with sugar until you get a lemon color mixture.
2. Then add orange juice, vanilla extract, cornflour, and orange zest. Whisk the mixture until smooth.
3. Pour the liquid in the Crock Pot and close the lid.
4. Cook the curd on low for 7 hours. Stir the curd every 1 hour.

per serving: 206 calories, 2.5g protein, 43.6g carbohydrates, 3.2g fat, 0.4g fiber, 140mg cholesterol, 6mg sodium, 185mg potassium.

Pumpkin Balls
Yield: 4 serving | **Prep time:** 15 minutes | **Cook time:** 2 hours

- ½ cup pumpkin puree
- ¼ cup of sugar
- 4 tablespoons flour
- 1 teaspoon olive oil

1. Mix pumpkin puree with sugar.
2. Then add flour and knead the soft dough.
3. Make the balls from the pumpkin mixture.
4. After this, brush the Crock Pot bottom with olive oil.
5. Put the pumpkin balls in the Crock Pot in one layer and close the lid.
6. Cook the pumpkin balls on High for 2 hours.

per serving: 96 calories, 1.2g protein, 20.9g carbohydrates, 1.3g fat, 1.1g fiber, 0mg cholesterol, 2mg sodium, 71mg potassium.

Apples with Raisins
Yield: 4 serving | **Prep time:** 15 minutes | **Cook time:** 5 hours

- 4 big apples
- 4 teaspoons raisins
- 4 teaspoons sugar
- ½ teaspoon ground cinnamon
- ½ cup of water

1. Core the apples and fill them with sugar and raisins.
2. Then arrange the apples in the Crock Pot.
3. Sprinkle them with ground cinnamon.
4. Add water and close the lid.
5. Cook the apples on low for 5 hours.

per serving: 141 calories, 0.7g protein, 37.4g carbohydrates, 0.4g fat, 5.7g fiber, 0mg cholesterol, 3mg sodium, 263mg potassium.

Berry Pudding
Yield: 2 servings | **Prep time:** 10 minutes | **Cook time:** 5 hours

- ¼ cup strawberries, chopped
- 2 tablespoons sugar
- 2 cups of milk
- 1 tablespoon corn starch
- 1 teaspoon vanilla extract

1. Mix milk with corn starch and pour liquid in the Crock Pot.
2. Add vanilla extract, sugar, and strawberries.
3. Close the lid and cook the pudding on low for 5 hours.
4. Carefully mix the dessert before serving.

per serving: 196 calories, 8.1g protein, 30.2g carbohydrates, 5.1g fat, 0.4g fiber, 20mg cholesterol, 115mg sodium, 171mg potassium.

Dump Cake
Yield: 8 servings | **Prep time:** 15 minutes | **Cook time:** 5 hours

- 1 cupcake mix
- 1 teaspoon vanilla extract
- ½ teaspoon ground nutmeg
- 1 tablespoon butter, melted
- 2 eggs, beaten
- 1 teaspoon lemon zest, grated
- ½ cup heavy cream
- 4 pecans, chopped

1. In the bowl mix all ingredients except pecans.

2. The line the Crock Pot with baking paper and pour the dough inside.
3. Flatten the batter and top with pecans.
4. Close the lid and cook the dump cake for 5 hours on Low.
5. Cook the cooked cake well before serving.

per serving: 245 calories, 3.8g protein, 27g carbohydrates, 13.9g fat, 1.1g fiber, 55mg cholesterol, 246mg sodium, 90mg potassium

Classic Apple Pie
Yield: 6 servings | **Prep time:** 15 minutes | **Cook time:** 2 hours

- 1 cup apples, chopped
- 1 cup flour
- 4 eggs, beaten
- 1 cup of sugar
- 1 tablespoon butter, melted
- 1 teaspoon vanilla extract

1. Blend the sugar with eggs until you get a lemon color mixture.
2. Then add flour, butter, vanilla extract, and mix until smooth.
3. Add apples and carefully stir the mixture until homogenous.
4. After this, line the Crock Pot bottom with baking paper and pour the dough inside.
5. Cook the pie on High for 2 hours on High.
6. Cook the cooked pie well.

per serving: 281 calories, 6g protein, 54.7g carbohydrates, 5.1g fat, 1.5g fiber, 114mg cholesterol, 56mg sodium, 103mg potassium.

Chocolate Fudge Cake
Yield: 6 servings | **Prep time:** 20 minutes | **Cook time:** 2 hours

- ¼ cup of sugar
- 1 cup flour
- 1 tablespoon cocoa powder
- 1 teaspoon baking powder
- 2 oz chocolate chips
- 1/3 cup coconut milk
- 1 tablespoon coconut oil, softened

1. Mix flour with sugar, cocoa powder, baking powder, and coconut milk.
2. Stir the mixture until smooth and place in the Crock Pot. (use the baking paper to avoid burning).
3. Then Cook the mixture on high for 2 hours.
4. Meanwhile, mix coconut oil and coconut chips and melt them in the microwave oven.
5. When the fudge is cooked, pour the chocolate chips mixture over it and leave to cool for 10-15 minutes as a minimum.
6. Cut the cake into servings.

per serving: 211 calories, 3.3g protein, 31.5g carbohydrates, 8.6g fat, 1.5g fiber, 2mg cholesterol, 11mg sodium, 199mg potassium.

Walnut Pudding
Yield: 4 servings | **Prep time:** 10 minutes | **Cook time:** 1.5 hours

- 3 cups of milk
- 2 oz walnuts, grinded
- 1 teaspoon vanilla extract
- 1 tablespoon butter
- 2 tablespoon cornstarch
- 1 tablespoon sugar

1. Mix milk with cornstarch and sugar and pour in the Crock Pot.
2. Add vanilla extract and butter.
3. Then add walnuts and close the lid.
4. Cook the pudding on High for 1 hour.
5. Then carefully mix it and cook it for 30 minutes on high more.

per serving: 234 calories, 9.5g protein, 17.2g carbohydrates, 15g fat, 1g fiber, 23mg cholesterol, 107mg sodium, 182mg potassium.

Red Muffins
Yield: 8 servings | **Prep time:** 15 minutes | **Cook time:** 2 hours

- 5 oz carrot, grated
- 2 eggs, beaten
- 3 tablespoons coconut oil, softened
- 2 tablespoons cream cheese
- 1 cup flour
- ¼ cup skim milk
- ¼ cup of sugar
- 1 teaspoon baking powder

1. In the bowl mix eggs, coconut oil, cream cheese, flour, skim milk, sugar, and baking powder.
2. Carefully stir the mixture until you get a smooth batter.
3. Then add carrot and stir the mixture with the help of the spoon.
4. Pour the batter in the muffin molds (fill ½ part of every mold) and place it in the Crock Pot.
5. Cook the muffins on high for 2 hours.

per serving: 159 calories, 3.6g protein, 20.8g carbohydrates, 7.2g fat, 0.9g fiber, 44mg cholesterol, 40mg sodium, 167mg potassium.

Lemon Apple Slices
Yield: 2 servings | **Prep time:** 10 minutes | **Cook time:** 3 hours

- 2 apples, sliced
- 2 tablespoons lemon juice
- 1 tablespoon maple syrup
- 2 tablespoons butter

1. Sprinkle the apples with lemon juice and put them in the Crock Pot.
2. Add butter and maple syrup.
3. Close the lid and cook the apples on low for 3 hours.

per serving: 248 calories, 0.8g protein, 37.8g carbohydrates, 12.1g fat, 5.5g fiber, 31mg cholesterol, 88mg sodium, 281mg potassium.

Mint Lava Cake
Yield: 6 servings | **Prep time:** 15 minutes | **Cook time:** 1 hour

- 1 cup fudge cake mix
- 1 teaspoon dried mint
- 4 tablespoons sunflower oil
- 2 eggs, beaten

1. Mix cake mix with dried mint, sunflower oil, and eggs.
2. When the mixture is smooth, pour it in the ramekins and place in the Crock Pot.
3. Cook the lava cakes on High for 1 hour.

per serving: 291 calories, 4.4g protein, 32g carbohydrates, 17.6g fat, 1.1g fiber, 55mg cholesterol, 381mg sodium, 165mg potassium.

Caramel Pie

Yield: 6 servings | **Prep time:** 15 minutes | **Cook time:** 2 hours

- 1 cup vanilla cake mix
- 4 eggs, beaten
- 1 teaspoon butter, melted
- 4 caramels, candy, crushed

1. Mix vanilla cake mix with eggs and butter.
2. Pour the liquid in the Crock Pot and sprinkle with crushed candies.
3. Close the lid and cook the pie on high for 2 hours.
4. Then cool it and remove from the Crock Pot.
5. Cut the pie into 6 servings.

per serving: 173 calories, 4g protein, 30.1g carbohydrates, 4.1g fat, 0.7g fiber, 111mg cholesterol, 355mg sodium, 54mg potassium.

Blueberry Tapioca Pudding

Yield: 4 servings | **Prep time:** 10 minutes | **Cook time:** 3 hours

- 4 teaspoons blueberry jam
- 4 tablespoons tapioca
- 2 cups of milk

1. Mix tapioca with milk and pour it in the Crock Pot.
2. Close the lid and cook the liquid on low for 3 hours.
3. Then put the blueberry jam in 4 ramekins.
4. Cool the cooked tapioca pudding until warm and pour over the jam.

per serving: 112 calories, 4.1g protein, 18.8g carbohydrates, 2.5g fat, 0.1g fiber, 10mg cholesterol, 58mg sodium, 71mg potassium.

Cottage Cheese Dip

Yield: 4 servings | **Prep time:** 10 minutes | **Cook time:** 4 hours

- 4 bananas, mashed
- 1 cup cottage cheese
- 1 tablespoon butter
- 1 egg, beaten
- ¼ cup milk

1. Put the bananas in the blender.
2. Add cottage cheese, butter, egg, and milk.
3. Blend the mixture until smooth and pour it in the Crock Pot.
4. Close the lid and cook it on Low for 4 hours.

per serving: 205 calories, 11g protein, 29.8g carbohydrates, 5.8g fat, 3.1g fiber, 54mg cholesterol, 274mg sodium, 501mg potassium.

Soft Thin Pie

Yield: 6 servings | **Prep time:** 15 minutes | **Cook time:** 2 hours

- 1 cup coconut flour
- ½ cup coconut flakes
- 3 eggs, beaten
- ¼ cup of sugar
- 1 teaspoon vanilla extract
- ¼ cup of coconut oil
- ½ teaspoon baking powder

1. In the bowl mix coconut flour, coconut flakes, eggs, sugar, vanilla extract, and baking powder.
2. Add coconut oil and stir the mixture until homogenous.
3. Then line the Crock Pot bowl with baking paper and put the dough inside.
4. Flatten it and close the lid.
5. Cook the pie on High for 2 hours.
6. Then cool it well and cut into serving bars.

per serving: 247 calories, 5.7g protein, 23.1g carbohydrates, 15.5g fat, 8.6g fiber, 82mg cholesterol, 33mg sodium, 97mg potassium.

Orange Cake

Yield: 12 servings | **Prep time:** 20 minutes | **Cook time:** 2 hours

- 2 cups of orange juice
- ½ cup poppy seeds
- ½ cup olive oil
- 2 cups semolina
- ½ cup of sugar

1. Mix orange juice with poppy seeds, olive oil, sugar, and semolina.
2. Then pour the liquid in the Crock Pot.
3. Cook it on High for 2 hours.
4. When the cooking time is finished, let the cake to cool to the room temperature, remove it from the Crock Pot and cut into servings.

per serving: 252 calories, 4.8g protein, 34.2g carbohydrates, 11.3g fat, 1.7g fiber, 0mg cholesterol, 2mg sodium, 174mg potassium.

Pavlova

Yield: 6 servings | **Prep time:** 15 minutes | **Cook time:** 3 hours

- 5 egg whites
- 1 cup of sugar powder
- 1 teaspoon lemon juice
- 1 teaspoon vanilla extract
- ½ cup whipped cream

1. Mix egg whites with sugar powder, lemon juice, and vanilla extract and whisk until you get firm peaks.
2. Then line the Crock Pot with baking paper and put the egg white mixture inside.
3. Flatten it and cook for 3 hours on low.
4. When the egg white mixture is cooked, transfer it in the serving plate and top with whipped cream.

per serving: 124 calories, 3.2g protein, 20.5g carbohydrates, 3.2g fat, 0g fiber, 11mg cholesterol, 32mg sodium, 57mg potassium.

Peach Bread Pudding

Yield: 6 servings | **Prep time:** 10 minutes | **Cook time:** 6 hours

- 5 oz white bread, chopped
- 2 eggs, beaten
- 1 cup heavy cream
- ½ cup peaches, chopped
- 1 teaspoon flour
- 1 teaspoon coconut oil
- 2 tablespoons sugar
1. Grease the Crock Pot bottom with coconut oil.
2. Then add white bread.
3. Mix heavy cream with eggs, flour, sugar, and pour over the bread.
4. Then add peaches and close the lid.
5. Cook the pudding on Low for 6 hours.

per serving: 181 calories, 4.2g protein, 18.1g carbohydrates, 10.4g fat, 0.8g fiber, 82mg cholesterol, 189mg sodium, 82mg potassium.

Almond Bars
Yield: 6 servings | **Prep time:** 15 minutes | **Cook time:** 2 hours

- 1 tablespoon cocoa powder
- ½ cup flour
- ½ cup coconut flour
- 4 tablespoons coconut oil
- 1 teaspoon baking powder
- 2 oz almonds, chopped
- ¼ cup of sugar
- 2 eggs, beaten
1. Mix all ingredients in the bowl and knead the smooth dough.
2. The put the dough in the Crock Pot, flatten it, and cut into bars.
3. Close the lid and cook the dessert on High for 2 hours.

per serving: 266 calories, 6.4g protein, 26g carbohydrates, 16.5g fat, 5.8g fiber, 55mg cholesterol, 22mg sodium, 206mg potassium.

Caramel
Yield: 10 servings | **Prep time:** 10 minutes | **Cook time:** 7 hours

- 1 cup of sugar
- 1 cup heavy cream
- 2 tablespoons butter
1. Put sugar in the Crock Pot.
2. Add heavy cream and butter.
3. Close the lid and cook the caramel on Low for 7 hours.
4. Carefully mix the cooked caramel and transfer it in the glass cans.

per serving: 137 calories, 0.3g protein, 20.3g carbohydrates, 6.7g fat, 0g fiber, 23mg cholesterol, 21mg sodium, 10mg potassium.

Granola Apples
Yield: 6 servings | **Prep time:** 10 minutes | **Cook time:** 2.5 hours

- 6 apples, cored
- 6 teaspoons granola
- 3 teaspoons maple syrup
- ½ cup of water
1. Mix maple syrup with granola.

2. Fill the apples with granola mixture and transfer in the Crock Pot.
3. Add water and close the lid.
4. Cook the apples on High for 2.5 hours.

per serving: 131 calories, 1.4g protein, 35.7g carbohydrates, 1.6g fat, 5.9g fiber, 0mg cholesterol, 4mg sodium, 273mg potassium.

Pineapple Upside Down Cake
Yield: 8 servings | **Prep time:** 15 minutes | **Cook time:** 2.5 hours

- ½ cup milk
- 3 tablespoons butter, melted
- 4 eggs, beaten
- 1/3 cup sugar
- 1 teaspoon vanilla extract
- 1 ½ cup flour
- 5 oz pineapple, sliced
- 1 teaspoon baking powder
1. In the bowl mix milk, butter, eggs, vanilla extract, sugar, and flour.
2. Then add baking powder and mix the mixture until you get a smooth batter.
3. After this, line the Crock Pot with baking paper.
4. Put the sliced pineapples in the Crock Pot in one layer.
5. Pour the batter over the pineapples and close the lid.
6. Cook the cake on High for 2.5 hours.

per serving: 205 calories, 5.8g protein, 29.8g carbohydrates, 7.1g fat, 0.9g fiber, 95mg cholesterol, 70mg sodium, 148mg potassium.

Pear Crumble
Yield: 2 servings | **Prep time:** 10 minutes | **Cook time:** 3 hours

- 4 tablespoons oatmeal
- 1 pear, chopped
- 2 tablespoons sugar
- 1 tablespoon coconut oil
- ½ teaspoon ground cardamom
- 1 tablespoon dried apricots, chopped
- ¼ cup of coconut milk
1. Mix oatmeal with chopped pear, sugar, coconut oil, ground cardamom, dried apricots, and coconut milk.
2. Then put the mixture in the Crock Pot and close the lid.
3. Cook the crumble on Low for 3 hours.

per serving: 255 calories, 2.4g protein, 32g carbohydrates, 14.8g fat, 4.1g fiber, 0mg cholesterol, 6mg sodium, 215mg potassium.

Coffee Pie
Yield: 6 servings | **Prep time:** 15 minutes | **Cook time:** 2.5 hours

- ½ cup brewed coffee
- 1 cup flour
- 2 tablespoons coconut flakes
- 1 egg, beaten
- 1 teaspoon baking powder
- 1 tablespoon apple cider vinegar
- ¼ cup sour cream

- 3 tablespoons sugar
- Cooking spray

1. Spray the Crock Pot bottom with cooking spray.
2. Then put all ingredients in the food processor and blend until homogenous.
3. Transfer the dough mixture in the Crock Pot and flatten it well.
4. Close the lid and cook the pie on High for 2.5 hours.
5. Then cook the pie well and remove it from the Crock Pot.
6. Cut the pie into servings.

per serving: 137 calories, 3.5g protein, 23g carbohydrates, 3.5g fat, 0.7g fiber, 31mg cholesterol, 17mg sodium, 147mg potassium.

Blondie Pie
Yield: 6 servings | **Prep time:** 15 minutes | **Cook time:** 2.5 hours

- 1 teaspoon vanilla extract
- 1 cup cream
- 1 cup flour
- 1 egg, beaten
- ¼ cup of sugar
- 1 teaspoon baking powder
- 2 oz chocolate chips
- 1 tablespoon coconut oil, softened

1. Mix vanilla extract, cream, flour, and egg.
2. Then add sugar, baking powder, and coconut oil.
3. When the mixture is smooth, add chocolate chips and mix them with the help of the spatula.
4. Then pour the mixture in the Crock Pot and close the lid.
5. Cook the pie on High for 2.5 hours.

per serving: 216 calories, 4.1g protein, 31.6g carbohydrates, 8.2g fat, 0.9g fiber, 37mg cholesterol, 32mg sodium, 167mg potassium.

Raspberry Biscuits
Yield: 8 servings | **Prep time:** 15 minutes | **Cook time:** 6.5 hours

- 4 eggs, beaten
- 1 cup of sugar
- 1 cup flour
- 1 teaspoon ground cinnamon
- 1 tablespoon coconut flakes
- 1 cup raspberries
- Cooking spray

1. Blend the eggs with sugar until you get a smooth and fluffy mixture.
2. Add flour, ground cinnamon, and coconut flakes. Mix the mixture until smooth.
3. Spray the Crock Pot with cooking spray and pour the dough inside.
4. Then sprinkle the dough with raspberries and close the lid.
5. Cook the meal on Low for 6.5 hours.
6. After this, remove the cooked dessert from the Crock Pot and cut into servings.

per serving: 193 calories, 4.6g protein, 39.3g carbohydrates, 2.7g fat, 1.6g fiber, 82mg cholesterol, 31mg sodium, 73mg potassium.

Lemon Bars
Yield: 4 servings | **Prep time:** 15 minutes | **Cook time:** 2 hours

- 4 tablespoons sugar
- 4 tablespoons butter
- 1 cup flour
- 2 tablespoons lemon curd
- 1 teaspoon baking powder
- 1 teaspoon vanilla extract

1. Mix sugar with butter, flour, baking powder, and vanilla extract.
2. When you get smooth and non-sticky dough, put it in the Crock Pot and flatten in the shape of the layer.
3. Close the lid and cook the dough on High for 2 hours.
4. Then remove the cooked dough from the Crock Pot and spread with lemon curd.
5. When the meal is cool, cut it into bars.

per serving: 295 calories, 3.9g protein, 38.6g carbohydrates, 14.8g fat, 0.9g fiber, 56mg cholesterol, 109mg sodium, 165mg potassium.

Cinnamon Butter
Yield: 6 servings | **Prep time:** 25 minutes | **Cook time:** 6 hours

- 2 cups apples, chopped
- ½ cup butter
- 1 teaspoon ground cinnamon
- 2 tablespoons sugar

1. Mix sugar with apples and put in the Crock Pot.
2. Leave the apples for 5-10 minutes or until they start to give the juice. Add ground cinnamon.
3. Then add butter and close the lid.
4. Cook the cinnamon butter on Low for 6 hours.
5. Then blend it with the help of the blender and transfer in the ramekins. Cool it.

per serving: 190 calories, 0.4g protein, 14.6g carbohydrates, 15.5g fat, 2g fiber, 41mg cholesterol, 110mg sodium, 86mg potassium.

Peanut Sweets
Yield: 8 servings | **Prep time:** 60 minutes | **Cook time:** 4 hours

- 1 cup peanuts, roasted, chopped
- 1 cup of chocolate chips
- ¼ cup heavy cream

1. Put chocolate chips and heavy cream in the Crock Pot.
2. Cook the mixture on low for 4 hours.
3. Then mix the mixture until smooth and add roasted peanuts.
4. Carefully mix the mixture again.
5. Line the baking tray with baking paper.
6. With the help of the spoon, make the medium size balls (sweets) and put on the baking paper.
7. Cool the sweets until they are solid.

per serving: 229 calories, 6.4g protein, 15.5g carbohydrates, 16.6g fat, 2.3g fiber, 10mg cholesterol, 21mg sodium, 210mg potassium.

Bounty

Yield: 6 servings | **Prep time:** 25 minutes | **Cook time:** 20 minutes

- 2 tablespoons condensed milk
- 1 tablespoon coconut oil
- 1 cup coconut shred
- 3 oz milk chocolate
- 2 tablespoons heavy cream

1. Mix heavy cream with milk chocolate and put it in the Crock Pot.
2. Cook the mixture on High for 20 minutes or until it is melted.
3. Meanwhile, mix condensed milk with coconut oil and coconut shred.
4. Make the small sweets and freeze them for 15 minutes.
5. Then sprinkle every coconut sweet with melted chocolate mixture.

per serving: 240 calories, 3g protein, 22.7g carbohydrates, 15.6g fat, 1.8g fiber, 12mg cholesterol, 21mg sodium, 80mg potassium.

Melon Pudding

Yield: 3 servings | **Prep time:** 10 minutes | **Cook time:** 3 hours

- 1 cup melon, chopped
- ¼ cup of coconut milk
- 2 tablespoons cornstarch
- 1 teaspoon vanilla extract

1. Blend the melon until smooth and mix with coconut milk, cornstarch, and vanilla extract.
2. Transfer the mixture in the Crock Pot and cook the pudding on low for 3 hours.

per serving: 88 calories, 0.9g protein, 10.4g carbohydrates, 4.9g fat, 1g fiber, 0mg cholesterol, 12mg sodium, 194mg potassium.

Stuffed Peaches

Yield: 4 servings | **Prep time:** 15 minutes | **Cook time:** 20 minutes

- 4 peaches, halved, pitted
- 4 pecans
- 1 tablespoon maple syrup
- 2 oz goat cheese, crumbled

1. Fill every peach half with pecan and sprinkle with maple syrup.
2. Then put the fruits in the Crock Pot in one layer and top with goat cheese.
3. Close the lid and cook the peaches for 20 minutes on High.

per serving: 234 calories, 7.2g protein, 19.7g carbohydrates, 15.5g fat, 3.8g fiber, 15mg cholesterol, 49mg sodium, 360mg potassium.

Milk Fondue

Yield: 3 servings | **Prep time:** 10 minutes | **Cook time:** 4 hours

- 5 oz milk chocolate, chopped
- 1 tablespoon butter

- 1 teaspoon vanilla extract
- ¼ cup milk

1. Put the chocolate in the Crock Pot in one layer.
2. Then top it with butter, vanilla extract, and milk.
3. Close the lid and cook the dessert on Low for 4 hours.
4. Gently stir the cooked fondue and transfer in the ramekins.

per serving: 301 calories, 4.3g protein, 29.3g carbohydrates, 18.3g fat, 1.6g fiber, 23mg cholesterol, 74mg sodium, 191mg potassium.

Sponge Cake

Yield: 6 servings | **Prep time:** 15 minutes | **Cook time:** 7 hours

- 2 egg yolks
- 4 egg whites
- 1 cup of sugar
- ½ cup flour
- 1 teaspoon vanilla extract
- Cooking spray

1. Spray the Crock Pot with cooking spray from inside.
2. Then whisk the egg whites until you get soft peaks.
3. After this, mix egg yolks with sugar and blend until smooth.
4. Add flour and vanilla extract.
5. Then add egg whites and carefully mix the mixture until homogenous.
6. Pour it in the Crock Pot and close the lid.
7. Cook the sponge cake on Low for 7 hours.

per serving: 194 calories, 4.4g protein, 41.7g carbohydrates, 1.6g fat, 0.3g fiber, 70mg cholesterol, 25mg sodium, 54mg potassium.

Semolina Pie

Yield: 4 servings | **Prep time:** 10 minutes | **Cook time:** 2 hours

- ½ cup cottage cheese
- 1 teaspoon vanilla extract
- 1 teaspoon corn starch
- 1 tablespoon flour
- ½ cup semolina
- 2 tablespoons butter, melted

1. Mix semolina with cottage cheese and vanilla extract.
2. Then add corn starch, flour, and butter.
3. Blend the mixture with the help of the blender until smooth and put in the Crock Pot. Flatten it.
4. Close the lid and cook the semolina pie for 2 hours on High.

per serving: 165 calories, 6.8g protein, 18.6g carbohydrates, 6.6g fat, 0.9g fiber, 18mg cholesterol, 156mg sodium, 71mg potassium.

Classic Banana Foster

Yield: 3 servings | **Prep time:** 10 minutes | **Cook time:** 3 hours

- 3 bananas, peeled chopped
- 2 tablespoons sugar

- 2 tablespoons butter, melted
- 1 teaspoon vanilla extract
- 1 tablespoon rum
- 3 ice cream balls
1. Put the bananas in the Crock Pot in one layer.
2. Then sprinkle them with sugar, butter, vanilla extract, and rum.
3. Close the lid and cook on Low for 3 hours.
4. Transfer the cooked bananas in the ramekins and top with ice cream balls.

per serving: 378 calories, 3.4g protein, 57.1g carbohydrates, 16.1g fat, 3.1g fiber, 40mg cholesterol, 106mg sodium, 532mg potassium.

Crème Brule
Yield: 4 servings | **Prep time:** 15 minutes | **Cook time:** 8 hours

- 6 egg yolks
- 1 ½ cup heavy cream
- ½ cup of sugar
- 1 teaspoon flour
1. Blend the egg yolks with sugar until you get a smooth lemon color mixture.
2. Add heavy cream and flour. Mix the liquid until smooth.
3. Pour the liquid in the ramekins and place in the Crock Pot.
4. Cover the ramekins with foil and close the lid of the Crock Pot.
5. Cook the dessert on Low for 8 hours.

per serving: 332 calories, 5g protein, 27.7g carbohydrates, 23.4g fat, 0g fiber, 376mg cholesterol, 29mg sodium, 62mg potassium.

Caramelized Bananas
Yield: 6 servings | **Prep time:** 10 minutes | **Cook time:** 2 hours 15 minutes

- 6 bananas, peeled
- 2 tablespoons butter
- 3 tablespoons caramel
1. Put butter in the Crock Pot.
2. Add bananas and cook them on High for 15 minutes.
3. Then add caramel and cook the dessert on Low for 2 hours.
4. Carefully mix the cooked dessert and transfer it into the plates.

per serving: 159 calories, 1.6g protein, 29.3g carbohydrates, 5.3g fat, 3.1g fiber, 10mg cholesterol, 28mg sodium, 424mg potassium.

Plum Pie
Yield: 6 servings | **Prep time:** 10 minutes | **Cook time:** 2 hours

- 1 cup flour
- ¼ cup butter, melted
- 2 eggs, beaten
- ¼ cup of sugar
- 1 teaspoon ground nutmeg
- ½ cup plums, pitted, chopped
1. Put flour, eggs, butter, and sugar in the food processor.
2. Blend the mixture until smooth.
3. Add ground nutmeg and stir it.

4. Then transfer the mixture in the Crock Pot and top with plums.
5. Close the lid and cook the pie on High for 2 hours.

per serving: 200 calories, 4.1g protein, 25.2g carbohydrates, 9.5g fat, 0.7g fiber, 75mg cholesterol, 76mg sodium, 54mg potassium.

Cherry Jam
Yield: 4 servings | **Prep time:** 10 minutes | **Cook time:** 3 hours

- 2 cups cherries, pitted
- ½ cup of sugar
- 1 tablespoon agar
- 3 tablespoons water
1. Mix sugar with cherries and put in the Crock Pot.
2. Then mix water and agar and pour the liquid in the Crock Pot too.
3. Stir well and close the lid.
4. Cook the jam on high for 3 hours.
5. Then transfer the jam in the glass cans and store it in the fridge for up to 2 months.

per serving: 139 calories, 0.5g protein, 36.1g carbohydrates, 0g fat, 1.5g fiber, 0mg cholesterol, 0mg sodium, 3mg potassium.

Raisin Bake
Yield: 4 servings | **Prep time:** 15 minutes | **Cook time:** 6 hours

- 1 cup cottage cheese
- 2 oz raisins, chopped
- 1 egg, beaten
- 3 tablespoons sugar, powdered
- 1 teaspoon vanilla extract
- 1 teaspoon peanuts, chopped
1. The Crock Pot with baking paper.
2. Then mix all ingredients in the bowl and mix until smooth.
3. Transfer the mixture in the Crock Pot and flatten the surface of it well.
4. Close the lid and cook the bake on Low for 6 hours.

per serving: 150 calories, 9.8g protein, 22.6g carbohydrates, 2.6g fat, 0.6g fiber, 45mg cholesterol, 247mg sodium, 182mg potassium.

Cheese Cake
Yield: 8 servings | **Prep time:** 10 minutes | **Cook time:** 8 hours

- 6 oz cookies, crushed
- 2 tablespoon butter, softened
- 2 cups cream cheese
- 1 teaspoon vanilla extract
- 3 eggs, beaten
- ¼ cup of sugar
- 1 cup of water
1. Mix cookies with butter and transfer the mixture in the cheesecake mold.
2. Flatten the cookies mixture in the shape of the pie crust.
3. Then blend sugar with eggs, vanilla extract, and cream cheese.

4.   Pour the cream cheese mixture over the pie crust.
5.   Then pour water in the Crock Pot and insert the mold with cheesecake inside.
6.   Close the lid and cook the dessert on Low for 8 hours.
 per serving: 357 calories, 7.4g protein, 25.8g carbohydrates, 25.3g fat, 0.3g fiber, 133mg cholesterol, 273mg sodium, 101mg potassium.

Pumpkin Spices Hot Chocolate
Yield: 4 servings | **Prep time:** 10 minutes | **Cook time:** 2 hours
- 3 cups of milk
- ½ cup of chocolate chips
- 1 teaspoon pumpkin spices
1.   Put all ingredients in the Crock Pot.
2.   Close the lid and cook the hot chocolate on high for 2 hours.
3.   Then stir the cooked dessert well and pour it into glasses.
 per serving: 205 calories, 7.6g protein, 21.8g carbohydrates, 10g fat, 0.8g fiber, 20mg cholesterol, 103mg sodium, 186mg potassium.

Sautéed Figs
Yield: 2 servings | **Prep time:** 10 minutes | **Cook time:** 5 hours
- 4 figs, chopped
- 1 oz peanuts, chopped
- 1 teaspoon butter
- ¼ cup milk
- 1 teaspoon ground cinnamon
1.   Put all ingredients in the Crock Pot and close the lid.
2.   Cook the figs on Low for 5 hours.
 per serving: 210 calories, 6g protein, 29g carbohydrates, 9.9g fat, 5.5g fiber, 8mg cholesterol, 34mg sodium, 381mg potassium.

Sweet Baked Milk
Yield: 5 servings | **Prep time:** 10 minutes | **Cook time:** 10 hours
- 4 cups of milk
- 3 tablespoons sugar
- ½ teaspoon vanilla extract
1.   Mix milk with sugar and vanilla extract and stir until sugar is dissolved.
2.   Then pour the liquid in the Crock Pot and close the lid.
3.   Cook the milk on Low for 10 hours.
 per serving: 126 calories, 6.4g protein, 16.9g carbohydrates, 4g fat, 3g fiber, 16mg cholesterol, 92mg sodium, 113mg potassium.

Cardamom Plums
Yield: 6 servings | **Prep time:** 10 minutes | **Cook time:** 5 hours
- 4 cups plums, pitted, halved
- 1 teaspoon ground cardamom
- ¼ cup of sugar
- 1 teaspoon lemon juice
- 1 cup of water

1.   Put plums in the Crock Pot and sprinkle them with ground cardamom, sugar, and lemon juice.
2.   Add water and close the lid.
3.   Cook the plums on Low for 5 hours.
4.   Carefully stir the cooked dessert and transfer in the serving ramekins.
 per serving: 52 calories, 0.4g protein, 13.9g carbohydrates, 0.2g fat, 0.7g fiber, 0mg cholesterol, 1mg sodium, 74mg potassium.

Chocolate Whipped Cream
Yield: 4 servings | **Prep time:** 15 minutes | **Cook time:** 2 hours
- ½ cup of chocolate chips
- 1 cup heavy cream
- 1 tablespoon sugar
- 1 teaspoon vanilla extract
- ½ teaspoon lime zest, sliced
1.   Mix chocolate chips with vanilla extract and put it in the Crock Pot.
2.   Close the lid and cook them on Low for 2 hours.
3.   Meanwhile, whip the heavy cream and mix it with sugar.
4.   Transfer the whipped cream in the serving ramekins.
5.   Then sprinkle it with melted chocolate chips.
6.   Top every serving with lime zest.
 per serving: 230 calories, 2.2g protein, 16.5g carbohydrates, 17.3g fat, 6.4g fiber, 46mg cholesterol, 28mg sodium, 103mg potassium.

Coconut Soufflé
Yield: 4 servings | **Prep time:** 15 minutes | **Cook time:** 6 hours
- 4 egg yolks
- 1 cup of sugar
- 2 cups of coconut milk
- 1 tablespoon cornstarch
- 1 tablespoon butter, softened
1.   Mix coconut milk with cornstarch and pour in the ramekins.
2.   Add sugar and butter in every ramekin and cover with foil.
3.   Pierce the foil and transfer the ramekins in the Crock Pot.
4.   Cook the soufflé on low for 6 hours.
 per serving: 550 calories, 5.5g protein, 59.1g carbohydrates, 36g fat, 2.7g fiber, 217mg cholesterol, 47mg sodium, 335mg potassium.

Jelly Bears
Yield: 4 servings | **Prep time:** 45 minutes | **Cook time:** 1 hour
- 1 cup of orange juice
- ¼ cup of water
- 3 tablespoons gelatin
1.   Pour orange juice in the Crock Pot and cook it on High for 1 hour.
2.   Meanwhile, mix water with gelatin and leave for 10-15 minutes.
3.   When the orange juice is cooked, cool it for 10-15 minutes and add gelatin mixture.
4.   Mix the liquid until smooth.

5. Then pour it in the jelly molds (in the shape of bears) and refrigerate for as minimum 40 minutes.
per serving: 46 calories, 4.9g protein, 6.5g carbohydrates, 0.1g fat, 0.1g fiber, 0mg cholesterol, 11mg sodium, 125mg potassium.

Chocolate Mango
Yield: 6 servings | **Prep time:** 10 minutes | **Cook time:** 4 hours
- 1-pound mango, puree
- 2 oz milk chocolate, chopped
- 1 cup coconut cream
1. Mix mango with coconut cream.
2. Then transfer the mixture in the ramekins.
3. Top every ramekin with chocolate and cover with foil.
4. Place the ramekins in the Crock Pot and close the lid.
5. Cook the meal on Low for 4 hours.
per serving: 188 calories, 2.3g protein, 19.2g carbohydrates, 12.6g fat, 2.4g fiber, 2mg cholesterol, 14mg sodium, 267mg potassium.

Matcha Shake
Yield: 4 servings | **Prep time:** 15 minutes | **Cook time:** 40 minutes
- 1 teaspoon matcha green tea
- 2 cups of coconut milk
- 2 bananas, mashed
- ¼ cup agave nectar
1. Mix agave nectar with coconut milk and matcha green tea. Mix the mixture until smooth and pour it in the Crock Pot.
2. Cook the mixture on high for 40 minutes.
3. Then transfer the mixture in the blender, add mashed bananas and blend the liquid until smooth.
4. Pour the cooked shake in the glasses and cool to room temperature.
per serving: 359 calories, 3.4g protein, 28.3g carbohydrates, 28.8g fat, 4.7g fiber, 0mg cholesterol, 19mg sodium, 527mg potassium.

Strawberry Marmalade
Yield: 8 servings | **Prep time:** 15 minutes | **Cook time:** 4 hours
- 2 cups strawberries, chopped
- 1 cup of sugar
- ¼ cup lemon juice
- 2 oz water
1. Put all ingredients in the Crock Pot and gently mix.
2. Then close the lid and cook the mixture on low for 4 hours.
3. Transfer the cooked mixture in the silicone molds and leave to cool for up to 8 hours.
per serving: 107 calories, 0.3g protein, 27.9g carbohydrates, 0.2g fat, 0.8g fiber, 0mg cholesterol, 2mg sodium, 65mg potassium.

Ginger Lemons
Yield: 6 servings | **Prep time:** 10 minutes | **Cook time:** 1.5 hours
- 4 lemons, sliced
- 1 teaspoon ground ginger
- ½ cup of water
- ½ cup of sugar
1. Mix the lemon with sugar and ginger and put it in the Crock Pot.
2. Add water and close the lid.
3. Cook the lemons on High for 1.5 hours.
4. Then transfer the hot lemons and all liquid in the glass cans and close the lid.
5. Store the dessert for up to 1 month in the fridge.
per serving: 75 calories, 0.5g protein, 20.5g carbohydrates, 0.1g fat, 1.1g fiber, 0mg cholesterol, 1mg sodium, 58mg potassium.

Vanilla and Cocoa Pudding
Yield: 2 servings | **Prep time:** 10 minutes | **Cook time:** 7 hours
- 1 cup of coconut milk
- 1 tablespoon cornflour
- 1 teaspoon vanilla extract
- 1 tablespoon brown sugar
- 1 tablespoon butter
- 2 tablespoons cocoa powder
1. Mix coconut milk with cocoa powder, brown sugar, vanilla extract, and cornflour.
2. Whisk the mixture until smooth and transfer in the Crock Pot.
3. Add butter and close the lid.
4. Cook the pudding on Low for 7 hours.
5. Then transfer it in the serving bowls and cool to the room temperature.
per serving: 375 calories, 4.1g protein, 17.1g carbohydrates, 35.2g fat, 4.5g fiber, 15mg cholesterol, 62mg sodium, 473mg potassium.

Fig Bars
Yield: 6 servings | **Prep time:** 15 minutes | **Cook time:** 2.5 hours
- 1 cup coconut flour
- ¼ cup of coconut oil
- 1 egg, beaten
- 1 teaspoon baking powder
- 5 oz figs, diced
- 1 teaspoon liquid honey
1. Mix coconut flour and coconut oil and egg.
2. Add baking powder and knead the soft dough.
3. Then line the Crock Pot bottom with baking paper.
4. Put the dough inside and flatten it in the shape of the pie crust.
5. After this, mix liquid honey with diced figs and transfer them on the dough. Flatten it well.
6. Close the lid and cook the fig bars on High for 2.5 hours.
per serving: 232 calories, 4.4g protein, 29.8g carbohydrates, 12g fat, 10.3g fiber, 27mg cholesterol, 13mg sodium, 255mg potassium.

Mascarpone with Strawberry Jelly
Yield: 6 servings | **Prep time:** 120 minutes | **Cook time:** 1 hour
- 2 cups strawberries, chopped
- 1 tablespoon gelatin

- 3 tablespoons sugar
- ¼ cup of water
- 1 cup mascarpone
1. Mix strawberries with sugar and blend the mixture until smooth.
2. Transfer it in the Crock Pot and cook on High for 1 hour.
3. Meanwhile, mix water with gelatin.
4. Whisk the mascarpone well.
5. When the strawberry mixture is cooked, cool it little and add gelatin. Carefully mix it.
6. Pour the strawberry mixture in the ramekins and refrigerate for 2 hours.
7. Then top the jelly with whisked mascarpone.
per serving: 125 calories, 9g protein, 11g carbohydrates, 5.5g fat, 1g fiber, 21mg cholesterol, 45mg sodium, 118mg potassium.

Coconut and Lemon Pie
Yield: 6 servings | **Prep time:** 10 minutes | **Cook time:** 4.5 hours
- 1 teaspoon baking powder
- 1 lemon, sliced
- 1 cup coconut flour
- 1 cup all-purpose flour
- 1 teaspoon vanilla extract
- 4 tablespoons sugar
- 1 cup skim milk
- 2 tablespoons coconut shred
- Cooking spray
1. Spray the Crock Pot with cooking spray from inside.
2. Then mix skim milk with sugar, vanilla extract, all types of flour, and baking powder.
3. When you get a homogenous mixture, pour it in the Crock Pot.
4. Then sprinkle the dough with sliced lemon and shredded coconut.
5. Close the lid and cook the pie on High for 4.5 hours.
per serving: 223 calories, 6.3g protein, 41.3g carbohydrates, 3.9g fat, 9.2g fiber, 1mg cholesterol, 24mg sodium, 184mg potassium.

Braised Pears
Yield: 6 servings | **Prep time:** 10 minutes | **Cook time:** 2.5 hours
- 6 pears
- 2 cups wine
- 1 tablespoon sugar
- 1 cinnamon stick
1. Cut the pears into halves and put them in the Crock Pot.
2. Add all remaining ingredients and close the lid.
3. Cook the pears on High for 2.5 hours.
4. Serve the pears with hot wine mixture.
per serving: 210 calories, 1.1g protein, 38g carbohydrates, 1.1g fat, 6.5g fiber, 0mg cholesterol, 29mg sodium, 320mg potassium.

Honey Pumpkin Cubes
Yield: 6 servings | **Prep time:** 10 minutes | **Cook time:** 6 hours
- 3 cups pumpkin, cubed

- 2 tablespoons of liquid honey
- ¼ cup of water
- 1 tablespoon brown sugar
- 1 teaspoon ground cinnamon
- 1 teaspoon ground cardamom
1. Put all ingredients in the Crock Pot and gently mix with the help of the spoon.
2. Close the lid and cook the dessert on Low for 6 hours.
per serving: 71 calories, 1.4g protein, 17.7g carbohydrates, 0.4g fat, 3.9g fiber, 0mg cholesterol, 7mg sodium, 263mg potassium.

Sweet Zucchini Pie
Yield: 6 servings | **Prep time:** 15 minutes | **Cook time:** 4 hours
- 2 cups zucchini, chopped
- ½ cup of sugar
- 2 cups all-purpose flour
- 1 teaspoon baking powder
- 4 eggs, beaten
- 1 tablespoon butter, melted
- 1 cup milk
- 1 teaspoon vanilla extract
1. Mix sugar with flour, baking powder, eggs, butter, milk, and vanilla extract.
2. Stir the mixture until smooth.
3. Then line the Crock Pot with baking paper and pour the smooth dough inside.
4. Top the dough with zucchini and close the lid.
5. Cook the pie on High for 4 hours.
per serving: 302 calories, 9.8g protein, 52.4g carbohydrates, 6.2g fat, 1.6g fiber, 118mg cholesterol, 79mg sodium, 291mg potassium.

Thick Pear Puree
Yield: 6 servings | **Prep time:** 10 minutes | **Cook time:** 2.5 hours
- 3 cups pears, chopped
- 3 tablespoons lemon juice
- 1 tablespoon sugar
- 1 teaspoon vanilla extract
- 1 tablespoon corn starch
- ¼ cup of water
1. Mix pears with lemon juice, sugar, vanilla extract, and water, and transfer in the Crock Pot.
2. Close the lid and cook the mixture on High for 2 hours.
3. Then blend it with the help of the immersion blender.
4. Add cornflour and stir until smooth.
5. Close the lid and cook the puree on High for 30 minutes.
6. Transfer the cooked dessert in the ramekins and cool to room temperature.
per serving: 64 calories, 0.4g protein, 16g carbohydrates, 0.2g fat, 2.5g fiber, 0mg cholesterol, 3mg sodium, 104mg potassium.

Cardamom Apple Jam
Yield: 4 servings | **Prep time:** 15 minutes | **Cook time:** 2.5 hours
- 1 cup apples, chopped
- 1 teaspoon ground cardamom

● 2 tablespoons brown sugar
● 1 teaspoon agar
1.   Mix apples with brown sugar and transfer in the Crock Pot.
2.   Leave the apples until they get the juice.
3.   Then add ground cardamom and agar. Mix the mixture.
4.   Close the lid and cook the jam on High for 2.5 hours.
5.   Then blend the mixture until smooth and cool to room temperature.
 per serving: 48 calories, 0.2g protein, 12.5g carbohydrates, 0.1g fat, 1.5g fiber, 0mg cholesterol, 2mg sodium, 72mg potassium.

Cinnamon Plum Jam
Yield: 6 servings | **Prep time:** 10 minutes | **Cook time:** 6 hours
● 4 cups plums, pitted, halved
● 1 tablespoon ground cinnamon
● ½ cup brown sugar
● 1 teaspoon vanilla extract
1.   Put all ingredients in the Crock Pot and gently mix.
2.   Close the lid and cook it on Low for 6 hours.
 per serving: 71 calories, 0.4g protein, 18.2g carbohydrates, 0.1g fat, 1.2g fiber, 0mg cholesterol, 4mg sodium, 91mg potassium.

Tarragon Peach Confiture
Yield: 6 servings | **Prep time:** 10 minutes | **Cook time:** 2.5 hours
● 1-pound peaches, pitted, halved
● ½ cup of sugar
● 1 teaspoon lemon zest, grated
● 1 teaspoon dried tarragon
● 1/3 cup water
1.   Put all ingredients in the Crock Pot and close the lid.
2.   Cook the dessert on high for 2.5 hours.
3.   Cool the cooked confiture well.
 per serving: 73 calories, 0.3g protein, 19.1g carbohydrates, 0.1g fat, 0.4g fiber, 0mg cholesterol, 0mg sodium, 52mg potassium.

Summer Fruits Compote
Yield: 6 servings | **Prep time:** 10 minutes | **Cook time:** 3 hours
● 1 cup apricots, pitted, chopped
● ½ cup cherries, pitted
● 1 cup strawberries
● ¼ cup blackberries
● ½ cup of sugar
● 8 cups of water
1.   Put all ingredients in the Crock Pot.
2.   Cook compote on High for 3 hours.
3.   Cool it and serve with ice cubes.
per serving: 93 calories, 0.7g protein, 23.9g carbohydrates, 0.3g fat, 1.4g fiber, 0mg cholesterol, 11mg sodium, 117mg potassium.

Rhubarb Jam
Yield: 6 servings | **Prep time:** 10 minutes | **Cook time:** 8 hours

● 2-pounds rhubarb, chopped
● 1 cup of sugar
● 1 teaspoon lime zest, grated
● ¼ cup of water
1.   Put all ingredients in the Crock Pot.
2.   Cook the jam on Low for 8 hours.
3.   Then transfer it in the glass jars and cool well.
 per serving: 157 calories, 1.4g protein, 40.2g carbohydrates, 0.3g fat, 2.8g fiber, 0mg cholesterol, 6mg sodium, 436mg potassium.

Lemon Zest Pudding
Yield: 2 servings | **Prep time:** 10 minutes | **Cook time:** 6 hours
● 1 teaspoon lemon zest, grated
● 2 cups of milk
● 1 tablespoon corn starch
● ¼ cup of sugar
● 1 teaspoon vanilla extract
1.   Put all ingredients in the Crock Pot and stir with the help of the hand whisker until corn starch is dissolved.
2.   Close the lid and cook the pudding on Low for 6 hours.
3.   The pudding is cooked, when it is thick.
 per serving: 240 calories, 8g protein, 42g carbohydrates, 5g fat, 0.1g fiber, 20mg cholesterol, 115mg sodium, 146mg potassium.

Berry Porridge with Syrup
Yield: 2 servings | **Prep time:** 10 minutes | **Cook time:** 1 hour
● 2 tablespoons agave syrup
● 1 cup raspberries
● 1 cup blackberries
● 1 cup strawberries
● ½ cup of water
● 1 tablespoon coconut shred
1.   Chop the strawberries roughly and put in the Crock Pot.
2.   Add raspberries and blackberries.
3.   Then add water and close the lid.
4.   Cook the mixture on High for 1 hour.
5.   Then transfer the berry mixture (porridge) in the serving bowls and top with coconut shred with agave syrup.
 per serving: 166 calories, 2.4g protein, 37.2g carbohydrates, 2.6g fat, 9.6g fiber, 0mg cholesterol, 19mg sodium, 333mg potassium.

Vegan Mousse
Yield: 3 servings | **Prep time:** 15 minutes | **Cook time:** 2 hours
● 1 cup of coconut milk
● 2 tablespoons corn starch
● 1 teaspoon vanilla extract
● 1 avocado, pitted, pilled
1.   Mix coconut milk and corn starch until smooth and pour in the Crock Pot.
2.   Add vanilla extract and cook it on High for 2 hours.
3.   Then cool the mixture till room temperature and mix with avocado.
4.   Blend the mousse until fluffy and smooth.

per serving: 348 calories, 3.1g protein, 16.4g carbohydrates, 32.1g fat, 6.3g fiber, 0mg cholesterol, 16mg sodium, 537mg potassium.

Sautéed Figs
Yield: 6 servings | **Prep time:** 10 minutes | **Cook time:** 2 hours

- 6 fresh figs
- 2 tablespoons butter
- 2 tablespoons maple syrup
- 1 tablespoon raisins
- 1 cup of water

1. Put butter and figs in the Crock Pot.
2. Add raisins and water.
3. Close the lid and cook the meal on High for 2 hours.
4. Then transfer the cooked figs in the plates and sprinkle with maple syrup.

per serving: 103 calories, 0.7g protein, 17.8g carbohydrates, 4g fat, 1.9g fiber, 10mg cholesterol, 31mg sodium, 156mg potassium.

Espresso Mousse Drink
Yield: 1 serving | **Prep time:** 10 minutes | **Cook time:** 1 hour

- ½ cup milk
- 1 teaspoon instant coffee
- ¼ cup of water

1. Mix instant coffee with water.
2. Then pour milk in the Crock Pot and cook it on High for 1 hour.
3. Meanwhile, blend the coffee mixture with the help of the hand blender until you get fluffy foam.
4. Transfer the blended mixture into the glass.
5. Add hot milk.

per serving: 61 calories, 4g protein, 6g carbohydrates, 2.5g fat, 0g fiber, 10mg cholesterol, 59mg sodium, 73mg potassium.

Glazed Carrot with Whipped Cream
Yield: 6 servings | **Prep time:** 10 minutes | **Cook time:** 2.5 hours

- 1 cup whipped cream
- 3 cups baby carrot
- 4 tablespoons maple syrup
- 1 teaspoon ground cinnamon
- 1 tablespoon lemon juice
- 1 teaspoon lime zest, grated
- ½ cup of water

1. Mix carrot with ground cinnamon, lemon juice, lime zest, and water.
2. Add maple syrup and transfer the mixture in the Crock Pot.
3. Cook the carrots on High for 2.5 hours.
4. Then cool the carrots and transfer them in the bowls.
5. Top the dessert with whipped cream.

per serving: 120 calories, 0.9g protein, 5.8g carbohydrates, 6.3g fat, 2.3g fiber, 22mg cholesterol, 64mg sodium, 220mg potassium.

Apricot Marmelade
Yield: 6 servings | **Prep time:** 15 minutes | **Cook time:** 2 hours

- 1 cup apricots, pitted, chopped
- 1 cup of sugar
- 1 teaspoon vanilla extract
- 1 tablespoon agar

1. Put all ingredients in the Crock Pot and close the lid.
2. Cook the mixture on High for 2 hours.
3. Then blend the mixture until smooth with the help of the immersion blender and pour in the silicone molds.
4. Cool the marmalade until solid.

per serving: 139 calories, 0.3g protein, 36.3g carbohydrates, 0.2g fat, 0.5g fiber, 0mg cholesterol, 0mg sodium, 68mg potassium.

Fluffy Vegan Cream
Yield: 6 servings | **Prep time:** 15 minutes | **Cook time:** 1.5 hours

- 1 cup coconut cream
- 1 avocado, pitted, peeled, chopped
- ½ cup of soy milk
- 1 tablespoon corn starch

1. Pour soy milk in the Crock Pot.
2. Add corn starch and stir until smooth.
3. Then close the lid and cook the liquid on high for 1.5 hours.
4. Meanwhile, whip the coconut cream and blend the avocado.
5. Mix the blended avocado with thick soy milk mixture and then carefully mix it with whipped coconut cream.

per serving: 363 calories, 4.2g protein, 14.5g carbohydrates, 33.7g fat, 2.8g fiber, 0mg cholesterol, 13mg sodium, 206mg potassium.

Prune Bake
Yield: 4 servings | **Prep time:** 15 minutes | **Cook time:** 3 hours

- 2 cups of cottage cheese
- 5 eggs, beaten
- 1 cup prunes, chopped
- 4 teaspoons butter

1. Mix cottage cheese with eggs and blend the mixture until smooth and fluffy.
2. Then put the butter into 4 ramekins.
3. Mix cottage cheese mixture with prunes and transfer in the ramekins with butter.
4. Transfer the ramekins in the Crock Pot and close the lid.
5. Cook the meal on High for 3 hours.

per serving: 316 calories, 23.4g protein, 31.7g carbohydrates, 11.6g fat, 3g fiber, 224mg cholesterol, 564mg sodium, 494mg potassium.

Sweet Pasta Bake
Yield: 6 servings | **Prep time:** 15 minutes | **Cook time:** 7 hours

- 5 oz macaroni, cooked
- 1 cup cottage cheese
- 5 eggs, beaten
- 3 tablespoon sugar
- 1 teaspoon vanilla extract
- Cooking spray

1. Mix cottage cheese with macaroni.

2. Add cottage cheese, sugar, and vanilla extract.
3. After this, spray the Crock Pot bottom with cooking spray and put the cottage mixture inside.
4. Flatten the surface of the mixture and close the lid.
5. Cook the meal on Low for 7 hours.

per serving: 198 calories, 12.9g protein, 25.4g carbohydrates, 4.7g fat, 0.8g fiber, 139mg cholesterol, 206mg sodium, 139mg potassium.

Cottage Cheese Ramekins
Yield: 4 servings | **Prep time:** 10 minutes | **Cook time:** 3 hours

- 4 teaspoons semolina
- 2 oz raisins, chopped
- 1 teaspoon vanilla extract
- 2 cups of cottage cheese
- 2 tablespoons butter, melted

1. Mix semolina with cottage cheese, vanilla extract, butter, and raisins.
2. Transfer the mixture into ramekins and place the ramekins in the Crock Pot.
3. Close the lid and cook the meal on High for 3 hours.

per serving: 211 calories, 16.5g protein, 18g carbohydrates, 8.1g fat, 0.7g fiber, 24mg cholesterol, 501mg sodium, 224mg potassium.

Ricotta Bake with Dates and Nuts
Yield: 3 servings | **Prep time:** 10 minutes | **Cook time:** 2.5 hours

- 2 oz nuts, chopped
- 2 dates, chopped
- 1 cup ricotta cheese
- 2 tablespoons of liquid honey
- 1 egg, beaten

1. Mix ricotta cheese with buts and eggs and transfer in the ramekins.
2. Put the ramekins in the Crock Pot and close the lid.
3. Cook the dessert on High for 2.5 hours.
4. Then top the ramekins with dates and liquid honey.

per serving: 305 calories, 14.7g protein, 24.8g carbohydrates, 17.7g fat, 2.2g fiber, 80mg cholesterol, 251mg sodium, 279mg potassium.

Avocado Jelly
Yield: 2 servings | **Prep time:** 15 minutes | **Cook time:** 1.5 hours

- 1 avocado, pitted, chopped
- 1 cup of orange juice
- 1 tablespoon gelatin
- 3 tablespoons brown sugar

1. Pour orange juice in the Crock Pot.
2. Add brown sugar and cook the liquid on High for 1.5 hours.
3. Then add gelatin and stir the mixture until smooth.
4. After this, blend the avocado until smooth, add orange juice liquid and mix until homogenous.
5. Pour it in the cups and refrigerate until solid.

per serving: 324 calories, 5.8g protein, 34.8g carbohydrates, 19.9g fat, 7g fiber, 0mg cholesterol, 18mg sodium, 754mg potassium.

Jelly Cake
Yield: 6 servings | **Prep time:** 20 minutes | **Cook time:** 2 hours

- 1 cup cream
- 1 cup apple juice
- 2 tablespoons gelatin
- ½ cup of sugar

1. Pour apple juice in the Crock Pot and cook it on High for 1 hour.
2. Then pour the liquid in the bowl, add 1 tablespoon of gelatin and stir until homogenous.
3. Pour the liquid in the ice molds and freeze until solid.
4. Meanwhile, pour the cream in the Crock Pot.
5. Add sugar and cook the liquid on High for 1 hour.
6. After this, add gelatin, stir the liquid until smooth and cool to the room temperature.
7. Then pour the liquid in the big bowl.
8. Add frozen apple jelly and refrigerate the cake until smooth.

per serving: 123 calories, 4.4g protein, 22.6g carbohydrates, 2.3g fat, 0.1g fiber, 8mg cholesterol, 24mg sodium, 57mg potassium.

Baked Camembert
Yield: 6 servings | **Prep time:** 15 minutes | **Cook time:** 1.5 hours

- 1-pound camembert
- 1 oz walnuts, chopped
- 2 tablespoons of liquid honey

1. Line the Crock Pot with baking paper.
2. Then put the camembert in the bottom of the Crock Pot and close the lid.
3. Cook the meal on High for 1.5 hours.
4. Then make the circle in the camembert with the help of the knife.
5. Sprinkle the cooked cheese with liquid honey and walnuts.

per serving: 277 calories, 16.1g protein, 6.6g carbohydrates, 21.1g fat, 0.3g fiber, 54mg cholesterol, 637mg sodium, 170mg potassium.

Honey Pasta Casserole
Yield: 6 servings | **Prep time:** 20 minutes | **Cook time:** 3 hours

- 8 oz pasta, cooked, chopped
- 3 tablespoons of liquid honey
- ½ cup plain yogurt
- 2 tablespoons ricotta cheese
- 2 eggs, beaten
- 1 teaspoon vanilla extract
- 1 tablespoon butter, melted

1. Mix pasta with eggs, yogurt, and vanilla extract.
2. Add ricotta cheese and stir it little.
3. Then pour butter in the Crock Pot.
4. Add pasta mixture and flatten it.
5. Close the lid and cook the casserole on High for 3 hours.

6.   Then cut the casserole into servings and top with honey.

per serving: 202 calories, 7.9g protein, 31.3g carbohydrates, 4.9g fat, 0g fiber, 31.3mg cholesterol, 65mg sodium, 149mg potassium.

Milky Custard
Yield: 6 servings | **Prep time:** 10 minutes | **Cook time:** 7 hours

● 3 cups of milk
● 3 tablespoons corn starch
● 1 teaspoon ground cardamom
● 1 cup of sugar

1.   Mix sugar with ground cardamom and corn starch.
2.   Add milk and whisk the mixture until smooth.
3.   After this, pour the liquid in the Crock Pot and cook it on Low for 7 hours. Stir the mixture every 1 hour.
4.   Then cool the cooked custard well and transfer in the ramekins.

per serving: 205 calories, 4g protein, 44.1g carbohydrates, 2.5g fat, 0.1g fiber, 10mg cholesterol, 58mg sodium, 74mg potassium.

Custard Tiramisu
Yield: 6 servings | **Prep time:** 15 minutes | **Cook time:** 1.5 hours

● 1 cup custard
● 5 oz savoiardi
● 1 cup of water
● 2 tablespoons instant coffee
● 1 tablespoon rum
● 2 tablespoons cocoa powder

1.   Pour water in the Crock Pot and cook it on high for 1.5 hours.
2.   Then add instant coffee and rub and stir the liquid until smooth and homogenous.
3.   Cool it.
4.   After this, dip savoiardi in the coffee mixture.
5.   Place ½ part of all savoiardi on the glass mold in one layer.
6.   Top it with ½ cup od custard.
7.   Then add remaining savoiardi and top them with custard.
8.   Sprinkle the dessert with cocoa powder.

per serving: 135 calories, 3.3g protein, 22.7g carbohydrates, 3.2g fat, 1.2g fiber, 6mg cholesterol, 46mg sodium, 67mg potassium.

Panna Cotta
Yield: 2 servings | **Prep time:** 15 minutes | **Cook time:** 1.5 hours

● 1 tablespoon gelatin
● 1 cup cream
● ¼ cup of sugar
● 2 tablespoons strawberry jam

1.   Pour cream in the Crock Pot.
2.   Add sugar and close the lid.
3.   Cook the liquid on High for 1.5 hours.
4.   Then cool it to the room temperature, add gelatin, and mix until smooth.

5.   Pour the liquid in the glasses and refrigerate until solid.
6.   Top every cream jelly with jam.

per serving: 270 calories, 7g protein, 47.4g carbohydrates, 6.7g fat, 0g fiber, 23mg cholesterol, 53mg sodium, 45mg potassium.

Sweet Corn Ramekins
Yield: 2 servings | **Prep time:** 10 minutes | **Cook time:** 5 hours

● 1 cup sweet corn kernels
● ½ cup coconut cream
● 2 tablespoons condensed milk
● 1 teaspoon butter, softened

1.   Mix corn kernels with coconut cream and condensed milk.
2.   Then grease the ramekins with softened butter.
3.   Put the corn kernels mixture in the ramekins.
4.   Transfer them in the Crock Pot and close the lid.
5.   Cook the meal on Low for 5 hours.

per serving: 283 calories, 5.1g protein, 29.1g carbohydrates, 18.6g fat, 2.9g fiber, 12mg cholesterol, 291mg sodium, 340mg potassium.

Flax Seeds Bars
Yield: 8 servings | **Prep time:** 15 minutes | **Cook time:** 4 hours

● 1 cup flax seeds
● 1 cup of chocolate chips
● ¼ cup cream
● 3 oz nuts, chopped
● 1 tablespoon coconut oil

1.   Line the Crock Pot bottom with baking paper.
2.   Then put all ingredients inside and close the lid.
3.   Cook the mixture on low for 4 hours.
4.   Then open the lid and make the mixture homogenous.
5.   Transfer it in the silicone mold and flatten well.
6.   Refrigerate it until solid and crush into bars.

per serving: 269 calories, 6.1g protein, 19.4g carbohydrates, 18.2g fat, 5.5g fiber, 6mg cholesterol, 94mg sodium, 258mg potassium.

Mint Summer Drink
Yield: 6 servings | **Prep time:** 10 minutes | **Cook time:** 3 hours

● 1 cup fresh mint, chopped
● 7 cups of water
● 1 orange, sliced
● 1 lemon, sliced
● 1 cup agave syrup
● 1 cup strawberries

1.   Put all ingredients in the Crock Pot.
2.   Close the lid and cook the drink on High for 3 hours.
3.   Then refrigerate the drink until cool.

per serving: 200 calories, 1.1g protein, 51.8g carbohydrates, 0.3g fat, 2.5g fiber, 0mg cholesterol, 51mg sodium, 211mg potassium.

Orange and Apricot Jam
Yield: 4 servings | **Prep time:** 15 minutes | **Cook time:** 3 hours

- 2 oranges, peeled, chopped
- 1 cup apricots, chopped
- 1 tablespoon orange zest, grated
- 4 tablespoons sugar
1. Put all ingredients in the bowl and blend them until smooth with the help of the immersion blender.
2. Then pour the mixture in the Crock Pot and cook it on High for 3 hours.
3. Transfer the hot jam in the glass cans and close with a lid.
4. Cool the jam well.
per serving: 108 calories, 1.4g protein, 27.4g carbohydrates, 0.4g fat, 3.1g fiber, 0mg cholesterol, 1mg sodium, 270mg potassium.

Passion Fruit Mousse
Yield: 6 servings | **Prep time:** 15 minutes | **Cook time:** 1.5 hours
- 1 cup milk
- 3 tablespoons corn starch
- 5 oz passion fruit, puree
- 3 tablespoons sugar
- 1 teaspoon vanilla extract
1. Mix milk with sugar, vanilla extract, and corn starch.
2. Then pour the liquid in the Crock Pot and cook it on High for 1.5 hours.
3. Cool the liquid well and transfer in the serving glasses.
4. Top every glass with passion fruit puree.
per serving: 85 calories, 1.9g protein, 18.1g carbohydrates, 1g fat, 2.5g fiber, 3mg cholesterol, 26mg sodium, 107mg potassium.

Coconut and Mango Mousse
Yield: 3 servings | **Prep time:** 15 minutes | **Cook time:** 7 hours
- 1 cup coconut cream
- 3 egg yolks
- 3 tablespoons sugar
- 1 teaspoon vanilla extract
- 1 mango, peeled, chopped, pureed
1. Mix egg yolks with sugar and blend until smooth.
2. Pour the liquid in the Crock Pot, add coconut cream, and stir carefully.
3. Close the lid and cook it on Low for 7 hours.
4. After this, stir the mixture well and pour in the glasses.
5. Add mango puree.
per serving: 354 calories, 5.5g protein, 34g carbohydrates, 24g fat, 3.6g fiber, 210mg cholesterol, 21mg sodium, 419mg potassium.

Sweet Milk Souffle
Yield: 4 servings | **Prep time:** 10 minutes | **Cook time:** 10 hours
- 2 cups of milk
- 1 cup condensed milk
- 5 eggs, beaten
1. Mix eggs with milk and pour the mixture in the Crock Pot.
2. Add condensed milk.
3. Carefully mix the mixture and close the lid.

4. Cook the soufflé on Low for 10 hours.
per serving: 385 calories, 17g protein, 48g carbohydrates, 14.6g fat, 0g fiber, 241mg cholesterol, 232mg sodium, 428mg potassium.

Banana Chia Seeds Pudding
Yield: 2 servings | **Prep time:** 15 minutes | **Cook time:** 5 hours
- 1 cup milk
- 4 tablespoons chia seeds
- 2 bananas, chopped
1. Mix milk with chia seeds and pour in the Crock Pot.
2. Cook the liquid on Low for 5 hours.
3. Meanwhile, put the chopped bananas in the bottom of glass jars.
4. When the pudding is cooked, pour it over the bananas.
per serving: 304 calories, 10g protein, 44.9g carbohydrates, 11.6g fat, 12.8g fiber, 10mg cholesterol, 63mg sodium, 608mg potassium.

Oatmeal Soufflé
Yield: 3 servings | **Prep time:** 10 minutes | **Cook time:** 2.5 hours
- 6 oz oatmeal
- 1 egg yolk
- 3 tablespoons sugar
- 1 cup milk
- 1 tablespoon butter
1. Whisk egg yolk with sugar until you get a lemon color mixture.
2. Then add milk and pour the liquid in the Crock Pot.
3. Add butter and oatmeal.
4. Cook the soufflé on High for 2.5 hours.
per serving: 352 calories, 11.1g protein, 54.6g carbohydrates, 10.7g fat, 5.7g fiber, 87mg cholesterol, 72mg sodium, 259mg potassium.

Sweet Chai Latte
Yield: 4 servings | **Prep time:** 10 minutes | **Cook time:** 4 hours
- 2 tablespoons black tea
- 2 tablespoons chai latte spices
- 2 cups of water
- 1 cup milk
- 4 teaspoons sugar
1. Put black tea in the Crock Pot.
2. Add water, milk, and sugar.
3. Close the lid and cook the mixture on High for 2 hours.
4. Then sieve the liquid and return in the Crock Pot.
5. Add spices and carefully mix them.
6. Cook the drink on Low for 2 hours.
per serving: 68 calories, 2.3g protein, 11g carbohydrates, 1.6g fat, 0g fiber, 5mg cholesterol, 38mg sodium, 39mg potassium.

Sliced Apples Pie
Yield: 6 servings | **Prep time:** 20 minutes | **Cook time:** 4 hours
- 1 cup flour

- ¼ cup butter, softened
- 2 tablespoons sugar
- 1 tablespoon lemon juice
- 3 apples, sliced
- 1 egg, beaten
- 1 teaspoon baking powder

1.   Mix flour with butter, egg, and baking powder. Knead the soft dough.
2.   Then line the Crock Pot bottom with baking paper and put the butter inside. Flatten it in the shape of the pie crust.
3.   Then top the pie crust with sliced apples.
4.   Sprinkle the apples with lemon juice and sugar.
5.   Close the lid and cook the pie on High for 4 hours.

per serving: 229 calories, 3.5g protein, 35.8g carbohydrates, 8.8g fat, 3.3g fiber, 48mg cholesterol, 67mg sodium, 241mg potassium.

Coconut Shaped Cake

Yield: 6 servings | **Prep time:** 120 minutes | **Cook time:** 1.5 hours

- 1 cup cream
- 4 tablespoons coconut shred
- ¼ cup condensed milk
- 2 tablespoons gelatin
- 2 tablespoons agar

1.   Pour cream in the Crock Pot. Add agar and mix it until smooth.
2.   Close the lid and cook it on high for 1.5 hours.
3.   When the time is finished, pour ½ part of all cream in the silicone mold and freeze it until solid.
4.   Then mix condensed milk with gelatin and microwave for 2 minutes.
5.   Carefully mix and cool the mixture.
6.   Pour it over the frozen cream and return in the freezer for 25 minutes.
7.   Pour the remaining cream over the condensed milk.
8.   Add coconut shred.
9.   Refrigerate the cake until solid.

per serving: 108 calories, 3.3g protein, 9.6g carbohydrates, 6.7g fat, 0.7g fiber, 12mg cholesterol, 36mg sodium, 66mg potassium.

Cardamom Rice Porridge

Yield: 2 servings | **Prep time:** 10 minutes | **Cook time:** 4 hours

- ¼ cup basmati rice
- 1 cup milk
- ½ cup of water
- 1 teaspoon butter
- 1 teaspoon ground cardamom

1.   Put all ingredients in the Crock Pot.
2.   Close the lid and cook the dessert on high for 4 hours.
3.   Cool the cooked meal and add sugar if desired.

per serving: 165 calories, 5.8g protein, 25.2g carbohydrates, 4.6g fat, 0.6g fiber, 15mg cholesterol, 74mg sodium, 109mg potassium.

Sweet Tabbouleh

Yield: 6 servings | **Prep time:** 15 minutes | **Cook time:** 2.5 hours

- 1 cup bulgur
- 2 cups of water
- 1 orange, peeled, chopped
- 3 dates, chopped
- 1 tablespoon coconut shred
- 2 tablespoons of liquid honey
- 1 tablespoon raisins

1.   Mix bulgur and water and transfer in the Crock Pot.
2.   Cook it on High for 2.5 hours.
3.   Then cool the bulgur and transfer in the mixing bowl.
4.   Add all remaining ingredients and carefully mix.

per serving: 140 calories, 3.3g protein, 31.7g carbohydrates, 1.2g fat, 5.6g fiber, 0mg cholesterol, 7mg sodium, 194mg potassium.

Lentil Pudding

Yield: 4 servings | **Prep time:** 10 minutes | **Cook time:** 6 hours

- ½ cup green lentils
- 3 cups of milk
- 2 tablespoons of liquid honey
- 1 teaspoon vanilla extract
- 1 teaspoon cornflour

1.   Put all ingredients in the Crock Pot and carefully mix.
2.   Close the lid and cook the pudding on Low for 6 hours.
3.   Cool the pudding to the room temperature and transfer in the serving bowls.

per serving: 213 calories, 12.3g protein, 32.7g carbohydrates, 4g fat, 7.4g fiber, 15mg cholesterol, 88mg sodium, 343mg potassium.

Amaranth Bars

Yield: 7 servings | **Prep time:** 40 minutes | **Cook time:** 1 hour

- ½ cup amaranth
- 4 oz peanuts, chopped
- ¼ cup of coconut oil
- 3 oz milk chocolate, chopped

1.   Put all ingredients in the Crock Pot and cook on High for 1 hour.
2.   Then transfer the melted amaranth mixture in the silicone mold, flatten it, and refrigerate until solid.
3.   Cut the dessert into bars.

per serving: 276 calories, 7.1g protein, 19.1g carbohydrates, 20.3g fat, 3.1g fiber, 3mg cholesterol, 15mg sodium, 210mg potassium.

Baked Goat Cheese Balls

Yield: 6 servings | **Prep time:** 15 minutes | **Cook time:** 1 hour

- 8 oz goat cheese
- 4 tablespoons sesame seeds
- 1 teaspoon of sugar powder
- 1 teaspoon butter
- 1 tablespoon breadcrumbs

1.   Mix goat cheese with sugar powder and breadcrumbs.
2.   Make the medium size balls and coat them in the sesame seeds.

3.   Melt the butter and pour it in the Crock Pot.
4.   Put the balls in the Crock Pot in one layer and close the lid.
5.   Cook the dessert on high for 1 hour.
per serving: 217 calories, 12.8g protein, 3.5g carbohydrates, 17.1g fat, 0.8g fiber, 41mg cholesterol, 144mg sodium, 49mg potassium.

Cinnamon Rice Milk Cocktail
Yield: 6 servings | **Prep time:** 15 minutes | **Cook time:** 1.5 hours
● 1 cup long-grain rice
● ½ cup agave syrup
● 3 cups of water
● 1 teaspoon ground cinnamon
● 1 banana, chopped
1.   Put rice in the food processor.
2.   Add water and blend the mixture until smooth.
3.   Then sieve the liquid and transfer it in the Crock Pot.
4.   Add agave syrup and ground cinnamon. Cook the liquid on High for 1.5 hours.
5.   After this, transfer the hot liquid in the food processor.
6.   Add banana and blend until smooth.
per serving: 215 calories, 2.4g protein, 51.5g carbohydrates, 0.3g fat, 1.1g fiber, 0mg cholesterol, 24mg sodium, 125mg potassium.

Banana Ice Cream
Yield: 2 servings | **Prep time:** 30 minutes | **Cook time:** 5 hours
● ½ cup cream
● 4 tablespoons sugar
● 4 bananas, chopped
● 2 egg yolks
1.   Mix sugar with egg yolks and blend until you get a lemon color mixture.
2.   After this, mix the cream with egg yolks and transfer in the Crock Pot.
3.   Cook the mixture on low for 5 hours. Stir the liquid from time to time.
4.   After this, mix the cream mixture with bananas and blend until smooth.
5.   Place the mixture in the plastic vessel and refrigerate until solid.
per serving: 392 calories, 5.8g protein, 80.4g carbohydrates, 8.6g fat, 6.1g fiber, 221mg cholesterol, 30mg sodium, 885mg potassium.

Caramel Apple Tart
Yield: 4 servings | **Prep time:** 15 minutes | **Cook time:** 3.5 hours
● 2 tablespoons salted caramel
● 2 apples, sliced
● 1 teaspoon butter
● 5 oz puff pastry
● 1 teaspoon olive oil
1.   Sprinkle the Crock Pot bowl with olive oil from inside.
2.   Then put the puff pastry inside and flatten it in the shape of the pie crust.
3.   Grease the pie crust with butter and top with sliced apples.

4.   Then sprinkle the apples with salted caramel and close the lid.
5.   Cook the apple tart on High for 3.5 hours.
per serving: 291 calories, 3.1g protein, 35.3g carbohydrates, 16.2g fat, 3.2g fiber, 3mg cholesterol, 108mg sodium, 152mg potassium.

Clove Pastry Wheels
Yield: 4 servings | **Prep time:** 25 minutes | **Cook time:** 3 hours
● 1 teaspoon ground clove
● 4 oz puff pastry
● 1 tablespoon brown sugar
● 1 tablespoon butter, softened
1.   Roll up the puff pastry into a square.
2.   Then grease the puff pastry with butter and sprinkle with ground clove.
3.   Roll it in the shape of a log and cut it into pieces (wheels).
4.   Put the baking paper at the bottom of the Crock Pot.
5.   Then put puff pastry wheels inside in one layer and close the lid.
6.   Cook the meal on High for 3 hours.
per serving: 192 calories, 2.1g protein, 15.3g carbohydrates, 13.8g fat, 0.6g fiber, 8mg cholesterol, 93mg sodium, 27mg potassium.

Orange Muffins
Yield: 4 servings | **Prep time:** 15 minutes | **Cook time:** 3 hours
● 1 egg, beaten
● 1 teaspoon orange zest, grated
● 1 tablespoon butter, melted
● ½ cup of orange juice
● 1 cup flour
● 1 teaspoon baking powder
1.   Mix egg with orange juice and butter.
2.   Then add baking powder and flour. Stir it until you get the smooth butter.
3.   Add orange zest and stir the batter with the help of the spoon.
4.   Transfer the batter in the muffin molds, filling ½ part of every mold.
5.   Then place them in the Crock Pot and close the lid.
6.   Cook the muffins on high for 3 hours.
per serving: 171 calories, 4.9g protein, 27.9g carbohydrates, 4.4g fat, 1g fiber, 49mg cholesterol, 38mg sodium, 238mg potassium.

Tender Bacon Cookies
Yield: 5 servings | **Prep time:** 30 minutes | **Cook time:** 3 hours
● 1 cup flour
● 3 tablespoons butter, softened
● 1 egg yolk
● 2 tablespoons sugar
● 2 tablespoons maple syrup
● 1 teaspoon baking powder
● 2 bacon slices, cooked, chopped
1.   Put all ingredients except bacon in the mixing bowl.

2. Stir the mixture until homogenous, add bacon. Knead the soft non-sticky dough.
3. Then cut the dough into pieces and roll them in the balls. Press the balls gently.
4. Line the Crock Pot bottom with baking paper.
5. Put the cookies inside in one layer and close the lid.
6. Cook the cooking on High for 3 hours.
per serving: 235 calories, 5.2g protein, 29.9g carbohydrates, 10.9g fat, 0.7g fiber, 66mg cholesterol, 157mg sodium, 150mg potassium.

Brownie Bars
Yield: 8 servings | **Prep time:** 10 minutes | **Cook time:** 5 hours
- ½ cup of cocoa powder
- ½ cup flour
- 1 teaspoon baking powder
- ¼ cup butter, melted
- 1 teaspoon vanilla extract
- 3 eggs, beaten
- ¼ cup of sugar
- 2 oz chocolate chips
1. Mix all ingredients in the bowl and stir until smooth.
2. Line the Crock Pot with baking paper and transfer the mixture inside.
3. Close the lid and cook the brownie on low for 5 hours.
4. When the brownie is cooked, let it cool little.
5. Cut the dessert into bars.
per serving: 178 calories, 4.5g protein, 19.9g carbohydrates, 10.3g fat, 2.1g fiber, 78mg cholesterol, 71mg sodium, 258mg potassium.

Peanut Cookies
Yield: 6 servings | **Prep time:** 30 minutes | **Cook time:** 2 hours
- 1/3 cup buttermilk
- 1 teaspoon baking powder
- 1 teaspoon vanilla extract
- ¼ cup peanuts, crushed
- 3 tablespoons peanut butter
- 1 ½ cup flour
- 2 tablespoons brown sugar
1. Mix all ingredients and knead the soft dough.
2. Then make the medium size balls from the dough and press them gently with the help of the hand palm to get the shape of cookies.
3. After this, line the Crock Pot bowl with baking paper.
4. Put the cookies inside in one layer.
5. Close the lid and cook the dessert on High for 2 hours.
6. Cool the cooked cookies well.
per serving: 215 calories, 7.3g protein, 30.5g carbohydrates, 7.5g fat, 1.9g fiber, 1mg cholesterol, 54mg sodium, 238mg potassium.

Banana Cookies
Yield: 4 servings | **Prep time:** 15 minutes | **Cook time:** 2 hours
- 2 bananas, mashed
- 1 egg, beaten
- 1 cup oatmeal
- 1 teaspoon ground cinnamon
- Cooking spray
1. Mix bananas with egg and ground cinnamon.
2. Add oatmeal and whisk the mixture until smooth.
3. Then spray the Crock Pot with cooking spray.
4. Make the cookies from the banana mixture with the help of the spoon and put them in the Crock Pot.
5. Cook the cookies on High for 2 hours.
per serving: 147 calories, 4.7g protein, 27.9g carbohydrates, 2.6g fat, 3.9g fiber, 41mg cholesterol, 17mg sodium, 302mg potassium.

Cranberry Cookies
Yield: 6 servings | **Prep time:** 20 minutes | **Cook time:** 2.5 hours
- 2 oz dried cranberries, chopped
- 3 tablespoons peanut butter
- 1 cup flour
- 1 teaspoon baking powder
- 3 tablespoons sugar
- 1 tablespoon cream cheese
1. Mix peanut butter with flour, baking powder, and sugar.
2. Add cream cheese and cranberries and knead the dough.
3. Make the small balls and press them gently to get the shape of the cookies.
4. After this, line the Crock Pot bowl with baking paper.
5. Put the cookies inside and close the lid.
6. Cook the cookies on high for 2.5 hours.
per serving: 157 calories, 4.3g protein, 24.8g carbohydrates, 4.8g fat, 1.4g fiber, 2mg cholesterol, 43mg sodium, 176mg potassium.

Coffee Cookies
Yield: 12 servings | **Prep time:** 30 minutes | **Cook time:** 4 hours
- 2 eggs, beaten
- 1 tablespoon coffee beans, grinded
- 1 teaspoon baking powder
- ½ cup butter, softened
- 2 cups flour
- ¼ cup of sugar
- 1 teaspoon sunflower oil
1. Brush the Crock Pot bowl with sunflower oil.
2. Then mix all remaining ingredients in the mixing bowl.
3. Knead the dough and cut it into small pieces.
4. Roll the dough pieces into small balls and make the small cut in the center of every ball (to get the shape of the cocoa bean).
5. Put the cocoa beans in the Crock Pot in one layer and close the lid.
6. Cook them on High for 2 hours.
7. Repeat the same steps with remaining cookies.
per serving: 174 calories, 3.2g protein, 20.3g carbohydrates, 9g fat, 0.6g fiber, 48mg cholesterol, 66mg sodium, 77mg potassium.

Soft Sable Cookies

Yield: 2 servings | **Prep time:** 15 minutes | **Cook time:** 2 hours
- 1 teaspoon sesame seeds
- 2 tablespoons butter, softened
- 1 egg yolk, whisked
- ½ teaspoon baking powder
- 2 teaspoons brown sugar
- 1/3 cup flour
- ½ teaspoon olive oil
1. Mix butter with baking powder, brown sugar, and flour.
2. Knead a soft dough and cut into 2 pieces.
3. Then roll the balls from the dough and press them gently.
4. Brush every ball with the help of the egg yolk and sprinkle with sesame seeds.
5. Brush the Crock Pot bowl with olive oil and put the cookies inside.
6. Cook them on High for 2 hours. Then cool the cookies well.

per serving: 236 calories, 3.9g protein, 20.1g carbohydrates, 15.9g fat, 0.8g fiber, 135mg cholesterol, 88mg sodium, 172mg potassium.

Coconut Clouds
Yield: 4 servings | **Prep time:** 15 minutes | **Cook time:** 2.5 hours
- 2 egg whites
- 1 cup coconut shred
- 2 tablespoons of sugar powder
1. Whisk the egg whites until you get firm peaks.
2. Add sugar powder and coconut shred and carefully mix the mixture.
3. Then line the Crock Pot with baking paper.
4. With the help of the spoon put the small amount of coconut mixture in the Crock Pot to get the cookies in the shape of clouds.
5. Cook them on High for 2.5 hours.

per serving: 246 calories, 3g protein, 12g carbohydrates, 22g fat, 4g fiber, 80mg cholesterol, 40mg sodium, 0mg potassium.

Glazed Bacon
Yield: 4 servings | **Prep time:** 7 minutes | **Cook time:** 2 hours
- 4 bacon slices
- 1 tablespoon butter
- 3 tablespoons water
- 5 tablespoons maple syrup
1. Put all ingredients in the Crock Pot.
2. Close the lid and cook the dessert on High for 2 hours.
3. Then transfer the bacon in the serving plates and top with maple syrup mixture from the Crock Pot.

per serving: 193 calories, 7.1g protein, 17g carbohydrates, 10.9g fat, 0g fiber, 29mg cholesterol, 462mg sodium, 159mg potassium.

Vanilla Buns
Yield: 4 servings | **Prep time:** 40 minutes | **Cook time:** 3 hours
- 1 cup flour
- ½ teaspoon fresh yeast
- 3 tablespoons sugar
- ¼ cup milk
- 2 tablespoons olive oil
- 1 teaspoon vanilla extract
1. Mix sugar with fresh yeast and leave for 5 minutes.
2. Then mix the mixture with milk, flour, and vanilla extract.
3. Knead it and add olive oil.
4. Knead the dough until smooth and cut into 4 buns.
5. Leave the buns for 30 minutes in a warm place to rise.
6. Then line the Crock Pot bowl with baking paper.
7. Put the buns inside and close the lid.
8. Cook them on High for 3 hours.

per serving: 220 calories, 3.9g protein, 33.9g carbohydrates, 7.6g fat, 1g fiber, 1mg cholesterol, 8mg sodium, 54mg potassium.

Mango Muffins
Yield: 2 servings | **Prep time:** 15 minutes | **Cook time:** 3 hours
- 3 tablespoons mango puree
- 1 tablespoon butter, softened
- 1 teaspoon vanilla extract
- 3 tablespoons flour
- ¼ teaspoon baking powder
1. Mix mango puree with butter, vanilla extract, flour, and baking powder.
2. Stir the mixture until you get a smooth batter.
3. Then fill the muffin molds with batter (fill ½ part of every muffin mold) and transfer them in the Crock Pot.
4. Close the lid and cook the muffins on High for 3 hours.

per serving: 110 calories, 1.4g protein, 11.8g carbohydrates, 5.9g fat, 0.6g fiber, 15mg cholesterol, 42mg sodium, 107mg potassium.

Rhubarb Muffins
Yield: 4 servings | **Prep time:** 15 minutes | **Cook time:** 3 hours
- 1 egg, beaten
- ½ cup skim milk
- ½ cup flour
- 1 teaspoon baking powder
- ½ cup rhubarb, diced
- 1 tablespoon olive oil
1. Put all ingredients except rhubarb in the mixing bowl.
2. Stir them carefully until you get a smooth mass.
3. After this, add rhubarb and mix.
4. Fill ½ part of every muffin mold with muffin batter and transfer in the Crock Pot.
5. Cook the muffin on High for 3 hours.

per serving: 118 calories, 4.1g protein, 14.8g carbohydrates, 4.8g fat, 0.7g fiber, 42mg cholesterol, 34mg sodium, 249mg potassium.

Cumin Cookies
Yield: 8 servings | **Prep time:** 15 minutes | **Cook time:** 3 hours
- 1 teaspoon cumin seeds

- 1 tablespoon water
- 1 egg, beaten
- ½ cup cream cheese
- 2 cups flour
- ¼ cup of sugar
- 1 teaspoon baking powder
- ¼ cup milk
- Cooking spray

1. Mix egg with cream cheese, flour, sugar, baking powder, and milk.
2. Knead the non-sticky dough and cut it into pieces.
3. Make balls.
4. Brush every ball with water and sprinkle with cumin seeds.
5. Line the Crock Pot bowl with baking paper.
6. Put the cumin cookies inside and close the lid.
7. Cook them on High for 3 hours.

per serving: 201 calories, 5.3g protein, 31.3g carbohydrates, 6.1g fat, 0.9g fiber, 37mg cholesterol, 56mg sodium, 131mg potassium.

Sugar Almonds

Yield: 2 servings | **Prep time:** 10 minutes | **Cook time:** 30 minutes

- ½ cup almonds
- ½ cup of sugar
- 1 tablespoon butter

1. Put butter in the Crock Pot.
2. Add almonds and close the lid.
3. Cook the almond on High for 20 minutes.
4. Then open the lid, mix the almonds, and add sugar.
5. Carefully mix the dessert and cook it for 10 minutes on high.

per serving: 376 calories, 5.1g protein, 55.1g carbohydrates, 17.6g fat, 3g fiber, 15mg cholesterol, 41mg sodium, 176mg potassium.

Snowballs

Yield: 2 servings | **Prep time:** 10 minutes | **Cook time:** 2 hours

- 2 tablespoons of sugar powder
- ¼ teaspoon vanilla extract
- ¼ teaspoon baking powder
- 4 tablespoons flour
- 1 tablespoon butter, softened
- 1 teaspoon oatmeal

1. Mix oatmeal with butter, flour, baking powder, and vanilla extract.
2. Knead the soft dough and make the small balls.
3. Coat the balls in the sugar powder carefully.
4. Transfer the balls in the Crock Pot and cook them on High for 2 hours.

per serving: 144 calories, 1.8g protein, 20.9g carbohydrates, 6g fat, 0.5g fiber, 15mg cholesterol, 42mg sodium, 86mg potassium.

Cracked Chocolate Cookies

Yield: 3 servings | **Prep time:** 15 minutes | **Cook time:** 2 hours

- ¼ cup of cocoa powder
- 4 tablespoons flour
- 1 tablespoon sugar

- 2 tablespoons butter
- ½ teaspoon baking powder
- 3 tablespoons of sugar powder

1. Mix cocoa powder with flour and sugar.
2. Add baking powder and butter. Knead the soft dough.
3. Make the medium-size balls from the dough and coat them in the sugar powder.
4. Put the coated cocoa balls in the Crock Pot and close the lid.
5. Cook the cookies on high for 2 hours.

per serving: 169 calories, 2.5g protein, 24.3g carbohydrates, 8.7g fat, 2.4g fiber, 20mg cholesterol, 57mg sodium, 277mg potassium.

Gingerbread

Yield: 4 servings | **Prep time:** 15 minutes | **Cook time:** 5 hours

- 4 tablespoons coconut oil
- 1 tablespoon gingerbread spices
- ½ cup flour
- ¼ cup of sugar

1. Mix all ingredients in the mixing bowl and knead the dough.
2. Roll it up and cut into the cookies with help of the cookie cutter.
3. Line the Crock Pot with baking paper.
4. Put the cookies in the Crock Pot in one layer and bake them on High for 2.5 hours.
5. Repeat the same steps with remaining cookies.

per serving: 221 calories, 1.6g protein, 24.4g carbohydrates, 13.8g fat, 0.4g fiber, 0mg cholesterol, 0mg sodium, 17mg potassium.

Mint Cookies

Yield: 6 servings | **Prep time:** 15 minutes | **Cook time:** 3.5 hours

- 1 teaspoon dried mint
- ½ cup buttermilk
- 1 tablespoon olive oil
- 2 eggs, beaten
- 1 cup flour
- 4 tablespoons brown sugar
- 4 tablespoons flax meal
- 1 teaspoon baking powder

1. Put all ingredients in the mixing bowl.
2. Knead the soft dough.
3. Then line the Crock Pot with baking paper.
4. Cut the dough into small pieces and roll them in the balls.
5. Put the balls in the Crock Pot one-by-one.
6. Close the lid and cook the cookies on High for 3.5 hours.

per serving: 169 calories, 5.7g protein, 24.6g carbohydrates, 5.8g fat, 1.9g fiber, 55mg cholesterol, 45mg sodium, 204mg potassium.

Pumpkin Bars

Yield: 6 servings | **Prep time:** 15 minutes | **Cook time:** 5 hours

- 1 teaspoon pumpkin spices
- ½ cup pumpkin puree
- 1 cup flour
- ½ teaspoon baking powder

- 1 teaspoon lime zest, grated
- ¼ cup of sugar
- 4 tablespoons flax meal
- 2 tablespoons olive oil
1. Put all ingredients in the mixing bowl. Mix the mixture until smooth.
2. Then line the Crock Pot with baking paper.
3. Transfer the pumpkin mixture in the Crock Pot.
4. Close the lid and cook it on Low for 5 hours.
5. Then cool the dessert and cut into bars.

per serving: 176 calories, 3.4g protein, 27.7g carbohydrates, 6.6g fat, 2.6g fiber, 0mg cholesterol, 2mg sodium, 147mg potassium.

Sweet Puffs
Yield: 3 servings | **Prep time:** 25 minutes | **Cook time:** 2.5 hours

- 1 tablespoon brown sugar
- 1 tablespoon butter, melted
- ½ teaspoon ground cinnamon
- 5 oz puff pastry
- Cooking spray
1. Make the small balls from the puff pastry.
2. In the shallow bowl mix ground cinnamon with brown sugar.
3. Dip every puff pastry ball in the butter and then coat in the sugar mixture.
4. Spray the Crock Pot bowl with cooking spray.
5. Put the balls in the Crock Pot and cook them on High for 2.5 hours.

per serving: 307 calories, 3.5g protein, 24.6g carbohydrates, 21.8g fat, 0.9g fiber, 10mg cholesterol, 146mg sodium, 36mg potassium.

Cottage Cheese Corners
Yield: 3 servings | **Prep time:** 30 minutes | **Cook time:** 3 hours

- 2 tablespoons cottage cheese
- 1 teaspoon sugar
- 1 teaspoon vanilla extract
- 1 egg, beaten
- 3 oz puff pastry
- Cooking spray
1. Mix cottage cheese with sugar, vanilla extract, and ½ of the beaten egg.
2. Stir the mixture until smooth.
3. Then roll up the puff pastry and cut it in the shape of squares.
4. Spread every dough square with a cottage cheese mixture.
5. Then wrap them in the shape of corners.
6. Spray the Crock Pot bowl with cooking spray.
7. Put the corners inside and close the lid.
8. Cook them on High for 3 hours.

per serving: 195 calories, 5.2g protein, 14.8g carbohydrates, 12.4g fat, 0.4g fiber, 55mg cholesterol, 130mg sodium, 48mg potassium.

Pecan Muffins
Yield: 5 servings | **Prep time:** 20 minutes | **Cook time:** 3 hours

- 4 pecans, chopped
- ½ cup plain yogurt
- 1 egg, beaten
- 1 teaspoon ground clove
- 1 cup flour
- 2 tablespoons olive oil
- 2 tablespoons brown sugar
1. Mix all ingredients except pecans in the mixing bowl.
2. When you get a smooth batter, add chopped pecans and carefully mix them with the help of the spoon.
3. Pour the muffin batter in the muffin molds (fill ½ part of every muffin mold) and transfer them in the Crock Pot.
4. Cook the dessert on High for 3 hours.

per serving: 262 calories, 6.3g protein, 26.3g carbohydrates, 15.1g fat, 2g fiber, 221mg cholesterol, 32mg sodium, 152mg potassium.

Avocado Bread with Maple Syrup
Yield: 6 servings | **Prep time:** 30 minutes | **Cook time:** 3 hours

- ½ cup flour
- 1 avocado, mashed
- 3 eggs, beaten
- 3 tablespoons sunflower oil
- 1 teaspoon baking powder
- 1 teaspoon vanilla extract
- ½ cup maple syrup
- Cooking spray
1. Mix eggs with mashed avocado, baking powder, vanilla extract, and flour.
2. Stir the mixture until smooth.
3. Then spray the Crock Pot bottom with cooking spray.
4. Pour the avocado mixture inside and close the lid.
5. Cook the bread on High for 3 hours.
6. Then pour the maple syrup over the hot avocado bread and leave it until the bread is cool.

per serving: 271 calories, 4.5g protein, 29.1g carbohydrates, 15.9g fat, 2.5g fiber, 82mg cholesterol, 36mg sodium, 342mg potassium.

Lime Tarts
Yield: 4 servings | **Prep time:** 30 minutes | **Cook time:** 3 hours

- 1 lime, sliced
- 7 oz puff pastry
- 1 egg, beaten
- 4 teaspoons sugar
- 4 teaspoons butter, soften
- Cooking spray
1. Roll up the puff pastry and cut it into 4 squares.
2. Then grease the puff pastry squares with butter and top with sliced lime.
3. Sprinkle lime with sugar and beaten egg. Lime tarts are prepared.
4. Spray the Crock Pot bowl with cooking spray.
5. Put the lime tarts in the Crock Pot in one layer and cook in High for 3 hours.

per serving: 343 calories, 5.2g protein, 28.2g carbohydrates, 23.8g fat, 1.2g fiber, 51mg cholesterol, 166mg sodium, 63mg potassium.

Seeds Cookies

Yield: 4 servings | **Prep time:** 25 minutes | **Cook time:** 2 hours

- ½ cup flax meal
- 1 teaspoon flax seeds
- 1 teaspoon sunflower seeds
- 4 tablespoons butter
- 1 egg, beaten
- 2 tablespoons flour
- 1 tablespoon maple syrup
- Cooking spray

1. Spray the Crock Pot with cooking spray from inside.
2. Then mix all ingredients from the list above in the mixing bowl and carefully stir until smooth. You should get soft non-sticky dough. Add more flour if needed.
3. Make the small cookies and put them in the Crock Pot.
4. Cook them on High for 2 hours.

per serving: 209 calories, 5.1g protein, 10.6g carbohydrates, 18g fat, 4.3g fiber, 71mg cholesterol, 98mg sodium, 152mg potassium.

Chia Muffins
Yield: 4 servings | **Prep time:** 20 minutes | **Cook time:** 2.5 hours

- 2 eggs, beaten
- ¼ cup plain yogurt
- 1 teaspoon ground nutmeg
- 1 tablespoon brown sugar
- ½ cup flour
- 1 tablespoon chia seeds
- 1 teaspoon butter, melted

1. Mix eggs with plain yogurt, ground nutmeg, brown sugar, flour, and butter.
2. Whisk the mixture until you get a smooth batter.
3. Then add chia seeds and mix the batter with the help of the spoon.
4. Pour the batter in the silicone muffin molds (fill ½ part of every mold).
5. Place the muffins in the Crock Pot.
6. Close the lid and cook them on High for 2.5 hours.

per serving: 136 calories, 5.9g protein, 17.2g carbohydrates, 4.8g fat, 1.8g fiber, 85mg cholesterol, 50mg sodium, 102mg potassium.

Banana Muffins
Yield: 2 servings | **Prep time:** 10 minutes | **Cook time:** 2.5 hours

- 2 eggs, beaten
- 2 bananas, chopped
- 4 tablespoons flour
- ½ teaspoon vanilla extract
- ½ teaspoon baking powder

1. Mash the chopped bananas and mix them with eggs.
2. Then add vanilla extract and baking powder.
3. Add flour and stir the mixture until smooth.
4. Pour the banana mixture in the muffin molds (fill ½ part of every muffin mold) and transfer in the Crock Pot.
5. Cook the muffins on High for 2.5 hours.

per serving: 229 calories, 84g protein, 39.9g carbohydrates, 4.9g fat, 3.5g fiber, 164mg cholesterol, 64mg sodium, 626mg potassium.

Caramel Cookies
Yield: 6 servings | **Prep time:** 25 minutes | **Cook time:** 3 hours

- 2 tablespoons salted caramel
- ½ cup butter
- 1 egg yolk
- 1 teaspoon baking powder
- 3 tablespoon sugar
- 1 ½ cup flour

1. Mix butter with egg yolk and baking powder.
2. Then add sugar and flour. Knead the soft non-sticky dough.
3. After this, line the Crock Pot bottom with baking paper.
4. Make the small balls from the dough and press them gently.
5. Put the dough balls in the Crock Pot in one layer and sprinkle with salted caramel.
6. Close the lid and cook the cookies on High for 3 hours.

per serving: 282 calories, 3.9g protein, 30.4g carbohydrates, 16.4g fat, 0.9g fiber, 76mg cholesterol, 112mg sodium, 125mg potassium.

S'mores Cake
Yield: 6 servings | **Prep time:** 25 minutes | **Cook time:** 2 hours

- 1 cup chocolate cake mix
- ¼ cup pudding mix
- 3 eggs, beaten
- ¼ cup plain yogurt
- 3 tablespoons butter, melted
- 3 oz marshmallows
- 3 oz graham crackers, crushed
- Cooking spray

1. Mix chocolate cake mix with pudding mix.
2. Add eggs, plain yogurt, and butter. Stir it until homogenous.
3. After this, add graham crackers and carefully mix them again.
4. Spray the Crock Pot bottom with cooking spray and put the chocolate mixture inside.
5. Cook it on high for 2 hours.
6. Then add marshmallows and broil the mixture.

per serving: 390 calories, 7.1g protein, 56.7g carbohydrates, 16.4g fat, 1.5g fiber, 98mg cholesterol, 579mg sodium, 219mg potassium.

Buttered Rum
Yield: 2 servings | **Prep time:** 20 minutes | **Cook time:** 2 hours

- 2 tablespoon butterscotch syrup
- 2 tablespoons butter
- 2 teaspoons brown sugar
- 1 teaspoon ground cinnamon
- 1 cup cream soda
- 3 cups of water
- ¼ cup rum

1. Put all ingredients except rum in the Crock Pot. Gently mix the liquid.

2. Close the lid and cook it on High for 2 hours.
3. Then add rum and cook for 10 minutes on high more.
4. Pour the hot drink in the serving glasses.
per serving: 340 calories, 0.2g protein, 44.3g carbohydrates, 11.5g fat, 0.6g fiber, 31mg cholesterol, 194mg sodium, 18mg potassium.

White Wine Chocolate
Yield: 2 servings | **Prep time:** 10 minutes | **Cook time:** 3 hours
- 1 tablespoon cocoa powder
- 2 teaspoons sugar
- 3 cups white wine
- ¼ cup of chocolate chips
- 1 teaspoon vanilla extract
1. Put all ingredients in the Crock Pot.
2. Close the lid.
3. Cook the dessert on Low for 3 hours.
4. Then carefully mix it and pour it in the glasses.

per serving: 289 calories, 1.6g protein, 18.6g carbohydrates, 4.4g fat, 1g fiber, 3mg cholesterol, 23mg sodium, 333mg potassium.

Marshmallow Hot Drink
Yield: 3 servings | **Prep time:** 10 minutes | **Cook time:** 5 hours
- ½ cup of chocolate chips
- 4 oz marshmallows
- 1 teaspoon butter
- 2 cups of milk
1. Put all ingredients in the Crock Pot and close the lid.
2. Cook the drink on Low for 5 hours. Stir it every 2 hours.
per serving: 364 calories, 7.8g protein, 54.g carbohydrates, 13g fat, 1g fiber, 23mg cholesterol, 138mg sodium, 200mg potassium.

Appendix:Recipes Index

Cheesy Fish Dip 114
Cherry Jam 161
Cherry Rice 46
Chia Muffins 176
Chicken and Cabbage Bowl 61
Chicken and Lentils Meatballs 66
Chicken and Noodles Soup 32
Chicken Bowl 52
Chicken Burger Meat 71
Chicken Cacciatore 59
Chicken Casserole 66
Chicken Chili 38
Chicken Cordon Bleu 68
Chicken Dip 48
Chicken Drumsticks with Zucchini 61
Chicken in Apricots 64
Chicken in Onion Rings 64
Chicken in Sweet Soy Sauce 57
Chicken Masala 53
Chicken Meatballs 22
Chicken Minestrone 53
Chicken Mix 59
Chicken Mole 58
Chicken Omelet 23
Chicken Pancake 67
Chicken Parm 59
Chicken Pasta Casserole 68
Chicken Pate 53
Chicken Pilaf 42
Chicken Pocket 70
Chicken Pockets 52
Chicken Sausages in Jam 64
Chicken Soufflé 68
Chicken Stuffed with Plums 69
Chicken Teriyaki 53
Chicken Wings in Vodka Sauce 71
Chicken with Figs 62
Chicken with Vegetables 60
Chickpea and Chicken Bowl 69
Chili Beef Ribs 78
Chili Beef Sausages 78
Chili Beef Strips 83
Chili Bigeye Jack (Tuna) 128
Chili Chicken 54
Chili Chicken Liver 68
Chili Dip 138
Chili Okra 139
Chili Perch 129
Chili Salmon 115
Chili Sausages 63
Chinese Style Cod Stew 41
Chipotle Beef Strips 88
Chocolate Fudge Cake 156
Chocolate Mango 163
Chocolate Oatmeal 17
Chocolate Rice 48
Chocolate Toast 16
Chocolate Whipped Cream 162
Chopped Balls 67
Chopped Chicken Liver Balls 68

Chorizo Eggs 27
Chorizo Soup 35
Cider Pork Roast 110
Cilantro Beef 73
Cilantro Beef Meatballs 83
Cilantro Haddock 119
Cilantro Meatballs 76
Cilantro Pork Chops 93
Cilantro Salmon 120
Cilantro Shrimp Bake 30
Cinnamon and Cumin Chicken
Drumsticks 63
Cinnamon Buckwheat 49
Cinnamon Butter 159
Cinnamon Catfish 112
Cinnamon Giant Cookie 154
Cinnamon Plum Jam 165
Cinnamon Rice Milk Cocktail 171
Cinnamon Turkey 58
Clam Soup 35
Clams in Coconut Sauce 111
Classic Apple Pie 156
Classic Banana Foster 160
Classic Huevos Rancheros 46
Clove Pastry Wheels 171
Coated Salmon Fillets 124
Cocktail Beef Meatballs 81
Cocoa Cake 154
Cocoa Chicken 56
Cocoa Pork Chops 98
Coconut and Lemon Pie 164
Coconut and Mango Mousse 169
Coconut Beef 75
Coconut Catfish 113
Coconut Cauliflower Florets 146
Coconut Clouds 173
Coconut Cod Stew 37
Coconut Curry Cod 124
Coconut Milk Lentils Bowl 143
Coconut Millet with Apples 49
Coconut Oatmeal 27
Coconut Pollock 128
Coconut Shaped Cake 170
Coconut Soufflé 162
Cod and Clams Saute 121
Cod Fingers 116
Cod in Lemon Sauce 123
Cod Sticks 114
Cod Sticks in Blankets 125
Coffee Cookies 172
Coffee Pie 158
Collard Greens Saute 141
Coriander Cod Balls 123
Corn and Chicken Saute 72
Corn Casserole 18
Corn Fritters 145
Corn Pudding 136
Corn Salad 139
Corned Beef 85
Cottage Cheese Corners 175

Thyme Whole Chicken 55
Tilapia Fish Balls 123
Tofu and Cauliflower Bowl 143
Tofu Curry 144
Tofu Eggs 29
Tofu Kebabs 147
Tofu Tikka Masala 149
Tomato and Turkey Chili 38
Tomato Beef Chowder 80
Tomato Bulgur 45
Tomato Chicken Sausages 63
Tomato Chickpeas Stew 36
Tomato Dal 46
Tomato Eggs 26
Tomato Fish Casserole 121
Tomato Ground Chicken 27
Tomato Hot Eggs 23
Tomato Okra 146
Tomato Pork Sausages 96
Tomato Seabass 129
Tomato Squid 117
Trout Cakes 115
Tuna Casserole 114
Turkey in Pomegranate Juice 57
Turkey Omelet 25
Turkey with Plums 60
Turkish Meat Saute 74
Turmeric Beef Brisket 77
Turmeric Mackerel 120
Turmeric Meatballs 66
Turmeric Parsnip 138
Turmeric Squash Soup 35
Turnip and Beans Casserole 47

V

Vanilla and Cocoa Pudding 163

Vanilla Applesauce 136
Vanilla Buns 173
Vanilla Quinoa 22
Vegan Kofte 147
Vegan Milk Clams 120
Vegan Mousse 165
Vegan Pepper Bowl 145
Vegetable Korma 149
Vegetable Pasta 49
Vinegar Chicken Wings 63

W

Walnut and Cheese Balls 31
Walnut Kale 140
Walnut Pudding 156
Warm Bean Salad 47
White Beans in Sauce 48
White Beef Chili 84
White Mushroom Soup 36
White Wine Chocolate 177
Wild Rice Medley 50
Wild Rice with Crumbled Cheese 44
Wine Chicken 66
Wine Pork Shoulder 98
Wine-Braised Beef Heart 90
Winter Pork with Green Peas 100

Y

Yam Fritters 142
Yogurt Casserole 105
Yogurt Soup 36

Z

Zucchini Caviar 137
Zucchini Chicken 63
Zucchini Latkes 142
Zucchini Mash 140
Zucchini Quinoa 17

CPSIA information can be obtained
at www.ICGtesting.com
Printed in the USA
BVHW011635220321
603177BV00013B/1136